a LANGE medical book

CURRENT
ESSENTIALS
PEDIATRICS

Judith M. Sondheimer, MD
Professor Emeritus
Department of Pediatrics
Section of Pediatric Gastroenterology, Hepatology and Nutrition
University of Colorado School of Medicine
The Children's Hospital
Denver, Colorado

D0753913

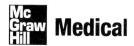 **Medical**

New York   Chicago   San Francisco   Lisbon   London   Madrid   Mexico City
Milan   New Delhi   San Juan   Seoul   Singapore   Sydney   Toronto

1 2 3 4 5 6 7 8 9 0   DOC/DOC   0 9 8 7

ISBN 978-0-07-141256-8
MHID 0-07-141256-5
ISSN 1940-0691

Notice

Medicine is an ever-changing science. As new research and clinical experience broaden our knowledge, changes in treatment and drug therapy are required. The authors and the publisher of this work have checked with sources believed to be reliable in their efforts to provide information that is complete and generally in accord with the standards accepted at the time of publication; however, in view of the possibility of human error or changes in medical sciences, neither the authors nor the publisher nor any other party who has been involved in the preparation or publication of this work warrants that the information contained herein is in every respect accurate or complete, and they disclaim all responsibility for any errors or omissions or for the results obtained from use of the information contained in this work. Readers are encouraged to confirm the information contained herein with other sources. For example and in particular, readers are advised to check the product information sheet included in the package of each drug they plan to administer to be certain that the information contained in this work is accurate and that changes have not been made in the recommended dose or in the contraindications for administration. This recommendation is of particular importance in connection with new or infrequently used drugs.

The book was set in Times by International Typesetting and Composition.
The editors were Anne M. Sydor and Kim J. Davis.
Project management was provided by Vastavikta Sharma at International Typesetting and Composition.
The cover designer was Mary McKeon.
The index was prepared by Vicki Boyle.
RR Donnelley was the printer and binder.

This book is printed on acid-free paper.

International Edition ISBN 978-0-07-111689-3; MHID 0-07-111689-3
Copyright © 2008. Exclusive rights by the McGraw-Hill Companies, Inc., for manufacture and export. The book cannot be re-exported from the country to which it is consigned by McGraw-Hill. The International Edition is not available in North America.

To Henry M. Sondheimer

Contents

Contributors

The topics covered in *Current Essentials: Pediatrics* are based on chapters from the eighteenth edition of *Current Diagnosis & Treatment: Pediatrics*, edited by William W. Hay, Jr., Myron J. Levin, Judith M. Sondheimer, Robin R. Deterding authored by the following:

Frank J. Accurso, MD
Professor, Department of Pediatrics
Head, Section of Pediatric Pulmonary Medicine
University of Colorado School of Medicine
The Children's Hospital
Denver, Colorado

Daniel R. Ambruso, MD
Professor, Department of Pediatrics
Section of Pediatric Hematology/Oncology/Bone Marrow Transplant
Associate Medical Director, Belle Bonfils Blood Center
University of Colorado School of Medicine
The Children's Hospital
Denver, Colorado

Marsha S. Anderson, MD
Associate Professor, Department of Pediatrics
Section of Pediatric Infectious Diseases
University of Colorado School of Medicine
The Children's Hospital
Denver, Colorado

Vivek Balasubramaniam, MD
Assistant Professor, Department of Pediatrics
Section of Pediatric Pulmonary Medicine
University of Colorado School of Medicine
The Children's Hospital
Denver, Colorado

F. Keith Battan, MD, FAAP
Attending Pediatrician, Colorado Permanent Medical Group
Denver, Colorado

Timothy A. Benke, MD, PhD
Assistant Professor, Departments of Pediatrics, Neurology, and
    Pharmacology
Director, Division of Child Neurology Residency Training Program
University of Colorado School of Medicine
The Children's Hospital
Denver, Colorado

Timothy J. Bernard, MD
Department of Pediatrics and Neurology
University of Colorado School of Medicine
The Children's Hospital
Denver, Colorado

Mark Boguniewicz, MD
Professor, Divisions of Pediatric Allergy-Immunology
Department of Pediatrics, National Jewish Medical and Research
    Center
University of Colorado School of Medicine
Denver, Colorado

Robert M. Brayden, MD
Associate Professor, Department of Pediatrics
Section of General and Academic Pediatrics
University of Colorado School of Medicine
The Children's Hospital
Denver, Colorado

Jeffrey M. Brown, MD, MPH
Professor, Department of Pediatrics
University of Colorado School of Medicine
Director, General Pediatrics Division
Denver Health Medical Center
Denver, Colorado

Joanna M. Burch, MD
Assistant Professor, Departments of Dermatology and Pediatrics
University of Colorado School of Medicine
Denver, Colorado

Todd C. Carpenter, MD
Associate Professor, Department of Pediatrics
Section of Pediatric Critical Care Medicine
University of Colorado School of Medicine
The Children's Hospital
Denver, Colorado

Keith Cavanaugh, MD
Assistant Professor, Department of Pediatrics
Section of Pediatric Pulmonary Medicine
University of Colorado School of Medicine
The Children's Hospital
Denver, Colorado

H. Peter Chase, MD
Professor, Department of Pediatrics
Clinical Director Emeritus, Barbara Davis Center for Childhood
    Diabetes
University of Colorado School of Medicine
Denver, Colorado

Matthew F. Daley, MD
Assistant Professor, Department of Pediatrics
Section of General and Emergency Medicine Pediatrics
University of Colorado School of Medicine
The Children's Hospital
Denver, Colorado

Richard C. Dart, MD, PhD
Professor, Department of Surgery
University of Colorado School of Medicine
Director, Rocky Mountain Poison and Drug Center
Denver, Colorado

Bert Dech, MD
Clinical Instructor, Department of Psychiatry
The Children's Hospital
Denver, Colorado

Robin R. Deterding, MD
Associate Professor, Department of Pediatrics
Section of Pediatric Pulmonary Medicine
University of Colorado School of Medicine
The Children's Hospital
Denver, Colorado

Emily L. Dobyns, MD
Associate Professor, Department of Pediatrics
Section of Pediatric Critical Care Medicine
University of Colorado School of Medicine
The Children's Hospital
Denver, Colorado

Arlene Drack, MD
Associate Professor, Departments of Ophthalmology and Pediatrics
University of Colorado School of Medicine
Rocky Mountain Lions Eye Institute
The Children's Hospital
Aurora, Colorado

Robert E. Eilert, MD
Clinical Professor, Department of Orthopedic Surgery
University of Colorado School of Medicine
Chairman, Department of Orthopedic Surgery
The Children's Hospital
Denver, Colorado

George S. Eisenbarth, MD, PhD
Professor, Department of Pediatrics
Executive Director, Barbara Davis Center for Childhood Diabetes
University of Colorado School of Medicine
Denver, Colorado

Ellen R. Elias, MD
Associate Professor, Departments of Pediatrics and Genetics
Section of Clinical Genetics and Metabolism
University of Colorado School of Medicine
Director, Special Care Clinic
The Children's Hospital
Denver, Colorado

Glenn Faries, MD
Assistant Professor, Department of Pediatrics
Co-Director, Core Clerkship Block in Urgent Care/Emergency
    Medicine
University of Colorado School of Medicine
Medical Director, Continuing Medical Education
The Children's Hospital
Denver, Colorado

Margaret A. Ferguson, MD
Clinical Assistant Professor, Department of Pediatrics
Section of Pediatric Critical Care Medicine
University of Colorado School of Medicine
The Children's Hospital
Denver, Colorado

Douglas M. Ford, MD
Professor, Department of Pediatrics
Section of Pediatric Renal Medicine
University of Colorado School of Medicine
The Children's Hospital
Denver, Colorado

Nicholas K. Foreman, MD
Professor, Department of Pediatrics
Section of Hematology/Oncology/Bone Marrow Transplant
University of Colorado School of Medicine
The Children's Hospital
Denver, Colorado

Norman R. Friedman, MD
Professor, Department of Otolaryngology
University of Colorado School of Medicine
The Children's Hospital
Denver, Colorado

Roger H. Giller, MD
Professor, Department of Pediatrics
Section of Pediatric Hematology/Oncology/Bone Marrow Transplant
Director, Pediatric BMT Program
University of Colorado School of Medicine
The Children's Hospital
Denver, Colorado

Neil A. Goldenberg, MD
Assistant Professor, Departments of Pediatrics and Medicine
Center for Cancer and Blood Disorders
Associate Director, Mountain States Regional Hemophilia and
    Thrombosis Center
Aurora, Colorado
University of Colorado at Denver and Health Sciences Center
The Children's Hospital
Denver, Colorado

Edward Goldson, MD
Professor, Department of Pediatrics
Section of Developmental and Behavioral Pediatrics
University of Colorado School of Medicine
The Children's Hospital
Denver, Colorado

Doug K. Graham, MD, PhD
Assistant Professor, Department of Pediatrics
Section of Pediatric Hematology/Oncology/Bone Marrow Transplant
University of Colorado School of Medicine
The Children's Hospital
Denver, Colorado

Eva N. Grayck, MD
Associate Professor, Department of Pediatrics
Section of Pediatric Critical Care Medicine
University of Colorado School of Medicine
The Children's Hospital
Denver, Colorado

Brian S. Greffe, MD
Associate Professor, Department of Pediatrics
Section of Pediatric Hematology/Oncology/Bone Marrow Transplant
University of Colorado School of Medicine
The Children's Hospital
Denver, Colorado

Jennifer Hagman, MD
Associate Professor, Department of Psychiatry
University of Colorado School of Medicine
Co-Director, Eating Disorders Treatment Program
The Children's Hospital
Denver, Colorado

Taru Hays, MD
Professor, Department of Pediatrics
Section of Pediatric Hematology/Oncology/Bone Marrow Transplant
University of Colorado School of Medicine
The Children's Hospital
Denver, Colorado

Francis Hoe, MD
Instructor, Department of Pediatrics
Section of Pediatric Endocrinology
University of Colorado School of Medicine
The Children's Hospital
Denver, Colorado

J. Roger Hollister, MD
Professor, Departments of Pediatrics and Medicine
Head, Section of Pediatric Rheumatology
University of Colorado School of Medicine
The Children's Hospital Senior Staff Physician, National Jewish
　Medical and Research Center
Denver, Colorado

Candice E. Johnson, MD, PhD
Professor, Department of Pediatrics
Section of General Academic Pediatrics
University of Colorado School of Medicine
The Children's Hospital
Denver, Colorado

Richard B. Johnston, Jr., MD
Professor of Pediatrics, Section of Immunology
Associate Dean for Research Development
Executive Vice President for Academic Affairs
National Jewish Medical and Research Center
University of Colorado School of Medicine
Denver, Colorado

Carol S. Kamin, MS, EdD
Associate Professor, Department of Pediatrics
Director, Medical Education Research & Development
Director, Project L.I.V.E (Learning through Interactive Video
　Education.)
University of Colorado School of Medicine
The Children's Hospital
Denver, Colorado

David W. Kaplan, MD, MPH
Professor, Department of Pediatrics
Head, Section of Adolescent Medicine
University of Colorado School of Medicine
The Children's Hospital
Denver, Colorado

Michael S. Kappy, MD, PhD
Professor, Department of Pediatrics
Head, Section of Pediatric Endocrinology
University of Colorado School of Medicine
The Children's Hospital
Denver, Colorado

Paritosh Kaul, MD
Assistant Professor, Department of Pediatrics
Director, Denver School Based Health Centers
Section of Adolescent Medicine
University of Colorado School of Medicine
The Children's Hospital
Denver Health Medical Center
Denver, Colorado

Amy K. Keating, MD
Fellow, Department of Pediatrics
Section of Pediatric Hematology/Oncology/Bone Marrow Transplant
Center for Cancer and Blood Disorders
The University of Colorado School of Medicine
The Children's Hospital
Denver, Colorado

Peggy E. Kelly, MD
Associate Professor, Department of Otolaryngology
University of Colorado School of Medicine
The Children's Hospital
Denver, Colorado

Gwendolyn S. Kerby, MD
Assistant Professor, Department of Pediatrics
Section of Pediatric Pulmonary Medicine
University of Colorado School of Medicine
The Children's Hospital
Denver, Colorado

Nancy F. Krebs, MD, MS
Professor, Department of Pediatrics
Head, Section of Nutrition
University of Colorado School of Medicine
The Children's Hospital
Denver, Colorado

Richard D. Krugman, MD
Professor, Department of Pediatrics
Dean, University of Colorado School of Medicine
Denver, Colorado

Myron J. Levin, MD
Professor, Departments of Pediatrics and Medicine
Section of Pediatric Infectious Diseases
University of Colorado School of Medicine
The Children's Hospital
Denver, Colorado

Andrew H. Liu, MD
Associate Professor, Department of Pediatrics
Section of Allergy & Clinical Immunology
National Jewish Medical & Research Center
University of Colorado School of Medicine
Denver, Colorado

Kathryn A. Love-Osborne, MD
Assistant Professor, Department of Pediatrics
Section of Adolescent Medicine
University of Colorado School of Medicine
The Children's Hospital
Denver, Colorado

Gary M. Lum, MD
Professor, Departments of Pediatrics and Medicine
Head, Section of Pediatric Renal Medicine
University of Colorado School of Medicine
The Children's Hospital
Denver, Colorado

Kelly Maloney, MD
Associate Professor, Department of Pediatrics
Section of Pediatric Hematology/Oncology/Bone Marrow Transplant
University of Colorado School of Medicine
The Children's Hospital
Denver, Colorado

David K. Manchester, MD
Professor, Department of Pediatrics
Section of Clinical Genetics and Metabolism
University of Colorado School of Medicine
Co-Director, Division of Genetic Services
The Children's Hospital
Denver, Colorado

Dennis J. Matthews, MD
Professor and Chairman, Department of Rehabilitation Medicine
University of Colorado School of Medicine
Chairman and Medical Director
The Children's Hospital Rehabilitation Center
Denver, Colorado

Elizabeth J. McFarland, MD
Associate Professor, Department of Pediatrics
Section of Pediatric Infectious Diseases
University of Colorado School of Medicine
The Children's Hospital
Denver, Colorado

Shelley D. Miyamoto, MD
Instructor, Department of Pediatrics
Section of Pediatric Cardiology
University of Colorado School of Medicine
The Children's Hospital
Denver, Colorado

Paul G. Moe, MD
Professor, Departments of Pediatrics and Neurology
Division of Child Neurology
University of Colorado School of Medicine
The Children's Hospital
Denver, Colorado

Joseph G. Morelli, MD
Professor, Departments Dermatology and Pediatrics
University of Colorado School of Medicine
Denver, Colorado

Peter M. Mourani, MD
Assistant Professor, Department of Pediatrics
Section of Pediatric Critical Care Medicine
University of Colorado School of Medicine
The Children's Hospital
Denver, Colorado

William A. Mueller, DMD
Clinical Associate Professor
University of Colorado School of Dentistry
The Children's Hospital
Denver, Colorado

Kristen Nadeau, MD
Assistant Professor, Department of Pediatrics
Section of Pediatric Endocrinology
University of Colorado School of Medicine
The Children's Hospital
Denver, Colorado

Michael R. Narkewicz, MD
Professor, Department of Pediatrics
Section of Pediatric Gastroenterology, Hepatology and Nutrition
The Pediatric Liver Center
University of Colorado School of Medicine
The Children's Hospital
Denver, Colorado

Ann-Christine Nyquist, MD, MSPH
Associate Professor, Department of Pediatrics
Section of Pediatric Infectious Diseases
University of Colorado School of Medicine
The Children's Hospital
Denver, Colorado

John W. Ogle, MD
Professor, Department of Pediatrics
Section of Pediatric Infectious Diseases
University of Colorado School of Medicine
The Children's Hospital Director, Department of Pediatrics
Denver Health Medical Center
Denver, Colorado

Christopher C. Porter, MD
Fellow, Section of Hematology/Oncology/Bone Marrow Transplant
Department of Pediatrics
University of Colorado School of Medicine
The Children's Hospital
Denver, Colorado

Laura E. Primak, RD, CNSD, CSP
Professional Research Assistant
Nutritionist, Section of Nutrition
Department of Pediatrics
University of Colorado School of Medicine
The Children's Hospital
Denver, Colorado

Ralph R. Quinones, MD
Associate Professor, Department of Pediatrics
Section of Pediatric Hematology/Oncology/Bone Marrow Transplant
Director, Pediatric Blood and Marrow Processing Laboratory
University of Colorado School of Medicine
The Children's Hospital
Denver, Colorado

Ann Reynolds, MD
Assistant Professor, Department of Pediatrics
Child Development Unit
University of Colorado School of Medicine
The Children's Hospital
Denver, Colorado

Adam Rosenberg, MD
Professor, Department of Pediatrics
Section of Neonatology, Medical Director of the Newborn Service
University of Colorado Hospital
Director, Pediatric Residency Training Program
University of Colorado School of Medicine
The Children's Hospital
Denver, Colorado

Barry H. Rumack, MD
Clinical Professor, Department of Pediatrics
University of Colorado School of Medicine
Director Emeritus, Rocky Mountain Poison and Drug Center
Denver Health Authority
Denver, Colorado

Scott D. Sagel, MD
Assistant Professor, Department of Pediatrics
Section of Pediatric Pulmonary Medicine
University of Colorado School of Medicine
The Children's Hospital
Denver, Colorado

Rebecca Sands, MD
Assistant Professor, Department of Ophthalmology
University of Colorado School of Medicine
Rocky Mountain Lions Eye Institute
Denver, Colorado

Kelly D. Sawczyn, MD
Fellow, Department of Pediatrics
Section of Pediatric Hematology/Oncology/Bone Marrow Transplant
University of Colorado School of Medicine
The Children's Hospital
Denver, Colorado

Eric J. Sigel, MD
Assistant Professor, Department of Pediatrics
Section of Adolescent Medicine
University of Colorado School of Medicine
The Children's Hospital
Denver, Colorado

Eric A. F. Simoes, MD, DCH
Professor, Department of Pediatrics
Section of Pediatric Infectious Diseases
University of Colorado School of Medicine
The Children's Hospital
Denver, Colorado

Georgette Siparsky, PhD
Supervisor, Clinical Chemistry Laboratory
Department of Pathology
The Children's Hospital
Denver, Colorado

Andrew P. Sirotnak, MD
Associate Professor, Department of Pediatrics
University of Colorado School of Medicine
Director, Kempe Child Protection Team
The Children's Hospital and Kempe Children's Center for the
    Prevention and Treatment of Child Abuse
Denver, Colorado

Ronald J. Sokol, MD
Professor and Vice-Chair Head, Department of Pediatrics
Section of Pediatric Gastroenterology, Hepatology and Nutrition
The Pediatric Liver Center
Director, Pediatric Clinical Translational Research Center
University of Colorado School of Medicine
The Children's Hospital
Denver, Colorado

Henry M. Sondheimer, MD
Professor, Department of Pediatrics
Section of Pediatric Cardiology
Associate Dean for Admissions
University of Colorado School of Medicine
The Children's Hospital
Denver, Colorado

Judith M. Sondheimer, MD
Professor Emeritus, Department of Pediatrics
Section of Pediatric Gastroenterology, Hepatology and Nutrition
University of Colorado School of Medicine
The Children's Hospital
Denver, Colorado

Kurt R. Stenmark, MD
Professor, Department of Pediatrics, Head
Section of Pediatric Critical Care Medicine
Director, Developmental Lung Biology Lab
University of Colorado School of Medicine
The Children's Hospital
Denver, Colorado

Catherine Stevens-Simon, MD
Professor, Department of Pediatrics
Section of Adolescent Medicine
University of Colorado School of Medicine
The Children's Hospital
Denver, Colorado

Lora J. Stewart, MD
Fellow, Department of Pediatrics
Section of Allergy & Clinical Immunology
National Jewish Medical & Research Center
University of Colorado School of Medicine
Denver, Colorado

Elizabeth Thilo, MD
Associate Professor, Department of Pediatrics
Section of Neonatology
University of Colorado School of Medicine
The Children's Hospital
Denver, Colorado

Janet A. Thomas, MD
Assistant Professor, Department of Pediatrics
Section of Clinical Genetics and Metabolism
University of Colorado School of Medicine
The Children's Hospital
Denver, Colorado

Sharon H. Travers, MD
Associate Professor, Department of Pediatrics
Section of Pediatric Endocrinology
University of Colorado School of Medicine
The Children's Hospital
Denver, Colorado

Chun-Hui (Anne) Tsai, MD
Associate Professor, Department of Pediatrics
Section of Clinical Genetics and Metabolism
University of Colorado School of Medicine
The Children's Hospital
Denver, Colorado

Johan L. K. Van Hove, MD, PhD, MBA
Associate Professor, Department of Pediatrics
Section of Clinical Genetics and Metabolism
University of Colorado School of Medicine
The Children's Hospital
Denver, Colorado

Adriana Weinberg, MD
Professor, Departments of Pediatrics and Medicine
Director of Clinical Virology Laboratory
Section of Pediatric Infectious Diseases
University of Colorado School of Medicine
The Children's Hospital
Denver, Colorado

Pamela E. Wilson, MD
Assistant Professor, Department of Rehabilitation Medicine
University of Colorado School of Medicine
The Children's Hospital Rehabilitation Center
Denver, Colorado

Angela T. Yetman, MD
Associate Professor, Department of Pediatrics
Section of Pediatric Cardiology
University of Colorado School of Medicine
The Children's Hospital
Denver, Colorado

Patricia L. Yoon, MD
Assistant Professor, Department of Otolaryngology
University of Colorado School of Medicine
The Children's Hospital
Denver, Colorado

Philip S. Zeitler, MD, PhD
Associate Professor, Department of Pediatrics
Section of Pediatric Endocrinology
University of Colorado School of Medicine
The Children's Hospital
Denver, Colorado

Preface

This is the first edition of *Current Essentials: Pediatrics*. Like the other books in this series, it has been created as a ready reference on pediatric disease for trainees and professionals caring for pediatric in and out patients. It is not a complete text of pediatric medicine. There is a great body of information on normal growth, nutrition, development, and behavior in children that is not included but is integral to good pediatric practice. There is much about pediatric disease management that has not been included.

Current Essentials: Pediatrics is a handbook of pediatric disorders. It is based on its best-selling parent text, *Current Diagnosis and Treatment: Pediatrics*, proudly referred to locally as the "Denver Green Book." Each page describes a single disorder with a list of its key clinical and laboratory features, disorders with similar features that require differentiation, and major components of treatment. I have not included detailed management instructions or drug doses as these vary with each child's size, age, and medical status and are better described in other references. Some of the "pearls" appended to each disorder have been abstracted from *Current Diagnosis and Treatment: Pediatrics* and some are derived from my own experience as a pediatric gastroenterologist. I hope that something telegraphically written on each page will raise more questions about the disorder and will lead to more in-depth investigation.

Inevitably, there were topics that could have been inserted in more than one chapter and I made a number of arbitrary decisions on placement. Check the index and table of contents if a topic doesn't appear in the chapter you anticipated. I welcome all suggestions that will make the second edition of *Current Essentials: Pediatrics* more complete and more useful.

I have been privileged to work for nearly 25 years with the authors of *Current Diagnosis and Treatment: Pediatrics*, all faculty members of the University of Colorado Health Sciences Center. You couldn't ask for smarter, more dedicated, and more generous colleagues. Their consistent effort to keep the Green Book current has made my work on the present handbook a pleasure. Many thanks for the helpful advice of Drs Robert Eilert, William Hay, Taru Hays, Francis Hoe, David Kaplan,

Michael Kappy, Myron Levin, Gary Lum, Kelly Maloney, Kristen Nadeau, John Ogle, Janet Thomas, Sharon Travers, Rachel Seay (MS3), Henry Sondheimer, Neal Sondheimer, and Philip Zeitler. Thanks also to Anne Sydor and Kim Davis at McGraw-Hill for their enthusiasm and persistence.

Judith M. Sondheimer, MD
Denver, Colorado
December 2007

Respipatory Tract

Croup

- **Essentials of Diagnosis**
  - Viral croup—inflammation of the larynx and upper airway structures causes sudden-onset barking cough, stridor, congestion, ± fever. Usually self-limited. Common in children <5 years
  - Viral organisms causing croup—parainfluenza, respiratory syncytial virus (RSV), influenza, rubeola, adenovirus, *Mycoplasma pneumoniae*
  - Bacterial infection of epiglottitis or trachea causes life-threatening stridor (see Chap. 16, Epiglottitis)
  - Spasmodic croup—recurrent episodes of stridor with/without viral infection, may be allergic in origin
  - Viral croup is a clinical diagnosis. Evaluation for other causes of stridor is important and may require imaging, bronchoscopy

- **Differential Diagnosis**
  - Laryngomalacia—common cause of stridor in newborns. Immaturity of cartilage supporting epiglottis and other supraglottic structures improves with time
  - Laryngeal cleft—failure of posterior cricoid fusion causes stridor and recurrent aspiration
  - Angioedema—histamine-mediated acute swelling of skin and/or multiple other systems may involve the larynx and trachea. Caused by allergy, C1 esterase deficiency, medications (angiotensin-converting enzyme [ACE] inhibitors), and cold exposure
  - Laryngeal/esophageal foreign body
  - Retropharyngeal abscess or tumor, mediastinal tumor
  - Subglottic stenosis—congenital or secondary to endotracheal intubation

- **Treatment**
  - Most viral croup is self-limited. Stridor usually lasts 3–5 days
  - Use humidified air especially at night. Maintain good hydration and food intake
  - Stridor at rest or hypoxia should be treated with oxygen; inhale nebulized racemic epinephrine or budesonide
  - Dexamethasone (single dose .6 mg/kg intramuscularly [IM] or .15 mg/kg orally) improves symptoms and reduces frequency of intubation
  - Severe dyspnea/hypoxia, exhaustion, and respiratory failure require endotracheal intubation

- **Pearl**

The younger the child, the smaller diameter of the trachea, the higher the chance that swelling of the airway caused by viral infection may produce respiratory obstruction. Monitor the young child with croup carefully!

Bronchiolitis

- **Essentials of Diagnosis**
  - Acute respiratory infection of young infants producing cough, tachypnea, dyspnea, expiratory wheeze, rhinorrhea, ± fever
  - Other symptoms include irritability, hypoxia, anorexia, vomiting (often post-tussive)
  - Most common cause is RSV. Other organisms—parainfluenza, influenza, adenovirus, *Mycoplasma, Chlamydia, Ureaplasma,* and *Pneumocystis*
  - Nasal washing for RSV and other respiratory pathogens confirms etiology
  - Chest x-ray typically shows hyperinflation, peribronchial cuffing, increased interstitial markings, and subsegmental atelectasis. May be helpful in unusual cases

- **Differential Diagnosis**
  - Reactive airways disease
  - Acute bacterial or viral pneumonitis
  - Atelectasis
  - Heart failure with pulmonary edema
  - Airway foreign body

- **Treatment**
  - Supportive treatment suffices in most healthy infants—humidity, fluids, removal of secretions
  - Respiratory distress may require oxygen, intravenous fluids, frequent suctioning of secretions
  - Bronchodilators and corticosteroids used in severely distressed infants
  - In at-risk patients (immunocompromised, cardiac disease, organ transplant, chronic lung disease), monoclonal RSV antibody prophylaxis reduces hospitalization rate and morbidity
  - Antiviral agents (ribavirin) sometimes used in immunocompromised patients

- **Pearl**

Chronic airway hyper-reactivity (asthma) may be a long-term result of RSV infection. RSV infection is also a significant cause of morbidity in infants with underlying lung and heart disease.

Bronchiectasis

1

- ■ Essentials of Diagnosis
  - • Permanent dilation of bronchi resulting from obstruction by mucus or inflammation. Numerous precipitants—infection (pertussis, tuberculosis, cystic fibrosis, any bacterial or viral pneumonia), immunodeficiency (ciliary dyskinesia, immunoglobulin G [IgG] or IgA deficiency, chronic aspiration), or obstruction (foreign body, cyst)
  - • Chronic cough, sputum production, ronchi and/or wheezes on auscultation of chest, digital clubbing, hemoptysis
  - • In end-stage disease, there is dilation, stricture, and overt destruction of lung structures
  - • Diagnosis confirmed by high-resolution computed tomography (CT) scan of the chest. Sputum cultures reveal normal oropharyngeal flora. Pulmonary function studies show airflow obstruction

- ■ Differential Diagnosis
  - • Pneumonia of any cause
  - • TB
  - • Lung abscess
  - • Recurrent pulmonary emboli
  - • Allergic bronchopulmonary aspergillosis

- ■ Treatment
  - • Avoid tobacco smoke and other environmental pulmonary toxins
  - • Regular pulmonary toilet and aggressive antibiotic therapy during exacerbation
  - • Inhaled mucolytics and bronchodilators may be useful
  - • Surgical removal of severely affected pulmonary segment

- ■ Pearl

Hemoptysis is less common in children with bronchiectasis than it is in adults.

1

Cystic Fibrosis (CF)

- **Essentials of Diagnosis**
  - Autosomal recessive defect in cystic fibrosis transmembrane conductance regulator (CFTR) gene which regulates chloride ion movements in pancreas, biliary tree, intestines, airway epithelium, sweat ducts, and vas deferens
  - Numerous mutations at this locus on chromosome 7 produce varying clinical manifestations
  - 15% of homozygotes have ileal obstruction at birth (meconium ileus)
  - Infants present with diarrhea and failure to thrive due to pancreatic insufficiency or lung infections due to *S aureus* or *Pseudomonas* lung infections
  - Other presentations—liver disease, male infertility, spontaneous pneumothorax, hypochloremic dehydration, nasal polyps, sinusitis, rectal prolapse. Heterozygotes are unaffected
  - Serum immunoreactive trypsinogen elevated in most neonates (except in meconium ileus)
  - Sweat chloride >60 mmol/L in most cases. Genotyping identifies specific *CFTR* mutations

- **Differential Diagnosis**
  - Asthma and bronchiectasis mimic CF
  - Primary ciliary dyskinesia (Kartagener syndrome) causes chronic bronchitis, sinusitis, and otitis starting at birth. Often associated with situs inversus. Males are infertile. Sweat test normal
  - Immunodeficiency syndromes including AIDS
  - Other causes of pancreatic exocrine insufficiency—Shwachman syndrome

- **Treatment**
  - Progressive lung disease is the most important cause of morbidity and mortality. Prevention/treatment of lung infections is key to survival
  - High-calorie, high-protein diet with exocrine pancreatic enzyme supplements and fat-soluble vitamins
  - Inhaled mucolytics, inhaled recombinant human DNAase, inhaled tobramycin and oral azithromycin (for *Pseudomonas* infection), bronchodilators, anti-inflammatory medications, all preserve pulmonary function

- **Pearl**

CF is the most common recessive lethal gene of Caucasians. Disease frequency is about 1:3000. The most common severe mutation is ΔF508. Median life expectancy is now in the mid-thirties because of early detection and aggressive pulmonary therapy.

Bacterial Pneumonia

- **Essentials of Diagnosis**
  - Inflammation of the lung with variable presentation depending on causative organism. Usually includes fever, cough, systemic toxicity, sputum production
  - Abnormal chest sounds—rales, decreased breath sounds, dullness to percussion, splinting, friction rub, tactile or vocal fremitus
  - White blood cells (WBC) usually >15,000/μL; chest x-ray shows infiltrates, atelectasis, hilar adenopathy, or pleural effusion. WBC <5000/μL carries poor prognosis
  - Predisposing factors—aspiration, immunodeficiency, congenital lung abnormalities, inadequate mucous clearance, congestive heart failure
  - Empyema may complicate infections with staphylococcus, pneumococcus, and group A β-hemolytic streptococcus

- **Potential Bacterial Pathogens**
  - Most common organisms are *Streptococcus pneumoniae, Haemophilus influenzae, S aureus, Legionella pneumophillia,* gram-negative rods
  - Acid-fast bacteria
  - *Chlamydia pneumoniae, Clamydia trachomatis, Clamydia psittaci* (inclusion conjunctivitis, eosinophilia, and elevated Ig's)
  - *M pneumoniae* (positive-cold hemagglutinins and polymerase chain reaction
  - *Coxiella burnetii* (Q fever)
  - *Pneumocystis* species
  - *Bordetella pertussis*

- **Treatment**
  - Empiric antibiotic therapy for likely organism suggested by history and x-ray
  - Culture sputum, tracheobronchial secretions, or pleural fluid, if available
  - Nonspecific therapy—oxygen, humidification, hydration, nutrition support, pulmonary toilet, ventilatory support
  - Presumed *S pneumoniae* lobar pneumonia treated with oral β-lactams. Persistent symptoms suggest resistant organism and may require quinolones, clindamycin, or vancomycin
  - Final antibiotic choices based upon specific culture and sensitivity
  - Hospitalization depends upon clinical severity, underlying medical condition, and need for isolation

- **Pearl**

Pneumococcal vaccines prevent or reduce the severity of disease in 90% of patients.

Viral Pneumonia

- **Essentials of Diagnosis**
  - Upper respiratory prodrome followed by persistent cough, coryza, hoarseness, fever, wheezing, tachypnea, scant sputum, systemic malaise, and myalgia (especially in older children)
  - Causative agents—RSV, parainfluenza, influenza A and B, human metapneumovirus, adenovirus, measles
  - WBC often normal or slightly elevated
  - Rapid diagnosis by fluorescent-antibody technique (FA) or enzyme-linked immunosorbent assay (ELISA) on nasopharyngeal secretions available for many organisms
  - Chest x-ray shows perihilar streaking, increased interstitial markings, peribronchial cuffing, patchy infiltrates. Lobar consolidation can occur
  - Necrotizing pneumonia with pneumatoceles may occur in adenoviral pneumonia

- **Differential Diagnosis**
  - Bacterial pneumonia
  - Asthma
  - Foreign body aspiration
  - Acute bacterial or viral tracheitis

- **Treatment**
  - Most children with viral pneumonia recover uneventfully
  - Supportive care—oxygen, humidity, fluid and nutrition support, pulmonary toilet, fever control, isolation to control spread
  - Newborns, patients with underlying lung, cardiac or immune disorders are at highest risk for severe infection or long-term adverse impact on lung function
  - Antiviral agents (ribavirin, amantidine, rimantadine, oseltamivir) in appropriate high-risk patients
  - In high-risk patients, empiric antibiotic therapy may be indicated if bacterial infection cannot be excluded
  - Vaccinate (influenza A and B) or prophylax (RSV monoclonal) high-risk patients

- **Pearl**

In immunosuppressed patients, other viruses (cytomegalovirus, Epstein-Barr virus) or combinations of viruses, bacteria, and fungi may be the cause of pneumonia.

Lung Abscess

- **Essentials of Diagnosis**
  - High fever, malaise, weight loss with/without symptoms referable to the chest most often in patients with immunocompromise, severe infections elsewhere (embolism), aspiration, malnutrition, or chest trauma
  - Elevated WBC and elevated erythrocyte sedimentation rate (ESR). Blood cultures rarely positive
  - Chest x-ray—thick-walled cavities with air fluid levels, compression atelectasis, pleural thickening, and adenopathy. CT scan required for accurate localization
  - Organisms include *S aureus, H influenzae, S pneumoniae,* and *Streptococcus viridans.* Immunocompromised hosts may harbor anaerobes, gram negatives, *Nocardia, Legionella, Candida,* and *Aspergillus.*
  - Sputum culture may be diagnostic, but direct aspiration of abscess is better

- **Differential Diagnosis**
  - Loculated pyopneumothorax
  - Echinococcus cyst
  - Neoplasm
  - Plasma cell granuloma
  - Infected congenital cyst or sequestration

- **Treatment**
  - Broad-spectrum coverage directed at *S aureus, H influenzae,* and streptococci for 3 or more weeks unless a specific organism is identified
  - Transthoracic drainage is sometimes possible with radiologic guidance
  - In severe cases, surgical drainage or lobectomy may be required
  - Aspiration-related abscesses or abscess in immunocompromised patients may require antibiotics to cover gram-negative and anaerobic organisms.
  - In healthy hosts, ultimate outcome usually good

- **Pearl**

Consider the possibility of a radiolucent foreign body in a previously healthy child with a lung abscess. Bronchoscopy may be indicated.

1

Pulmonary Embolism

- **Essentials of Diagnosis**
  - Occurs in sickle cell anemia, rheumatic fever, bacterial endocarditis, schistosomiasis, bone fracture, dehydration, polycythemia, nephrotic syndrome, atrial fibrillation, contraceptive use, cancer chemotherapy, shock
  - Risk of embolism increased if there is underlying hypercoagulability—inflammatory bowel disease, antiphospholipid antibodies, protein S or protein C deficiency, factor V Leiden
  - Symptoms—acute-onset dyspnea, tachypnea, pleuritic pain, splinting, cyanosis, tachycardia
  - Radiographs often normal. May show peripheral infiltrate, pleural effusion, elevated hemidiaphragm, or unilateral increase in pulmonary artery size and flow (in large emboli)
  - Ventilation/perfusion scan, spiral CT, and pulmonary angiography are confirmatory

- **Differential Diagnosis**
  - Pneumonia and/or pleural effusion
  - Myocardial infarction
  - Atelectasis
  - Other causes of acute respiratory distress, eg, asthma, pneumothorax

- **Treatment**
  - Acute care—supplemental oxygen, sedation, anticoagulation with heparin to maintain activated partial thromboplastin time (PTT) of 1.5 normal for 24 hours
  - Intravenous (IV) urokinase or tissue plasminogen activator for 36 hours may dissolve embolus
  - Warfarin therapy for at least 6 weeks to keep the international normalized ratio (INR) >2
  - With lower extremity deep vein thrombosis inferior vena cava interruption may be necessary

- **Pearl**

Pulmonary embolism is relatively rare in children and symptoms are less severe than in adults. It is probably underdiagnosed for these reasons.

Sudden Infant Death Syndrome (SIDS)

■ Essentials of Diagnosis
- Death of an infant <1 year unexplained despite complete autopsy, review of the death scene, and thorough clinical history
- Peak age 2–4 months, most often occurring between midnight and 8 AM
- Risk factors—low socioeconomic status, prone sleeping, low birth weight, teenage or drug-addicted mothers, maternal smoking, family history of SIDS
- Decreased arousal during sleep or hypoxia and rebreathing of exhaled gases in the setting of autonomic immaturity appear to be key to pathogenesis
- Pathologic findings—intrathoracic petechiae, mild respiratory tract inflammation and congestion, brainstem gliosis, increased periadrenal brown fat

■ Differential Diagnosis
- Drug overdose
- Cardiac disease
- Child abuse
- Neurologic disease

■ Treatment
- Preventative measures include firm sleeping surface without fluffy bedding, supine sleep position, avoid cosleeping with parents, eliminate environmental smoke, pacifier at bed and nap, avoid overheating, educate all caregivers about sleep position
- Thorough evaluation may reveal an organic cause in up to 20% of SIDS cases
- Home respiratory and cardiac monitors do not decrease the risk of SIDS
- Family support and education are critical to recovery from this tragedy

■ Pearl

Histories in infants dying of SIDS rarely reveal a previous history of apparent life-threatening events (ALTEs). Childhood immunizations have not been linked to SIDS.

Pneumothorax

- ■ Essentials of Diagnosis
  - • Air leak from lung into pleural space can occur spontaneously but more often occurs after birth trauma, positive pressure ventilation, underlying obstructive/restrictive lung disease, emphysema, cystic lung disease
  - • Air may dissect into mediastinum, pericardium, subcutaneous tissue, peritoneal serosa, and intestinal mesenteries from the pleural space
  - • Symptoms variable. May include dyspnea, pain, cyanosis, decreased breath sounds, and hyper-resonance. Cardiac output may be impaired in large pneumothoraces
  - • Cross-table lateral and decubitus chest x-rays are helpful. CT is very sensitive

- ■ Differential Diagnosis
  - • Most common cause of acute deterioration of ventilated patient is pneumothorax, but dislodged or obstructed endotracheal tube should be ruled out by chest x-ray
  - • Diaphragmatic hernia
  - • Lung cyst, congenital lobar emphysema, cystic adenomatoid malformation, or pneumatocele may have similar physical and x-ray appearance
  - • Ball valve bronchial obstruction with hyperinflation due to extrinsic mass, foreign body, mucous plug

- ■ Treatment
  - • Assess underlying cause
  - • Small or asymptomatic pneumothorax (<15%), does not require treatment
  - • Large or symptomatic pneumothorax requires needle aspiration to relieve tension
  - • Chest tube or pigtail catheter may be placed to provide ongoing air removal
  - • In older patients with spontaneous pneumothorax, recurrences may require pleural sclerosing procedure (video-assisted thoracoscopic surgery [VATS])

- ■ Pearl

Tall, lean adolescent males have an increased risk of spontaneous pneumothorax. Pneumothorax may be the first manifestation of CF or Marfan syndrome.

Pulmonary Sequestration

- ■ Essentials of Diagnosis
  - • Nonfunctional pulmonary tissue lacking communication with the tracheobronchial tree
  - • *Extralobar*—mass of pulmonary tissue separate from normal lung with its own pleural covering. Blood supply from systemic or pulmonary circulation. May communicate with esophagus or stomach. Usual location near left diaphragm. 50% associated with other anomalies—congenital diaphragmatic hernia, bronchogenic cysts, heart defects
  - • *Intralobar*—isolated lung segment within the normal pleura. Blood supply from branches of aorta. Usual location in left lower lobe. No associated congenital abnormalities
  - • Presents with mass, cough, wheezing, recurrent pneumonia, hemoptysis

- ■ Differential Diagnosis
  - • Pneumonia
  - • Lung mass
  - • Diaphragmatic hernia
  - • Cystic adenomatoid malformation of the lung
  - • Respiratory distress of the newborn caused by heart or lung disease

- ■ Treatment
  - • Careful evaluation of blood supply by angiography
  - • Surgical resection if possible

- ■ Pearl

Intralobar sequestrations are rarely seen in newborn infants. This, plus the rarity of associated anomalies, suggests that these sequestrations may be acquired lesions resulting from chronic infection.

Eventration of the Diaphragm

- **Essentials of Diagnosis**
  - Striated musculature of the diaphragm replaced by connective tissue causes elevation of the diaphragm during inspiration
  - *Congenital*—incomplete in utero development of diaphragmatic muscle anlagen, may be unilateral or bilateral
  - *Acquired*—denervation and atrophy of diaphragm muscles secondary to pre- or postnatal phrenic nerve injury (trauma, tumor, surgery)
  - When large, paradoxical movement of diaphragm causes respiratory distress, pain, increased work of breathing, respiratory failure
  - Neonates with large eventrations may have a scaphoid abdomen with unilateral decreased basilar breath sounds
  - Often diagnosed postoperatively when patient cannot be extubated. Chest fluoroscopy is usually diagnostic

- **Differential Diagnosis**
  - Diaphragmatic hernia
  - Lung mass
  - Large basal pleural effusion or consolidation
  - Lateral chest x-rays may suggest anterior mediastinal mass

- **Treatment**
  - Spontaneous recovery occurs in ~50% of surgical or perinatal phrenic injuries within 3–4 months
  - No therapy required for small asymptomatic eventration. Eventrations may become larger with age and should be monitored
  - When symptomatic, surgical plication of the diaphragm prevents excessive paradoxical movement

- **Pearl**

The only symptom of congenital eventration in neonates may be dyspnea and distress during feedings. Listen carefully to both sides of the chest as well as the heart in babies who tire easily with feedings but seem normal otherwise.

Pulmonary Hypoplasia

- ■ Essentials of Diagnosis
  - • Incomplete development of one or both lungs with ↓numbers of alveoli and small airways
  - • Most common cause is diaphragmatic hernia. Other causes— intrathoracic mass, ↓ thoracic size, ↓fetal breathing, ↓pulmonary blood flow, primary mesodermal defect
  - • Advanced bronchopulmonary dysplasia is the most common post-natal cause of bilateral pulmonary hypoplasia
  - • Variable presentation relates to the severity of hypoplasia and related abnormalities
  - • Chest x-ray may be normal or show volume loss on affected side. CT scan is the optimal diagnostic imaging. Ventilation/perfusion scan, angiography, and bronchoscopy may be helpful

- ■ Differential Diagnosis
  - • Pulmonary agenesis usually affects left side. Mediastinum shifted to left. Often associated with vertebral abnormalities, rib fusion, and renal anomalies

- ■ Treatment
  - • Mainly supportive—prevention and treatment of infection, supplemental oxygen, ventilatory support
  - • Early surgical treatment of underlying causes (tumor, diaphragmatic hernia/eventration, pulmonary sequestration, chest cage abnormalities, cardiac lesions) may improve prognosis
  - • Monitor and treat subsequent pulmonary hypertension

- ■ Pearl

Consider pulmonary hypoplasia in a neonate with a "spontaneous" pneumothorax.

Acute Respiratory Distress Syndrome (ARDS)

- **Essentials of Diagnosis**
  - Acute respiratory failure with ↑pulmonary capillary permeability, pulmonary edema, refractory hypoxemia, and ↓lung compliance
  - Tachypnea, respiratory alkalosis are early signs followed by tachycardia, cyanosis, irritability, and dyspnea
  - Diagnosis requires absence of left ventricular failure and ratio of arterial oxygen (Pao_2) to inspired oxygen (Fio_2) concentration <200
  - Bilateral diffuse alveolar infiltrates on chest x-ray. CT shows areas of collapse and overaeration
  - Direct precipitants are lung injury from aspiration, hydrocarbon, heat, contusion, infection, near drowning
  - Indirect precipitants—sepsis, shock, pancreatitis, burns, trauma, fat embolism, drug overdose, transfusion reaction

- **Differential Diagnosis**
  - $Pao_2 : Fio_2$ between 200 and 300 with other ARDS criteria is usually called acute lung injury
  - Late phase of ARDS may be complicated by pulmonary fibrosis, pneumothorax, cor pulmonale, persistent infiltrates, all of which are characteristic of other chronic interstitial lung diseases

- **Treatment**
  - Precise identification of underlying cause is essential to effective therapy
  - Multiorgan system monitoring mandatory
  - Intensive cardiopulmonary and hemodynamic monitoring and support including pulmonary artery catheterization
  - Reduce intravascular volume to prevent pulmonary fluid accumulation
  - Ventilator strategies to recruit areas of dependent alveolar collapse and prevent overdistension of noncollapsed areas
  - Prone positioning may improve oxygenation
  - Inhaled nitric oxide reduces pulmonary artery pressure and improves ventilation/perfusion ratio
  - Surfactant replacement may improve lung compliance.
  - Corticosteroids may reduce late-stage inflammation and fibrosis
  - Extracorporeal membrane oxygenation (ECMO) may not have any advantage over careful ventilator strategies

- **Pearl**

Nonpulmonary organ failures are the leading cause of death in pediatric and adult ARDS patients. Mortality is about 40%.

Bronchiolitis Obliterans with Organizing Pneumonia (BOOP)

- ■ Essentials of Diagnosis
  - Obstruction of bronchi and bronchioles by fibrous tissue following damage to the lower respiratory tract
  - Causes include inhalation of toxic gases, infections, connective tissue diseases, AIDS, organ transplantation, aspiration, Stevens-Johnson syndrome, idiopathic
  - Persistent cough, wheezing, sputum production after an episode of acute pneumonia. Digital clubbing rare
  - Restrictive abnormalities tests of pulmonary function
  - Chest x-ray findings nonspecific. Diagnosis confirmed by lung biopsy

- ■ Differential Diagnosis
  - Reactive airways disease
  - CF
  - Bronchopulmonary dysplasia
  - Severe pneumonia due to bacteria, fungi, or TB

- ■ Treatment
  - Supplemental oxygen if needed. Antibiotics for documented infection
  - Prevent further airway damage from aspiration, environmental toxins, infection
  - Bronchodilators may be helpful if there is a reactive component
  - Corticosteroids may be used

- ■ Pearl

Prognosis depends upon underlying cause and age of onset. The course may progress to end-stage lung disease despite therapy.

1

Asthma—Reactive Airways Disease

- **Essentials of Diagnosis**
  - Most common chronic disease of childhood
  - Episodic wheezing, cough, dyspnea, chest tightness often in a setting of atopy, previous pulmonary viral infection, environmental allergen exposure or cold stress
  - Underlying airway hyper-responsiveness to specific and nonspecific stimuli produces inflammation with reversible expiratory airflow limitation

- **Differential Diagnosis**
  - Viral bronchiolitis or other pulmonary infection
  - Aspiration
  - Air flow obstruction—laryngotracheomalacia, vascular ring, airway stenosis, mediastinal mass, foreign body, vocal cord dysfunction
  - Bronchopulmonary dysplasia, obliterative bronchiolitis
  - CF
  - Chronic congestive heart failure with "cardiac asthma"

- **Treatment**
  - Decrease allergen exposure at home, especially in the bedroom
  - Avoid tobacco smoke, air pollution, suspected allergens, β-blockers, sulfite containing foods
  - Immunize against influenza. Treat respiratory illness aggressively
  - Assess peak flow rates daily to anticipate exacerbations
  - Mild intermittent symptoms respond to short-course corticosteroids, short-acting inhaled β_2-agonists
  - Moderate persistent symptoms may be treated with cromolyn, leukotriene modifiers, sustained release theophylline, longer course corticosteroids, β_2-agonists, anticholinergics

- **Pearl**

Mortality and morbidity (measured by hospital admissions) of asthma in the United States are three to four times higher in African American children than other ethnic groups. The cause(s) of this dramatic disparity is not clear but high incidence of atopy, poor access to medical services, and increased exposure to inhaled allergens may be important.

Pulmonary Tuberculosis (Pulmonary TB)   `1`

- ■ Essentials of Diagnosis
  - • Increasing frequency in United States and worldwide
  - • Variable clinical presentations—positive TB skin test, primary asymptomatic infection, Ghon complex, bronchial obstruction, segmental lesions, calcified nodules, pleural effusion, primary cavitary lesions, miliary pulmonary infection, local or metastatic spread to other organs (mediastinal nodes, bones, meninges, kidneys, adrenals, intestine)
  - • Poverty, malnutrition, homelessness, travel in endemic areas, contact with infected adults, and immunodeficiency are risk factors
  - • Diagnosis by positive skin test, x-ray findings, positive acid fast stain or culture of sputum, pleural biopsy, or gastric washings
  - • Chronic cough, anorexia, weight loss, failure to gain, unexplained fever suggest evaluation for TB

- ■ Differential Diagnosis
  - • Atypical mycobacterial infections. Routine TB skin test may be falsely positive. Culture may be required to differentiate
  - • Lymphadenitis, lymphoma
  - • Lung tumor
  - • Fungal infection
  - • Sarcoid
  - • Metastatic TB infection may present as isolated bacterial meningitis, osteomyelitis, enteritis, peritonitis, nephritis, otitis, dermatitis, adrenal insufficiency, sepsis, and multiorgan failure

- ■ Treatment
  - • Spontaneous healing is the usual course of primary infection in normal children
  - • Isoniazid is drug of choice for newly positive TB skin test
  - • Isoniazid plus rifampin for 6 months with pyrazinamide for first 2 months used for primary pulmonary infection
  - • Corticosteroids used for mediastinal lymphadenopathy compressing the airways, massive pleural effusion with mediastinal shift and miliary TB
  - • Increasingly, multiple drug-resistant strains require changes in antibiotic regimens. Check the AAP *Red Book* for updates.

- ■ Pearl

BCG immunization given to infants in endemic areas may cause false-positive tuberculin skin tests. Very malnourished or immunocompromised children may be anergic to intradermal antigens causing a false-negative TB skin test.

2

Cardiovascular Disorders

Atrial Septal Defect (ASD)

- ■ **Essentials of Diagnosis**
  - • Congenital opening in the interatrial septum
  - • Small ASD, often asymptomatic. Large ASD may cause fatigue and failure to thrive in children, and pulmonary hypertension with atrial arrhythmias in adults
  - • *Ostium secundum*—most common type, located in midseptum
  - • *Ostium primum defect*—located low in the septum, is a form of atrioventricular septal defect
  - • *Sinus venosus type defect*—located high in the septum, often associated with partial anomalous pulmonary venous return
  - • Physical examination—right ventricular heave
  - • Auscultation—fixed wide split S_2, systolic ejection murmur at left upper sternal edge, ± diastolic murmur at lower left sternal edge
  - • Electrocardiogram (ECG)—rSR′ in lead V_1
  - • Diagnosis confirmed by echocardiography

- ■ **Differential**
  - • Holt-Oram syndrome—autosomal dominant NKX2-5 mutation with variable penetration. Narrow shoulders, absent thumbs, upper limb anomalies, ostium secundum ASD
  - • Partial anomalous pulmonary venous return
  - • Ebstein anomaly of the tricuspid valve

- ■ **Treatment**
  - • Many ASDs close spontaneously
  - • In symptomatic children 1–3 years old, close ASD surgically or place occluding device during cardiac catheterization
  - • Bacterial endocarditis prophylaxis during dental work not required

- ■ **Pearl**

Ostium secundum ASDs <4 mm diameter usually close spontaneously.

Ventricular Septal Defect (VSD)

2

- **Essentials of Diagnosis**
  - Congenital opening in the interventricular septum accounts for 35% of congenital heart disease
  - Oxygenated blood shunts from left ventricle (LV) (high pressure) to right ventricle (RV) (low pressure)
  - *Small/moderate shunt*—acyanotic, asymptomatic, pansystolic murmur maximal along the lower left sternal border, normal P_2
  - *Large shunt*—acyanotic, easy fatigability, heart failure, pansystolic murmur at the lower left sternal border, accentuated P_2, apical diastolic murmur, biventricular enlargement
  - *Chronic left-to-right shunt* causes gradual ↑pulmonary vascular pressure, ↓gradient between ventricles, and ↓shunt volume, right ventricular lift, palpable P_2, systolic ejection murmur at left sternal border, arterial desaturation, right-sided heart failure
  - Murmur may not appear in neonates until the normal decrease in pulmonary vascular resistance at 4-6 weeks of age
  - Diagnosis confirmed by echocardiography. Cardiac catheterization only required to measure pulmonary artery pressure and resistance

- **Differential Diagnosis**
  - VSD is often associated with more complex congenital heart diseases such as transposition of the great arteries (TGA) or tricuspid atresia

- **Treatment**
  - VSDs <3 mm close spontaneously. 85% of VSDs are <3 mm
  - VSDs 3–5 mm rarely develop pulmonary hypertension. When left-to-right shunt ratio is >2:1, heart failure may be severe enough to require VSD closure by surgical patching
  - VSDs >6 mm always require surgery to prevent chronic left-to-right shunt and pulmonary hypertension
  - Most defects can be closed in infancy with mortality <2%
  - American Heart Association recommendation (2007)—no antibiotic prophylaxis for bacterial endocarditis in unrepaired or completely repaired VSD. Prophylaxis recommended for patients with residual VSD postsurgery.

- **Pearl**

Because surgery is now performed in young infants with VSD, Eisenmenger syndrome (suprasystemic pulmonary hypertension with right-to-left shunt) has almost disappeared.

Atrioventricular Septal Defect (AV Septal Defect)

■ Essentials of Diagnosis

- Incomplete fusion of embryonic endocardial cushions causes conjoined defect of lower atrial and upper ventricular septum with defects in tricuspid and mitral valve leaflets
- Murmur often inaudible in newborns. Loud pulmonary component of S_2
- Left axis deviation on ECG
- 4% of all congenital heart disease. Common in Down syndrome
- Small AV septal defects may act hemodynamically like an isolated ostium primum ASD
- Large, complete AV septal defect causes heart failure, failure to thrive, recurrent pneumonia, cardiac hypertrophy, diastolic flow murmur at lower left sternal border, pulmonary vascular hypertension
- Partial forms of AV septal defect have intermediate symptom severity
- Diagnosis confirmed by echocardiography. Cardiac catheterization only to measure pulmonary artery pressure

■ Differential Diagnosis

- Other causes of congestive heart failure—VSD, single ventricle

■ Treatment

- Surgery always required for AV septal defects
- Repair of partial defects is very successful with 1–2% mortality
- After repair of partial defects, monitor patients for late mitral valve dysfunction and LV outflow obstruction
- Repair complete defects in first year of life to avoid development of irreversible pulmonary hypertension
- Bacterial endocarditis prophylaxis is not required either pre- or postsurgery unless there is a residual VSD postoperatively

■ Pearl

Patients with Down syndrome have a lower incidence of mitral valve insufficiency after surgical repair of AV septal defect and less frequently require reoperation than children with normal chromosomes.

Patent Ductus Arteriosus (PDA)

- **Essentials of Diagnosis**
  - Postnatal persistence of the ductus arteriosus connecting pulmonary artery and aorta during fetal life
  - Variable murmur (premature neonates) or continuous murmur (term neonates) with active precordium and full pulses
  - Increased incidence of PDA at high altitude, in females, and preterms <1500 g
  - PDA causes left-to-right shunt, pulmonary volume overload, increased oxygen requirement, and deteriorating pulmonary status in premature infants with respiratory distress syndrome
  - Diagnosis confirmed by echocardiography

- **Differential Diagnosis**
  - ASD and VSD in neonates may have similar findings
  - Benign, loud venous hum in older children may sound like the continuous murmur of PDA

- **Treatment**
  - Spontaneous closure occurs in term neonates at 3–5 days of age
  - Hypoxia retards spontaneous closure
  - Medical closure with indomethacin or ibuprofen is 80–90% effective in infants >1000 g
  - In children >1 year, close small PDA with normal pulmonary artery pressure by inserting coil into ductus during cardiac catheterization
  - Surgically ligate large PDA with significant left-to-right shunt before age 1 year
  - Bacterial endocarditis prophylaxis not required in unrepaired PDA. After closure, prophylaxis needed only if closure is not complete.

- **Pearl**

The characteristic murmur of PDA—continuous "machinery" murmur radiating to the back—is rarely heard before 6 months of age.

Cardiac Malformations Causing Right-Sided Obstruction

2

- ■ Essentials of Diagnosis
  - Major entities—pulmonary valve stenosis (PS) with intact ventricular septum (most common); infundibular, supravalvular, and peripheral PS; Ebstein malformation of the tricuspid valve; absent pulmonary artery or vein
  - Peripheral pulmonic stenosis murmur—present in many healthy newborn infants. Resolves gradually
  - Severe right-sided obstruction causes—cyanosis, right-sided heart failure
  - Wide split S_2 and quiet P_2. Systolic murmur maximal in pulmonary area, systolic ejection click heard in valvular stenosis
  - Diagnosis by echocardiography. ECG and cardiac catheterization needed to fully define anatomy

- ■ Associated Syndromes
  - Supravalvular pulmonary stenosis—Noonan syndrome
  - Peripheral pulmonary stenosis—Williams syndrome, Alagille syndrome, congenital rubella
  - Ebstein malformation with minimal valve displacement may present in adults with tachyarrhythmias from progressive right atrial dilation
  - Tetralogy of Fallot (T of F)—absence of pulmonary artery (right or left) and absence of the pulmonary valve

- ■ Treatment
  - Immediate surgical repair if right ventricular systolic pressure is equal to or greater than systemic pressure
  - Elective surgical repair if right ventricular systolic pressure is two-thirds systemic
  - Repair infundibular stenosis surgically if there is significant right ventricular outflow obstruction
  - Significant peripheral pulmonic stenosis surgical repair is repaired using balloon angioplasty
  - Neonates with Ebstein malformation—prostaglandin E maintains pulmonary flow temporarily in very cyanotic infants. Surgery often needed
  - No antibiotic prophylaxis for endocarditis needed in these abnormalities (American Academy of Pediatrics, 2007)

- ■ Pearl

There are 5 Ts for cyanotic congenital heart disease: T of F, TGA, total anomalous pulmonary venous drainage, tricuspid atresia, and truncus arteriosus. But severe PS can present with cyanosis too.

Aortic Malformations with Left-Sided Obstruction

2

- ■ Essentials of Diagnosis
  - *Aortic coarctation*—pulse lag in lower extremities, systolic blood pressure ≥20 mm Hg higher in upper than lower extremities, blowing systolic murmur in left axilla
  - *Aortic stenosis*—systolic ejection murmur at upper right sternal border. Palpable thrill over carotid arteries, systolic click auscultated at cardiac apex, dilated ascending aorta on x-ray
  - Mild coarctation or stenosis causes no symptoms. Severe abnormalities cause left-sided heart failure
  - Diagnosis confirmed by echocardiography. Doppler ultrasound can estimate the transvalvular pressure gradients accurately

- ■ Associated Syndromes
  - Aortic coarctation—Turner syndrome, Shone syndrome (coarct with associated mitral stenosis and left heart hypoplasia)
  - Valvular aortic stenosis—more common in males
  - Supravalvular aortic stenosis—constriction of ascending aorta (can be familial). Associated with Williams syndrome (infantile hypercalcemia and mental retardation)

- ■ Treatment
  - Immediate surgical repair or balloon aortoplasty/valvuloplasty during cardiac catheterization for neonates with severe coarctation/stenosis and left heart failure
  - Elective surgery or balloon valvuloplasty for aortic stenosis if resting gradient is 60–80 mm Hg or if there is aortic insufficiency. Recurrence occurs in >25% of patients with subvalvular disease
  - Elective repair of aortic coarctation by balloon aortoplasty or surgery. Recurrences (10–15% of cases) treatable with stent or balloon
  - Surgical repair of coarctation repair after age 5 carries ↑risk of systemic hypertension, myocardial dysfunction, and sudden death from hypertension
  - Endocarditis prophylaxis needed after valve replacement surgery

- ■ Pearl

All forms of LV outflow tract obstruction tend to get worse as growth requires larger cardiac output through the same sized outflow tract.

Mitral Valve Prolapse

- ■ Essentials of Diagnosis

  - Redundant mitral valve tissue prolapses back into the left atrium during ventricular contraction causing mitral insufficiency
  - Most common in thin adolescent females
  - Symptoms—usually mild or none. Patients may have chest pain, palpitations, dizziness, weakness. Symptoms often mistaken for anxiety or depression
  - Midsystolic click best heard while patient stands or during Valsalva. Late systolic "whoop" or "honking" murmur
  - Continuous ECG monitoring may show ventricular ectopy and brief runs of ventricular tachycardia
  - Echocardiography shows posterior movement of the mitral valve leaflets to the atrium during systole, shows the extent of mitral insufficiency and degree of myxomatous change in mitral valve

- ■ Associated Conditions

  - Marfan syndrome
  - Ehlers-Danlos syndrome
  - Fragile X syndrome

- ■ Treatment

  - Treat associated arrhythmias with propranolol
  - As an isolated condition in childhood it is usually benign
  - Teenaged girls may benefit from increased fluid and salt intake to increase intravascular volume
  - Surgery for mitral insufficiency rarely needed
  - Endocarditis prophylaxis not required

- ■ Pearl

Cardiac ultrasonography may overdiagnose this condition.

2

Anomalous Origin of the Left Coronary Artery from the Pulmonary Artery

- **Essentials of Diagnosis**
  - Left coronary artery arises from the pulmonary artery rather than the aorta. Myocardial perfusion poor, secondary to low pulmonary pressure
  - Symptoms appear as neonate's pulmonary artery pressure falls (2–4 months) causing poor perfusion and oxygenation of the LV myocardium
  - Ischemia and infarction of the LV cause angina, poor feeding, pallor, sweating, colic, tachypnea, and cardiac failure
  - Pansystolic murmur of mitral regurgitation with large heart
  - ECG shows ischemic changes with inverted T waves in I, aVL, and precordial leads. Prominent Q waves in I, aVL, and V_{4-6}
  - Echocardiography is diagnostic
  - Prognosis is guarded, even with immediate surgery

- **Differential Diagnosis**
  - Other causes of LV failure—aortic disease, large VSD, cardiomyopathy
  - Food refusal
  - Infantile colic
  - Failure to thrive
  - Sepsis

- **Treatment**
  - Institute diuretics and afterload reduction
  - Immediate surgery to reimplant the coronary artery at the aortic root
  - Mitral valve may have to be replaced

- **Pearl**

An increase in cardiac output of 20% occurs after feeding in infants. This increased demand causes true angina in infants with anomalous left coronary syndrome and they refuse to eat.

Hypoplastic Left Heart Syndrome

2

- ■ Essentials of Diagnosis
  - • Underdeveloped LV musculature occurs in 1.3–3.8% of infants with congenital heart disease
  - • Mild cyanosis at birth; minimal auscultatory findings; rapid onset of profound left heart failure as ductus arteriosus closes at 3–5 days of age
  - • Associated abnormalities—mitral atresia, aortic atresia
  - • Uniformly fatal without treatment
  - • Diagnosis often made prenatally by ultrasonography at 18–20 weeks. Diagnosis confirmed by echocardiogram. ECG shows right axis deviation and paucity of LV forces

- ■ Differential Diagnosis
  - • Other causes of heart failure in the first month—coarctation, cardiomyopathy
  - • Severe acute pulmonary disease
  - • Multiorgan failure from septicemia

- ■ Treatment
  - • Continuous IV prostaglandin E_1 maintains patency of ductus arteriosus
  - • Nitrogen added to inhaled air lowers inspired O_2 to <21%, increases pulmonary vascular tone, and improves systemic perfusion
  - • Surgical palliation—Norwood operation uses the RV as the systemic ventricle with an aortopulmonary shunt for pulmonary blood flow
  - • Cardiac transplantation is a second surgical option
  - • Prophylaxis for endocarditis required after the Norwood operation

- ■ Pearl

Only 50% of children with hypoplastic left heart in the United States are diagnosed prenatally by in utero ultrasound.

Tetralogy of Fallot (T of F)

2

■ Essentials of Diagnosis

- Most common cyanotic cardiac lesion. 10% of all congenital heart disease
- Constellation of defects—large membranous VSD with overriding aorta, obstructed right ventricular outflow tract (pulmonary valve and infundibular hypoplasia), right ventricular hypertrophy
- Cyanosis due to right-to-left shunting through the VSD appears by age 4 months. May be mild if right ventricular outflow obstruction is mild
- Systolic ejection murmur at upper left sternal border
- Hypoxemic spells (Tet spells) start during infancy—sudden deep cyanosis, dyspnea, alteration in consciousness, syncope, decrease in murmur
- Echocardiography is diagnostic

■ Differential Diagnosis

- Other cyanotic congenital conditions can be ruled out by echocardiography
- Deletion of long arm of chromosome 22 (22q11) is found in 15% of cases

■ Treatment

- Treatment of Tet spells—correct acidosis, administer oxygen, increase pulmonary flow by placing child in knee-chest position. Propranolol and morphine sometimes helpful to increase pulmonary flow
- Prevention of Tet spells temporarily with oral propranolol
- Surgically created shunt from subclavian artery to pulmonary (Blalock-Taussig shunt) to palliate cyanosis, Tet spells, right heart failure
- Corrective open heart surgery performed early may make shunting unnecessary
- Endocarditis prophylaxis required in unrepaired or shunted T of F. None required after surgical correction

■ Pearl

Right-sided aortic arch is present in 25% of patients and ASD in 15%.

Transposition of the Great Arteries (TGA)

■ Essentials of Diagnosis

- Abnormal division of the truncus arteriosus in utero. Aorta arises from the RV and the pulmonary artery from the LV
- Cyanotic newborns without respiratory distress. Big babies. Male/female ratio 3:1
- *Type 1*—intact ventricular septum, ± pulmonary valvular or subvalvular stenosis
- *Type 2*—VSD, ± pulmonary stenosis or pulmonary vascular obstruction
- Cyanosis not relieved by increase in inspired O_2—hyperoxic test
- Murmur only present if there is a VSD
- Echocardiography is diagnostic

■ Differential Diagnosis

- Congenitally corrected TGA
- Other forms of cyanotic congenital heart disease can be differentiated by echocardiography

■ Treatment

- Balloon atrial septostomy (Rashkind) is performed at cardiac catheterization to provide intracardiac shunt in very cyanotic infants
- Early corrective open heart surgery is preferred
- Corrective arterial switch operation before 2 weeks in type 1, at 1–3 months in type 2
- Early relief of cyanosis improves developmental outcome
- No endocarditis prophylaxis is required

■ Pearl

Although the arterial switch operation requires moving the coronary arteries to the neo-aorta, the incidence of coronary artery insufficiency after the switch operation is low.

2

Tricuspid Atresia

- **Essentials of Diagnosis**
  - Complete atresia of the tricuspid valve with no direct blood flow from right atrium to RV
  - In the absence of VSD to provide right ventricular blood flow in utero, the RV is hypoplastic
  - All systemic blood return shunts from right atrium to left atrium through the foramen ovale with complete mixing of systemic and pulmonary return
  - Cyanosis at birth. Delayed growth and development. Exhaustion with feedings. VSD murmur may be present
  - ECG—left axis deviation, large right atrium, LV hypertrophy
  - Echocardiogram is diagnostic

- **Differential Diagnosis**
  - Other cyanotic congenital heart disease
  - Lung disease

- **Treatment**
  - If there is high pulmonary artery flow—anticongestive therapy with diuretics pulmonary banding to reduce pulmonary artery flow
  - If there is decreased pulmonary flow—PGE_1 used to keep ductus arteriosus open until aortopulmonary shunt (Blalock-Taussig) restores pulmonary flow
  - Ultimately, all children require a Fontan procedure (inferior and superior vena cava connected to pulmonary artery) to ensure pulmonary blood flow without a functioning RV
  - Prognosis after Fontan is best in those with low pulmonary artery pressure preoperatively
  - Antibiotic prophylaxis for endocarditis required after surgical shunting or pulmonary banding

- **Pearl**

Outcome depends upon how well one achieves a balance between adequate and excessive pulmonary flows by medication, banding, or surgery.

Total Anomalous Pulmonary Venous Return (TAPVR)

- ■ Essentials of Diagnosis
  - Abnormal connection of pulmonary veins to the right atrium or venae cavae causing mixture of oxygenated pulmonary blood and systemic deoxygenated blood with high pulmonary blood flow
  - Anatomic variants of TAPVR may allow some pulmonary venous return to the left atrium
  - With *unobstructed pulmonary venous drainage to the right atrium,* there is high pulmonary blood flow, cardiomegaly, congestive heart failure, and mild cyanosis
  - With *obstructed pulmonary return* (venous return into a systemic vein above or below the diaphragm), infants have small heart with severe cyanosis
  - Systolic ejection murmur with rumble and accentuated P_2 at the lower left sternal border. Right atrial and right ventricular hypertrophy
  - Echocardiography with color flow Doppler can suggest this anomaly but definitive diagnosis may still require cardiac catheterization

- ■ Differential Diagnosis
  - Other cyanotic congenital heart disease
  - Persistent fetal circulation

- ■ Treatment
  - Immediate surgery required if pulmonary venous return is obstructed
  - In unobstructed patients surgery may be delayed for weeks to months
  - Balloon atrial septostomy may be a palliative maneuver to improve mixing at the atrial level
  - Surgical outcome is very good. 5% develop late stenosis of the pulmonary veins, which has a poor prognosis

- ■ Pearl

Newborns with obstructed TAPVR frequently have a small heart on x-ray with "whited out" lungs. They are sometimes mistakenly thought to have hyaline membrane disease.

Truncus Arteriosis

2

- **Essentials of Diagnosis**
  - Failed division of the embryonic truncus produces a heart with a single great artery supplying systemic, pulmonary, and coronary circulations
  - VSD is always present. Truncal valve may be competent, incompetent, or stenotic
  - Symptoms depend on magnitude of pulmonary flow, which depends on truncal valve function and the size of the pulmonary arteries
  - High pulmonary flow is most common—presents like a VSD with congestive failure
  - Low pulmonary flow patients do poorly with cyanosis, poor growth, fatigue, dyspnea, and congestive failure
  - X-ray shows boot-shaped heart, no main pulmonary artery segment, large aorta with right arch in 30%
  - Echocardiogram is diagnostic. Color flow Doppler quantitates pulmonary flow and truncal valve function

- **Differential Diagnosis**
  - High-flow truncus arteriosus may be mistaken for a large VSD based on symptoms

- **Treatment**
  - Anticongestive treatment with diuretics for high pulmonary flow
  - Surgery for high-flow states should be performed before 6 months of age to avoid the development of pulmonary vascular obstructive disease
  - Surgery for high-flow state—closure of VSD, separation of pulmonary arteries from the truncus with conduit from RV to pulmonary arteries (often an allograft)
  - Children almost always outgrow their original conduit and need revision in childhood

- **Pearl**

Truncus arteriosus is the least common of the 5 cyanotic "Ts."

Rheumatic Fever

- **Essentials of Diagnosis**
  - Group A β-hemolytic streptococcus (GAS) infection causes B lymphocytes to make anti-GAS antibodies
  - Carditis—immune complexes cross-react with cardiac sarcolemma causing carditis, mitral and aortic insufficiency, and congestive heart failure
  - Polyarthritis—large joints are swollen, red, and extremely tender
  - Chorea—emotional lability, involuntary movements, ataxia, slurred speech, and weakness; sometimes onset is after acute stage of disease
  - Subcutaneous nodules—nontender, moveable, present in severe disease
  - Major Jones criteria—carditis, polyarthritis, Sydenham chorea, erythema marginatum, subcutaneous nodules
  - Minor Jones criteria—previous rheumatic fever, polyarthralgia, fever, high sedimentation rate, prolonged PR interval suggestive of carditis
  - Diagnosis requires 2 major or 1 major and 2 minor Jones criteria plus evidence of GAS infection (antistreptolysin O, positive throat culture)

- **Differential Diagnosis**
  - Other polyarthritis/arthralgia—juvenile rheumatoid arthritis, systemic lupus erythematosus, and other autoimmune disorders
  - Pyogenic arthritis—*Haemophilus influenza type B, Neisseria gonorrhoeae, Staphylococcus aureus, Streptococcus pyogenes, Kingella kingae*
  - Dystonia from medications, brain tumor
  - Other myocarditis—Kawasaki disease, adenovirus, coxsackie A and B, echovirus, cytomegalovirus, parvovirus, influenza A virus, human immunodeficiency virus
  - Mitral and aortic insufficiency due to bacterial endocarditis

- **Treatment**
  - Treat GAS infection with penicillin and arthritis with aspirin
  - Treat heart failure with diuretics, angiotensin-converting enzyme inhibitors
  - Treat carditis with aspirin or corticosteroid until acute phase inflammatory tests resolve
  - Prevent future GAS with monthly intramuscular benzathine penicillin. Erythromycin or sulfadiazine in children with penicillin allergy
  - Lifelong GAS prophylaxis in patients with heart disease. Prophylaxis for 3–5 years with no residual heart disease
  - Late development of mitral stenosis may require surgical replacement

- **Pearl**

Some patients have only Sydenham chorea or idiopathic chronic carditis with no obvious acute rheumatic fever episode. These patients have rheumatic fever is made in these patients even without tests proving recent streptococcal infection.

Cardiomyopathy

- ■ Essentials of Diagnosis
  - *Dilated cardiomyopathy*—usually idiopathic but also caused by acute or chronic carditis, chronic tachyarrhythmia, left heart obstruction, coronary artery disease, anthracycline toxicity, mitochondrial and fatty acid oxidation defects
  - Early symptoms of dilated cardiomyopathy may resemble upper respiratory infection
  - *Hypertrophic myopathy*—familial, leading cause of sudden cardiac death in children, mutations in several cardiac sarcomere proteins
  - *Restrictive myopathy*—rare, presents with heart failure, prominent S_4, jugular venous distension, may mimic constrictive pericarditis
  - Echocardiogram, ECG, and biopsy distinguish the three forms of cardiomyopathy

- ■ Associated Syndromes
  - Dilated cardiomyopathy—older children with Duchenne and Becker muscular dystrophy, carnitine deficiency, left-sided cardiac obstructive lesions, congenital coronary artery disease, fatty acid oxidation defects, mitochondrial oxidative phosphorylation defects
  - Hypertrophic cardiomyopathy—Noonan syndrome, Friedreich ataxia, mitochondrial disease, Pompe disease (type II glycogen storage), mitochondrial oxidation defects
  - Restrictive cardiomyopathy—endocardial fibroelastosis

- ■ Treatment
  - Treat dilated myopathy with digoxin, diuretics, afterload reduction, anticoagulants, antiarrhythmics, supplemental carnitine
  - Treat hypertrophic myopathy with restricted physical activity, β-blockers, verapamil or disopyramide for LV outlet obstruction, surgical myectomy, implanted cardiac defibrillator (ICD)
  - Cardiac transplantation is sometimes needed

- ■ Pearl

Ventricular tachycardia/fibrillation is the usual cause of death in hypertrophic cardiomyopathy.

Infective Endocarditis and Pericarditis

2

- ■ Essentials of Diagnosis
  - Endocarditis—underlying heart disease, fever, new or changing murmur, splenomegaly, septic emboli, dyspnea, and tachypnea, ↑white blood cell count (WBC), ↑erythrocyte sedimentation rate (ESR), hematuria. Blood culture grows *Streptococcus viridans* (50%), *S aureus* (30%), and fungus (10%)
  - Pericarditis—retrosternal pain, fever, shortness of breath, pericardial friction rub, tachycardia, hepatomegaly, jugular vein distension, ECG with elevated ST segment, muffled heart sounds
  - Endocarditis most common in persons with aortic valve disease, aorticopulmonary shunts, prosthetic valves. Dental procedure, nonsterile surgery, or cardiovascular surgery precedes onset in 30%
  - Pericarditis—effusion may cause cardiac tamponade and right heart failure
  - Chest x-ray and echocardiography confirm diagnosis

- ■ Differential Diagnosis
  - Acute rheumatic fever—immune-mediated pancarditis
  - Pericarditis—occurs in rheumatoid arthritis, uremia, tuberculosis (TB), autoimmune disorders, infection with TB, coxsackie B, influenza virus
  - Bacterial pericarditis—GAS, *Streptococcus pneumoniae, S aureus, Haemophilus influenzae* often cause severe disease with later restrictive pericardopathy
  - Postpericardiotomy—autoimmune pericarditis 1–2 weeks after open heart surgery with fever, friction rub, chest pain, elevated ST segments
  - Bacterial endocarditis in the normal heart—immunodeficiency, indwelling central venous catheters, drug abuse

- ■ Treatment
  - Endocarditis—empiric therapy is indicated in an at-risk setting even when cultures are negative. Use specific antibiotics based on culture results obtained
  - Monitor with ultrasound for valve damage and valvular vegetations
  - Pericarditis—treatment depends on cause. Cardiac tamponade requires immediate pericardiocentesis
  - Postpericardiotomy syndrome—aspirin or corticosteroids
  - Endocarditis antibiotic prophylaxis—required for some types of congenital heart defects in high-risk situations, especially dental work and surgery. American Heart Association updated the indications and drug recommendations in 2007

- ■ Pearl

The most common agent of bacterial endocarditis in IV drug users is S aureus.

Common Arrhythmias

- **Essentials of Diagnosis**
  - *Premature atrial contractions*—ectopic atrial focus, often in newborns. Conducted or nonconducted to the ventricle
  - *Premature ventricular contractions*—originate in either ventricle. QRS lasts >80 msec in newborns, >120 msec in adolescents
  - Supraventricular tachycardia—Re-entry rhythm may cause symptoms if prolonged
  - *Atrial flutter/fibrillation*—rare in children usually associated with organic heart disease and open heart surgery
  - *Ventricular tachycardia*—usually associated with myocardial disease, drug toxicity, and open heart surgery
  - *Long QT syndrome*—may be congenital. Ventricular repolarization irregular, QTc interval >.44–.46 msec. Associated with syncope, seizure, or death during exercise

- **Differential Diagnosis**
  - Sinus tachycardia occurs with fever, anemia, shock, heart failure. ECG normal
  - Sinus arrhythmia—acceleration/deceleration of heart rate with inspiration/expiration. Often exaggerated in infants and children
  - Sinus bradycardia—hypoxia, central nervous system (CNS) damage, eating disorder, medications, athletes. ECG normal
  - Multifocal premature ventricular contractions (PVCs) associated with drug toxicity (digoxin, taurocholate, electrolyte imbalance, myocarditis, hypoxia

- **Treatment**
  - PACs only require treatment if they trigger tachyarrhythmias or bradycardia because of nonconduction
  - Unifocal PVCs—usually benign and are suppressed during exercise. No treatment needed
  - Supraventricular tachycardia—correct electrolytes, hypoxia and acidosis, vagal maneuvers, adenosine, overdrive pacing, cardioversion. Prevent with digoxin, β-blocker, calcium channel antagonist, radiofrequency ablation
  - Ventricular tachycardia—cardioversion, lidocaine, antiarrhythmia drugs
  - Long QT syndrome—implanted cardiac defibrillator, exercise restriction, β-blockers

- **Pearl**

Wolff-Parkinson-White, a re-entrant supraventricular tachycardia, occurs more frequently in tricuspid atresia, Ebstein anomaly, hypertrophic cardiomyopathy, and corrected transposition of the great vessels than in other congenital malformations.

3

Gastrointestinal Tract

3

Gastroesophageal Reflux (GER) in Infants

■ Essentials of Diagnosis

- Postprandial regurgitation affects 40% of healthy infants <6 months
- Less common symptoms are fussiness, coffee ground emesis, feeding refusal, cough, wheezing, rumination, apnea
- Vomiting can be effortless, occasionally forceful, but never bilious
- Diagnosis is clinical in healthy infants. Upper gastrointestinal (GI) series will rule out obstruction. Endoscopy usually normal. Esophageal pH monitoring is a more sensitive test

■ Differential Diagnosis

- Upper GI obstruction—esophageal atresia, vascular ring, esophageal duplication, intestinal atresia, gastric outlet obstruction
- Food allergy
- Increased intracranial pressure
- Drug toxicity
- Urinary tract infection
- Metabolic disorders
- Chronic lung or heart disease

■ Treatment

- Usually self-limited in infants, diminishing between 6 and 12 months
- Small-volume, frequent feedings thickened with rice cereal
- Acid blockers—H2-receptor antagonists and proton pump inhibitors may help fussy behavior but do not stop reflux

■ Pearl

In a healthy thriving baby, even if with very frequent spitting and vomiting, the chance of finding organic disease is so slim that invasive tests are not indicated.

Gastroesophageal Reflux (GER) in Children

3

- **Essentials of Diagnosis**
  - Heartburn more common in children than infants
  - Effortless regurgitation, vomiting, and rumination are common
  - May worsen during intercurrent illness
  - Upper endoscopy rules out complications of reflux but does not make the diagnosis. Upper GI series has many false positives
  - Esophageal pH or impedance monitoring can confirm the diagnosis and can document the association between repetitive symptoms and reflux episodes
  - Children with developmental disabilities are at higher risk

- **Differential Diagnosis**
  - Eosinophilic esophagitis—most common in adolescent males
  - Chronic lung disease
  - Increased central nervous system (CNS) pressure
  - Emotional issues, eating disorder
  - Severe tonsillar enlargement
  - Herpetic esophagitis and candida esophagitis cause acute onset of symptoms. May occur in children with normal immune status
  - Pill, ulcer, or impacted foreign body cause sudden esophageal pain

- **Treatment**
  - Acid blockers reduce pain and heal esophagitis. Relapse is common when therapy discontinued
  - Promotility agents have limited benefit
  - Fundoplication may be required in children with esophageal stricture or relapsing esophagitis

- **Pearl**

An adolescent male with a single food impaction or chronic dysphagia should be suspected of having chronic reflux esophagitis or eosinophilic esophagitis even if he has never had heartburn. Such patients require diagnostic endoscopy.

Caustic Burns of the Esophagus

■ Essentials of Diagnosis

- Ingestion of solid or liquid of pH $\geq$12 produces lesions ranging from superficial inflammation to coagulative necrosis and perforation
- Very strong acids (pH <1) also cause coagulative necrosis and perforation
- Accurate identification of ingested material is critical to care
- Esophagoscopy within 24 hours to assess extent of esophageal damage
- Mouth and chest pain may be severe, drooling common, airway obstruction may occur
- Chest x-ray to detect perforation in severe cases. Immediate upper GI series usually not indicated

■ Differential Diagnosis

- Bleach, permanent wave solutions, and common household detergents rarely cause early or late complications
- Commercial dishwashing detergents occasionally produce coagulative necrosis and stricture
- Alkaline foreign bodies—retained button batteries, Clinitest tablets

■ Treatment

- Do not induce vomiting. Intravenous (IV) fluids for patients with dysphagia
- IV corticosteroids may reduce oral and laryngeal swelling. Admit for intensive care and antibiotics for perforation, mediastinitis, or peritonitis
- Antibiotics in absence of perforation may not be helpful
- In all cases of confirmed caustic ingestion, a follow-up esophagram 2–3 months postingestion is indicated

■ Pearl

The severity of the mouth burns in caustic ingestion may not reflect the severity of the esophageal damage. If there is any immediate question about the state of the esophagus, endoscopy is the only accurate test.

Hiatal Hernia

3

- ■ Essentials of Diagnosis
  - • Classified as paraesophageal—gastric cardia herniated into the chest to the left of the lower esophageal sphincter; or sliding—gastric cardia and gastroesophageal junction both herniated through the esophageal hiatus
  - • Sliding hernias are common and usually produce no symptoms. They may cause symptoms of reflux, burping, vomiting, and hiccups
  - • Large paraesophageal hernias cause pain, esophageal obstruction, respiratory compromise, and recurrent respiratory infection
  - • Diagnosed by upper GI series

- ■ Differential Diagnosis
  - • GER
  - • Lobar pneumonia mimics some symptoms
  - • Congenital diaphragmatic hernia
  - • Sliding and paraesophageal hernias may occur after fundoplication surgery
  - • Congenital or acquired esophageal stricture may produce sliding hernia

- ■ Treatment
  - • Most sliding hernias require no treatment
  - • Symptoms of heartburn may improve with acid blockade, upright position after meals, and avoidance of large meals
  - • Large or symptomatic hernias require surgical repair

- ■ Pearl

The vast majority of hiatus hernias cause no symptoms. Seeing a hiatus hernia by endoscopy or x-ray is common and is not a realistic explanation for chronic abdominal pain.

Achalasia

■ **Essentials of Diagnosis**

- Uncommon in childhood
- Typical symptoms include retrosternal pain or fullness with a sensation of food "sticking"
- Patients eat slowly and drink a lot of fluid with meals. They may have self-induced vomiting, night-time cough, wheezing, recurrent pneumonia, poor weight gain, and anemia
- Chest x-ray may show esophageal air-fluid level. Esophagram shows dilated esophagus with poor peristalsis and tapered gastroesophageal junction (bird beak)
- Esophageal manometry shows failure of lower esophageal relaxation after swallowing and nonperistaltic esophageal body motor function

■ **Differential Diagnosis**

- Esophageal obstruction or stricture—peptic stricture, eosinophilic esophagitis stricture, tight vascular ring, scleroderma, mediastinal mass
- Allgrove syndrome—inherited condition with alacrima, adrenal insufficiency, and achalasia
- Familial dysautonomia
- Eating disorder may mimic many symptoms of achalasia

■ **Treatment**

- Pneumatic dilation of the lower esophageal sphincter relieves obstruction for variable time
- Botulinum toxin injected into the lower esophageal sphincter gives temporary relief (3–4 months)
- Surgical lower esophageal sphincter myotomy often required
- Abnormal esophageal peristalsis is permanent regardless of therapy and may cause symptoms of obstruction

■ **Pearl**

The younger the child with achalasia, the less dramatic the esophageal dilation, and the less dramatic the x-ray findings. Early diagnosis and therapy may delay the development of esophageal dysmotility symptoms.

Pyloric Stenosis

■ Essentials of Diagnosis

- 1 in 1000 live births. 4:1 male predominance. Cause unknown
- Onset of nonbilious vomiting between 2 and 4 weeks. Rapid progression to complete gastric outlet obstruction
- Weight loss, dehydration, mild jaundice, coffee ground emesis, visible gastric contraction waves, palpable olive-shaped mass in the right upper abdomen
- Hypochloremic alkalosis with hypokalemia
- Upper GI series shows gastric retention, long narrow pyloric channel with semilunar impressions on gastric antrum from enlarged pyloric muscle.
- Ultrasonography shows thickened hypoechoic ring of pyloric muscle

■ Differential Diagnosis

- Other gastric outlet obstructions—gastric web, duodenal hematoma, pyloric channel ulcer, gastric or duodenal duplication
- Intestinal obstruction—malrotation with volvulus, intestinal atresia, intestinal stricture or stenosis, intestinal polyps, all characterized by bilious emesis
- Vomiting from increased intracranial pressure
- Vomiting associated with urinary tract or other infections, metabolic disease, child neglect

■ Treatment

- Surgical pyloromyotomy
- Treat and correct hydration and electrolyte imbalance before surgery, even if it requires a delay of 1–2 days

■ Pearl

Postoperative x-rays often remain abnormal despite resolution of obstruction.

Acid/Peptic Disease

- **Essentials of Diagnosis**

  - Peptic ulcer occurs at any age. More common in boys
  - Most ulcers are secondary to underlying illness (burns, CNS, shock, hypoxia, multiorgan failure), toxin, or drugs (alcohol, aspirin, caffeine, and nonsteroidal anti-inflammatory agents)
  - Infection with *Helicobacter pylori* causes gastritis, gastric and duodenal ulcers. Diagnosed by urease testing of gastric mucosa, histology, culture of gastric mucosa, or stool antibody testing. Serum antibody titers inadequate for diagnosis
  - Symptoms are pain, vomiting, hematemesis, and sometimes obstruction
  - Upper GI series insensitive. Endoscopy is required for accurate diagnosis

- **Differential Diagnosis**
  - Chronic recurrent abdominal pain (RAP) of childhood
  - GER
  - Hypergastrinemia (Zollinger-Ellison syndrome)
  - Cholecystitis
  - Celiac disease

- **Treatment**
  - Treat identified primary cause of ulcer/gastritis
  - Acid blockade with H2-receptor antagonists or proton pump inhibitors
  - Antibiotic therapy to eradicate *H pylori*

- **Pearl**

Bland diets do not cure ulcers. A positive serum titer for H pylori *does not prove active infection.*

3

Intestinal Volvulus

- **Essentials of Diagnosis**
  - Accounts for 10% of neonatal intestinal obstruction
  - Occurs in infants with intestinal malrotation, a developmental abnormality of the intestines. Most cases of malrotation do not cause disease
  - Most common presentation is recurrent bilious emesis or acute small bowel obstruction in the first 3 weeks of life
  - If untreated, volvulus causes occlusion of the superior mesenteric artery resulting in upper intestinal ischemia, perforation, and peritonitis
  - Upper GI series shows incomplete rotation of the intestines with ligament of Treitz and upper small bowel to the right of the midline and sometimes a left-sided cecum

- **Differential Diagnosis**
  - Other causes of small bowel obstruction including intussusception, internal hernia, tumor
  - Severe gastroenteritis may cause bilious emesis in infants and children
  - Abdominal infections and inflammatory disease (appendicitis, inflammatory bowel disease, necrotizing enterocolitis) cause bilious emesis
  - Volvulus secondary to malrotation occurs more rarely in older children

- **Treatment**
  - Surgical exploration is mandatory when volvulus is suspected
  - Resection of necrotic bowel may result in short-bowel syndrome
  - Resection of necrotic bowel may be delayed for 24 hours after exploratory laparotomy and devolving the intestine (second-look operation) in order to salvage as much intestinal length as possible
  - Surgical repair of malrotation (Ladd's procedure) is performed even in nonsymptomatic infants <12 months. Recommendation for prophylactic surgery is not established for older children

- **Pearl**

Bilious emesis in infants is either yellow or green. In infants, emesis of either color requires immediate assessment by appropriate x-rays to prevent a loss of bowel by volvulus.

Meckel Diverticulum

- ■ Essentials of Diagnosis
  - Meckel diverticulum is an omphalomenteric duct remnant on the antimesenteric border of the distal ileum
  - Occurs in 1.5% of the population and the majority cause no symptoms
  - In diverticula containing gastric mucosa, acid secretion may produce a contiguous ulcer with bleeding. Usual age for bleeding is 6–24 months
  - Other presentations of Meckel diverticula—volvulus around the remnant, intussusception, acute diverticulitis, and rarely recurrent abdominal pain of childhood
  - Technetium pertechnetate scan identifies diverticula containing gastric mucosa

- ■ Differential Diagnosis
  - Acute appendicitis
  - GI bleeding from vascular anomalies, duplications, bleeding disorder, sloughed juvenile polyp, other intestinal polyps
  - Intussusception

- ■ Treatment
  - Once diagnosed, treatment is surgical removal of the diverticulum
  - Prognosis is excellent

- ■ Pearl

Bleeding from a Meckel diverticulum is painless, large volume, purple or maroon, and often causes significant acute anemia. These features help differentiate the rectal bleeding of diverticula from that of a juvenile polyp or fissure.

Aganglionic Megacolon—Hirschsprung Disease

3

- **Essentials of Diagnosis**
  - Absence of ganglion cells in colon mucosa and muscularis produced by failure of neural crest cell migration during development
  - Normal bowel relaxation in response to proximal distension does not occur and defecation is prevented
  - May present with enterocolitis, sepsis, and perforation
  - Most present at <30 days of life with constipation and intestinal obstructive symptoms. Short segment involvement may present later
  - Familial forms caused by mutations in the RET proto-oncogene
  - Common in Down syndrome
  - Rectal biopsy is best diagnostic test. Barium enema and rectal manometry are helpful in older children

- **Differential Diagnosis**
  - Other congenital causes of lower intestinal obstruction are colon duplication, anorectal atresia or agenesis, imperforate anus
  - Chronic retentive constipation
  - Intestinal motility disorders
  - Small left colon syndrome in newborn infants of diabetic mothers
  - Hypothyroidism can cause constipation in neonates

- **Treatment**
  - Surgical diversion of intestinal flow proximal to the aganglionic segment is the first step in neonates
  - Definitive surgery requires removal of the aganglionic segment and re-establishment of GI continuity by colo- or ileoanal anastomosis

- **Pearl**

Distinguishing Hirschsprung disease from retentive constipation in older children is usually easy. Patients with Hirschsprung disease do not have encopresis and often appear generally unwell with a distended, tympanitic abdomen.

Peritonitis

- **Essentials of Diagnosis**
  - Most commonly the result of intestinal perforation, chronic peritoneal dialysis, or trauma
  - Spontaneous peritonitis accounts for <2% of cases
  - *Escherichia coli* is the most common organism
  - Fever, abdominal pain and distension, vomiting, rigid abdomen, acidosis, and prostration
  - Peritoneal tap reveals >500 WBC/μL. Total peripheral white blood cell count (WBC) usually >20,000/μL

- **Differential Diagnosis**
  - Acute appendicitis, intestinal obstruction with perforation
  - Enteric infections
  - Chylous ascites
  - Cirrhosis with portal hypertension and ascites
  - Abdominal tumor, intestinal or abdominal lymphangiectasia

- **Treatment**
  - Children with peritonitis are often critically ill. They require intensive care setting for support and antibiotics
  - Chronic peritonitis associated with peritoneal dialysis does not always produce critical illness

- **Pearl**

When in doubt, perform a diagnostic peritoneal tap using a small gage needle with ultrasound guidance if necessary. The fluid obtained may confirm the diagnosis and allow for speedy therapy.

Appendicitis

3

- ■ Essentials of Diagnosis
  - Most common cause of emergency abdominal surgery in childhood
  - Peak incidence in teenage years
  - Usually presents acutely with fever, right lower quadrant abdominal pain, signs of obstruction or peritoneal irritation, constipation or diarrhea, and vomiting
  - Monitoring with repeated examinations over 24–48 hours is essential in questionable cases
  - Increased white count, pyuria, guaiac-positive stool
  - Plain abdominal film may show a fecalith
  - Abdominal computed tomography (CT) scan with rectal contrast is the most sensitive diagnostic test

- ■ Differential Diagnosis
  - Acute enteric infection, especially *Salmonella* and *Yersinia*
  - Acute or chronic inflammatory bowel disease, especially Crohn disease
  - Urinary tract infection
  - Other causes of acute abdomen—pelvic inflammatory disease (PID), Henoch-Schönlein purpura, cholecystitis, pseudomembranous enterocolitis, peritonitis, pancreatitis, pneumococcal pneumonia, diabetic acidosis, mesenteric adenitis

- ■ Treatment
  - Surgical removal of the inflamed appendix
  - Drainage of abscess if perforation has occurred
  - Antibiotics used if perforation has occurred

- ■ Pearl

In children <2 years, the abdominal symptoms of appendicitis are poorly localized and the incidence of perforation is therefore high. A high index of suspicion must be maintained in these cases.

Intussusception

- **Essentials of Diagnosis**

  - Most frequent cause of intestinal obstruction in the first 2 years of life
  - More common in males
  - Usually ileocolonic producing characteristic waves of pain and bilious emesis with interval periods of lethargy
  - Swelling of the intussuscepted bowel may result in vascular occlusion and bowel necrosis
  - Typical symptoms include gradual development of pain, bilious emesis, diarrhea followed by bloody diarrhea (current jelly stool), fever, sausage-shaped mass in the right lower quadrant
  - Plain abdominal x-ray may show intestinal obstruction. Barium or air enema study will reveal the intussusception

- **Differential Diagnosis**

  - Lead points for intussusception include polyps, lipomas, lymphoma, swollen lymph nodes, bowel wall hematoma (Henoch-Schönlein purpura), parasites, foreign bodies, or hypertrophied Peyer patches (associated with infection)
  - Other causes of intestinal obstruction should be ruled out by appropriate testing
  - Rarely, cystic fibrosis, celiac disease, or small bowel tumors may cause small bowel intussusception

- **Treatment**

  - Reduction of the intussusception may occur during diagnostic barium or air enema
  - Surgical reduction of the intussusception is indicated when radiologic attempts fail or when perforation is suspected

- **Pearl**

Intussusception recurs within 24 hours in 3–4% of patients with uncomplicated reduction via air or barium enema. Parents should be advised of this possibility.

Inguinal Hernia

3

- Essentials of Diagnosis
    - Peritoneal sac descends into the scrotum during development and if persistent may contain residual fluid (hydrocele)
    - If the peritoneal sac remains patent after birth, fluid or abdominal contents may drop into the sac forming an indirect inguinal hernia—most common type
    - Male/female ratio 9:1. Found in 30% of premature males <1000 g birth weight
    - Most common presentation is mass in the scrotum or inguinal canal. Often retractable

- Differential Diagnosis
    - Inguinal lymphadenopathy
    - Undescended testicle
    - Testicular mass, orchitis, testicular torsion
    - Hydroceles may be very large. Can be differentiated from hernia by careful transillumination

- Treatment
    - Intermittently apparent or very easily reduceable inguinal hernias in young infants may close spontaneously
    - Hernias that cannot be reduced require surgical treatment (incarceration)
    - Hydroceles usually resolve spontaneously

- Pearl

Inguinal hernias that the mother sees at home are often not seen in the stressful environment of the doctor's office. Sometimes taking a picture at home is a good idea.

Umbilical Hernia

- ### Essentials of Diagnosis
  - More common in premature than term newborns
  - More common in black than white babies
  - Most regress spontaneously if fascial defect <1 cm diameter

- ### Differential Diagnosis
  - Omphalocele or gastroschisis
  - Discharge from the umbilicus suggests persistence of omphalomesenteric or urachal duct
  - Redness, swelling, or induration of the skin around the newborn umbilicus should be considered omphalitis until proven otherwise and is an emergency

- ### Treatment
  - Small defects persisting after age 4 years should be treated surgically
  - Large defects may require surgery before 4 years of age

- ### Pearl
  Taping a quarter over an umbilical hernia does not hasten its resolution.

Juvenile Colonic Polyps

- **Essentials of Diagnosis**
  - Common, benign, hyperplastic pedunculated polyps contain normal colon mucosal and vascular elements with cystic spaces. Most are single but the diagnosis is not changed unless >10 are found. 80% located in rectosigmoid
  - Most children present at 3–5 years with intermittent, small-volume, painless, red rectal bleeding upon defecation. Low rectal polyps may prolapse
  - Generalized juvenile polyposis syndrome—many juvenile polyps in colon (>10) and small bowel. Very slight malignancy risk
  - Colonoscopy is diagnostic test of choice. Histologic examination of removed polyps is diagnostic

- **Differential Diagnosis**
  - Other sources of small-volume red rectal bleeding include anal fissure, hemorrhoids, vascular anomalies of the rectum
  - Ulcerative colitis bleeding may suggest juvenile polyp especially at onset
  - Genetic polyposis syndromes—familial adenomatous polyposis and Peutz-Jeghers syndrome may have rectal bleeding from colon polyps, but histologic findings are distinct
  - Rectal foreign body

- **Treatment**
  - No treatment is required and many polyps will autoamputate in time
  - Colonoscopy is usually performed. It is therapeutic and clarifies for diagnosis by providing pathologic evaluation

- **Pearl**

Routine surveillance colonoscopy after removal of a single juvenile polyp is not required.

Acute Infectious Diarrhea

- ■ Essentials of Diagnosis

  - Rotavirus is the most common cause in children <2 years
  - Norovirus in older children produces 2-day diarrhea
  - Viral agents usually produce watery voluminous stool with low sodium content
  - Diagnostic tests not always indicated in obvious cases but immuno staining of stool or electron microscopy can identify most viral agents
  - Acute bacterial infections (Shigella, Salmonella, Campylobacter, Yersinia) characterized by invasion of small bowel or colon, fever, small volume, bloody diarrhea. Culture of stool indicated
  - Enterotoxigenic *E coli* and *Vibrio cholera* secrete enterotoxin causing intestinal secretion of high-volume diarrhea with sodium content usually >90 mEq/L stool
  - Other infectious agents causing high-volume diarrhea—*Giardia lamblia*, Cryptosporidium, enteric adenoviruses, and other enteric viruses

- ■ Differential Diagnosis

  - Neuroendocrine tumors (VIPoma, gastrinoma, occasionally neuroblastoma, carcinoid) produce watery diarrhea
  - Accidental or intentional laxative abuse
  - High intake of sorbitol in diet foods causes osmotic diarrhea
  - Ingested toxins (food poisoning) usually cause more rapid-onset diarrhea, vomiting without prodrome

- ■ Treatment

  - Uncomplicated viral gastroenteritis requires no specific treatment except attention to fluid and electrolyte replacement
  - Some bacterial agents require antibiotic therapy (see Chapter 27, Bacterial and Spirochetal infections)
  - Treatment with antidiarrheal preparations is generally not indicated especially in young infants

- ■ Pearl

High-volume diarrhea without blood in a previously healthy child is likely to be viral. Low-volume diarrhea with blood may be bacterial.

Chronic Diarrhea

3

- **Essentials of Diagnosis**
  - Stool output continuously >15 g/kg/day raises the suspicion of organic disease
  - Mechanisms include abnormal salt and water transport, loss of mucosal surface area, increased intestinal motility, osmotic agents, increased intestinal permeability, and secretory stimulants
  - Most common cause in healthy infants is antibiotic use followed by chronic nonspecific diarrhea
  - Diagnosis rests on a combination of history, general physical examination, stool examination, followed by specific testing

- **Differential Diagnosis**
  - Antibiotic use
  - Nonspecific diarrhea of toddlers. Often associated with excess intake of fruit juices
  - Infection/infestation
  - Malabsorption syndromes—celiac disease, a-beta-lipoproteinemia, lactase deficiency
  - Malnutrition may be associated with a chronic diarrhea because of inefficient digestion/absorption and because of increased risk of infections
  - Allergy is a rare cause of diarrhea outside of infancy. When present there is usually small amount of gross or occult blood in the stool
  - Inflammatory disease
  - Secretory tumors

- **Treatment**
  - Chronic diarrhea should not be treated until its etiology has been thoroughly investigated
  - Empiric treatment with antidiarrheal agents is not recommended without specific diagnosis

- **Pearl**

A healthy toddler with an intermittent history of frequent loose stools is likely to have "toddler diarrhea." This can often be "cured" by decreasing juice intake and increasing the fat in the diet. Once this diagnosis is secure through eliminating other causes, Imodium can be used.

Celiac Disease—Gluten Enteropathy

■ Essentials of Diagnosis

- Intestinal sensitivity to the gliadin fraction wheat, rye, barley, and sometimes oat gluten causes local immune destruction of absorbing cells
- Insidious onset typically at 15–30 months with failure to thrive, large pasty stools (parents may not describe diarrhea), and poor energy
- Can present at any age. Family history is positive in 10% of cases
- Complications include deficiencies of vitamin D (rickets), vitamin K (bleeding), vitamin E (neuropathy), and rarely, vitamin A
- May present with isolated short stature or delayed puberty in rare cases
- Stool examination shows unabsorbed fatty acids
- Serum tissue transglutaminase antibodies very sensitive and specific
- Diagnosis confirmed by small intestinal mucosal biopsy

■ Differential Diagnosis

- Giardia infestations often have severe fat malabsorption
- Cystic fibrosis
- Chronic liver disease
- Intestinal lymphangiectasia
- Endocrine causes of short stature

■ Treatment

- Lifelong avoidance of gluten is the only treatment
- Nutritional rehabilitation immediately after diagnosis may require fat-soluble vitamin supplementation
- Very malnourished children may require in-hospital monitoring during nutritional rehabilitation
- Complete recovery may take several months of high-calorie, gluten-free diet

■ Pearl

All untreated celiac patients are somewhat lactose intolerant until mucosal recovery is complete. If milk is all a toddler will take however, it does not harm the patient to drink it.

Disaccharidase Deficiency

3

- ■ **Essentials of Diagnosis**
  - Intestinal mucosal lactase and sucrase/isomaltase are the 2 most important disaccharidases
  - Genetic lactase deficiency affects >90% of Asians and Native Americans, about 70% of African Americans, and 30–60% of Caucasian Americans
  - Genetic sucrase deficiency is rare but affects 10% of Native Alaskans
  - Symptoms are nausea, diarrhea, abdominal pain, flatulence upon ingesting lactose or sucrose
  - Diagnosis usually clinical. Confirmed by measurement of enzyme activity in mucosal biopsy, breath hydrogen excretion after oral administration of suspect sugar. Reducing substances present in stool after lactose ingestion

- ■ **Differential Diagnosis**
  - Food allergy, especially milk allergy
  - Secondary disaccharidase deficiency is associated with many small bowel disorders, especially celiac disease, inflammatory bowel disease, infections, drugs, malnutrition, radiation

- ■ **Treatment**
  - Avoidance of offending dietary disaccharide(s)
  - Exogenous enzyme preparations available for both lactase and sucrase
  - Secondary causes often improve with treatment of the primary disorder

- ■ **Pearl**

Regardless of race or ethnicity, all infants have adequate lactase. Genetic lactase deficiency begins to appear after age 3–4 years.

Glucose-Galactose Malabsorption

- Essentials of Diagnosis
  - Rare autosomal recessive disorder in which sodium-glucose transport protein is defective
  - Presents at birth with osmotic diarrhea upon ingestion of any food that contains or can be broken down to yield glucose or galactose (milk, sucrose, starches)
  - Renal tubular glucose transport is decreased causing glycosuria at normal serum glucose concentration
  - Reducing substances are present in stool after glucose or galactose ingestion
  - Intestinal biopsy looks normal but transporter proteins abnormal

- Differential Diagnosis
  - Rare genetic diarrhea syndromes—microvillus inclusion disease, autoimmune enteropathy, chloride-losing diarrhea
  - Dietary overload of starch in infants causes diarrhea due to relative deficiency of pancreatic amylase
  - Secondary monosaccharide intolerance may follow severe enteric infection in infants <12 months
  - Iatrogenic osmotic diarrhea

- Treatment
  - This is a lifelong deficiency
  - Fructose is well tolerated and is used to supplement carbohydrate-free formulas in infants
  - Secondary monosaccharide intolerance usually resolves with nutrition support and diet low in sucrose, lactose, and glucose
  - Tolerance to glucose and galactose seems to improve with age and some starches and sugar are acceptable

- Pearl

Watery diarrhea, profound acidosis, and fecal reducing substances that disappear when newborn is fasting should suggest this rare diagnosis.

Cow's Milk Allergy

3

- **Essentials of Diagnosis**
  - Estimated prevalence of 0.5–1% of healthy infants <6 months. Much less common in older children
  - Typical symptoms are fussiness, frequent mucoid stools with blood streaks
  - Family history of atopy common
  - Usually a clinical diagnosis confirmed by resolution of symptoms on milk protein-free diet
  - Sigmoidoscopy shows mild superficial colitis
  - In older children, milk allergy may cause a celiac-like syndrome with protein-losing enteropathy, occult intestinal blood loss, edema, anemia, and failure to thrive
  - Anaphylactic shock after milk ingestion is rare but can be life threatening

- **Differential Diagnosis**
  - Low-volume blood loss due to anal stenosis, anal fissure, hemorrhoid, juvenile polyp does not respond to a milk protein-free diet
  - Celiac disease
  - Crohn disease
  - Severe diaper dermatitis may produce very similar symptoms of fussiness and small-volume rectal bleeding
  - Peri-anal streptococcal infection produces small volume rectal bleeding and fussiness

- **Treatment**
  - Milk protein-free diet for infants is helpful
  - If symptoms are minor in young infants with rectal bleeding, no therapy is required as the problem will resolve spontaneously

- **Pearl**

The infant with anal stenosis is fussy, has mucoid stools with blood streaks, and is often thought to be milk allergic. A careful rectal examination will differentiate this common problem from allergy.

Chronic Retentive Constipation

- **Essentials of Diagnosis**
  - Common GI problem of infants and children. Male/female ratio 4:1
  - Typical symptoms are infrequent or difficult defecation. Stools large but not necessarily hard
  - Older boys develop overflow incontinence
  - Infants and toddlers display retentive behavior
  - Complications in girls include urinary tract infection
  - Diagnosis is clinical. X-rays and colon mucosal biopsy rarely needed

- **Differential Diagnosis**
  - Hirschsprung disease—rare diagnosis beyond the neonatal period
  - Painful anal conditions such as fissure, perianal streptococcal infection
  - Hypothyroidism
  - Skeletal muscle weakness prevents Valsalva maneuver needed during defecation
  - Drugs—narcotics and antihistamines
  - Poor fluid and fiber intake are rarely the primary cause of constipation

- **Treatment**
  - Dietary manipulation and fluid intake rarely are sufficient to cure this problem
  - Medication to evacuate collected stool and induce daily complete rectal emptying usually needed for an extended period
  - Psychological issues are often secondary to constipation and soiling and improve with adequate treatment of constipation

- **Pearl**

Parents often think their child with retentive constipation has diarrhea because of the fecal leakage.

Short-Gut Syndrome

- **Essentials of Diagnosis**

  - May be congenital but usually a result of surgical treatment of conditions such as necrotizing enterocolitis, volvulus, intussusception, gastroschisis, or trauma
  - Symptoms of short bowel (diarrhea, malabsorption, failure to thrive, dependence on IV nutrition) appear when 50% of small bowel length has been resected
  - Most common causes of death in patients with neonatal short bowel disease are infection and liver failure

- **Differential Diagnosis**

  - Complications which aggravate diarrhea in patients with resection of bowel—small bowel bacterial overgrowth, antibiotic medications, infection, liver disease, intestinal dilation, dysmotility, intestinal stricture, overfeeding
  - Other congenital diarrheas

- **Treatment**

  - Nutritional support is the key to recovery. IV nutrition may be required for several years
  - Increase in body length is associated with a proportional increase in gut length, which results in improved absorption
  - Retention of the colon in short-gut syndrome is a major advantage in fluid salvage and some calorie salvage
  - The most significant complication of short-bowel syndrome is the liver disease associated with infections and long-term IV nutrition

- **Pearl**

Infants with as little as 15 cm of residual small bowel may after several years be independent of IV nutrition if growth has been well supported and the liver stays healthy.

Recurrent Abdominal Pain (RAP)

■ **Essentials of Diagnosis**

- Occurs in about 30% of school-aged children at some time
- Recurrent bouts of abdominal pain over at least 3 months. Variable intensity and duration, no obvious precipitant. Child may describe "continuous" pain. Daily activity, especially school attendance, is impacted
- Patient looks healthy with normal physical examination but may become pale during attacks, doubled over, anxious, verbal complaints of pain
- Fever, weight loss, diarrhea are rare. Nonbilious emesis occurs in 30%
- Blood tests are normal
- Upper endoscopy sometimes indicated. Colonoscopy not indicated unless there is diarrhea or rectal bleeding

■ **Differential Diagnosis**

- Very few organic disorders cause pain for 3 months with no impact on general health or change in physical examination
- Possible organic causes—urinary tract infection, ulcer, GER, gall stones, constipation, inflammatory bowel disease
- Cyclic vomiting syndrome, sometimes called abdominal migraine, is a rare cause of episodic abdominal pain and emesis
- Lactose intolerance is often associated but is not the cause of RAP
- School phobia is often a precipitant as is family stress

■ **Treatment**

- If screening examinations—complete blood count (CBC), urinalysis, stool examination for occult blood, and (in teenaged girls) abdominal ultrasound—are negative, no further diagnostic testing is needed
- Treat organic diseases identified, especially constipation or peptic disease
- Educate patient and family, reassure, return to regular activity, especially school
- Antispasmodic medications occasionally helpful. Low-dose amitriptyline occasionally used in teenaged girls

■ **Pearl**

Dramatic wincing and anticipation of tenderness are often seen on physical examination of the abdomen.

Crohn Disease

- **Essentials of Diagnosis**
  - Inflammatory disease of unknown etiology causing transmural inflammation and ulceration in any segment of the gastrointestinal tract
  - Median age of onset in second decade. Equal sex distribution
  - Insidious-onset weight loss, failure of linear growth, delayed puberty, diarrhea, abdominal pain, joint pain, aphthous oral ulcers, peri-anal abscess or fissures, amenorrhea
  - Microcytic anemia, low serum iron and iron binding capacity, and hypoalbuminemia
  - X-ray or endoscopy of upper and lower tracts is necessary for diagnosis. Esophagus, stomach, large and small bowel may have affected segments. Ileocolonic distribution is most common
  - Anti-saccharomyces cerevisiae antibodies (ASCA) found in up to 60% of patients but test not sufficiently sensitive or specific to confirm the diagnosis
  - Diagnosis rests on typical segmental distribution of full thickness inflammation of the GI tract with noncaseating granulomas on histologic specimens

- **Differential Diagnosis**
  - Celiac disease
  - Intestinal lymphoma
  - Crohn disease isolated to the colon can mimic ulcerative colitis
  - Appendiceal abscess
  - Endocrine causes of growth failure and pubertal delay
  - Anorexia nervosa

- **Treatment**
  - Nutritional support if necessary
  - Anti-inflammatory agents—corticosteroids, sulfasalazine, and mesalamine
  - Azathioprine or 6-mercaptopurine (6-MP) used in resistant cases
  - Infliximab indicated for peri-anal and fistulizing disease
  - Remission can be induced with enteral elemental diet alone

- **Pearl**

A therapeutic balance must be found between the suppression of linear growth and pubertal development associated with active Crohn disease and the similar effects of corticosteroid therapy.

Ulcerative Colitis

- ■ Essentials of Diagnosis
  - Chronic inflammatory disease characterized by superficial inflammation of the colon
  - More acute onset than Crohn disease with bloody diarrhea, cramps, tenesmus. Weight loss, growth failure, and pubertal delay not as prominent. Migratory arthralgia, uveitis, sclerosing cholangitis may occur
  - Elevated WBC, high erythrocyte sedimentation rate (ESR) and C-reactive protein (CRP). Anemia and hypoalbuminemia sometimes present
  - Perinuclear antineutrophil cytoplasmic antibody (pANCA) (neutrophil cytoplasmic antigen located in a perinuclear distribution) positive in ~60% of patients but not sensitive or specific enough to confirm diagnosis
  - Colonoscopy and biopsy essential for confirmation of disease
  - Colon cancer risk increases after the first 10 years of disease

- ■ Differential Diagnosis
  - Infectious colitis, especially shigella, *E coli* 0157, campylobacter, *N gonorrhoeae*
  - Toxin-mediated colitis—*Clostridium difficile, Staphylococcus* species
  - β-Hemolytic streptococcus can cause peri-anal infection and bleeding
  - Juvenile polyps or other colon polyps
  - Allergic colitis

- ■ Treatment
  - Anti-inflammatory therapy similar to Crohn disease—corticosteroids, sulfasalazine, mesalamine
  - Diet therapy is less helpful than in Crohn disease
  - Rectal administration of corticosteroid or mesalamine useful in proctitis
  - 6-MP, azathioprine, and infliximab sometimes effective
  - Colectomy is curative in cases resistant to medical therapy

- ■ Pearl

Because rectal bleeding is a common and dramatic presenting symptom, the time between onset of symptoms and diagnosis in chronic ulcerative colitis is usually <6 months. In contrast, the average time between onset and diagnosis in Crohn disease is 18 months.

Liver and Pancreas

4

Neonatal Infectious Hepatitis

- ■ Essentials of Diagnosis
  - Elevation of total and conjugated bilirubin, elevated transaminases
  - Hepatomegaly and dark urine
  - Patent extrahepatic biliary tree
  - Intrauterine or peripartum viral agents—herpes simplex, vari-
    cella, cytomegalovirus (CMV), rubella, adenovirus, parvovirus,
    human herpesvirus type 6, enterovirus, hepatitis B (HB) virus,
    human immunodeficiency virus (HIV), syphilis, toxoplasmosis
  - Bacterial agents acquired peripartum—Group B streptococci,
    Escherichia coli, Listeria monocytogenes, Staphylococcus aureus
    (associated with omphalitis)
  - Culture and biopsy required to confirm diagnosis

- ■ Differential Diagnosis
  - Bacterial sepsis, urosepsis, necrotizing enterocolitis, and other
    serious infections produce cholestasis
  - Shock liver
  - Cholestasis associated with intravenous (IV) nutrition or drug
    toxicity
  - Extrahepatic biliary atresia
  - Idiopathic neonatal hepatitis
  - Metabolic diseases—galactosemia, tyrosinemia, cystic fibrosis,
    hypopituitarism, fructose intolerance, neonatal hemochromato-
    sis, peroxisomal diseases, Alagille syndrome, Gaucher disease,
    glycogen storage disease type IV
  - Severe hemolysis may produce cholestatic phase

- ■ Treatment
  - Specific therapy for bacterial agents and for diagnosed viral agents
    (if available)
  - Supportive care includes vitamin K supplementation, adequate
    glucose administration
  - Perinatal HB transmission can be prevented by immediately giving
    the newborn HB immune globulin and first dose of HB vaccine

- ■ Pearl

Hepatitis C is rarely transmitted transplacentally or perinatally.

Intrahepatic Neonatal Cholestasis

■ Essentials of Diagnosis

- Elevated total and direct serum bilirubin, with or without elevated transaminase and hepatomegaly
- Dark urine and frequently very pale stools
- Intact extrahepatic biliary structures by ultrasound (US)

■ Differential Diagnosis

- Infections
- Genetic/metabolic diseases—galactosemia, fructose intolerance, tyrosinemia, cystic fibrosis, hypopituitarism, α_1-antitrypsin deficiency, Gaucher disease, Niemann-Pick disease, glycogen storage disease type IV, neonatal iron storage disease, peroxisomal disorders, bile acid synthesis defects, Byler disease, MDR_3 deficiency, Alagille syndrome
- Ischemia-hypoxia
- Prolonged parenteral nutrition
- Inspissated bile syndrome secondary to hemolytic disease
- Idiopathic neonatal hepatitis (giant cell hepatitis)
- Paucity of interlobular bile ducts (Alagille syndrome)
- Progressive familial intrahepatic cholestasis (Byler disease)
- Extrahepatic biliary atresia

■ Treatment

- Specific treatment varies with primary cause of cholestasis
- Cholestatic infants often require fat-soluble vitamin (A, D, E, K) supplements
- Diet high in medium-chain triglycerides (MCTs) may be better absorbed by cholestatic infants

■ Pearl

If total serum bile acids are low in a jaundiced infant there must be a bile acid synthetic or transport defect.

Extrahepatic Neonatal Cholestasis

- **Essentials of Diagnosis**
  - Elevated direct serum bilirubin with intermediate elevations of transaminases
  - Hepatomegaly, acholic stools
  - Lack of patency of extrahepatic tree must be confirmed by radionuclide excretion, biopsy, or exploratory laparotomy with operative cholangiogram before 2 months of age
  - Abdominal US helps with diagnosis of choledochal cyst but is not sensitive enough to evaluate the rest of the biliary tree in small infants
  - Diseases causing intrahepatic cholestasis must be ruled out (see section Intrahepatic Neonatal Cholestasis)

- **Differential Diagnosis**
  - Extrahepatic biliary atresia
  - Choledochal cyst
  - Spontaneous perforation of the extrahepatic ducts
  - Intrinsic obstruction of the extrahepatic tree by tumor, web, or stone
  - Extrinsic obstruction of biliary tree by tumor
  - Intrahepatic cholestatic diseases

- **Treatment**
  - Extrahepatic biliary atresia requires surgical palliation (Kasai portoenterostomy) before 60 days of life to prevent progressive cirrhosis and liver failure
  - Surgical palliation is ineffective in extrahepatic biliary atresia diagnosed after 4 months of life. Liver transplant is the primary therapy
  - Choledochal cysts require surgical cystectomy or bypass with cyst mucosectomy
  - Choledochal cyst—5–15% risk of biliary carcinoma in adulthood
  - Low fat diet, MCT formula, fat-soluble vitamin supplementation

- **Pearl**

In a thriving infant with "acholic" stools but normal bilirubin and transaminase enzymes, suspect excess intake of whole cow's milk.

Gilbert Syndrome

- ■ Essentials of Diagnosis
  - • 3–7% of the population affected. Male/female ratio 4:1
  - • Unconjugated hyperbilirubinemia caused by reduced hepatic bilirubin uridine diphosphate-glucuronyl transferase
  - • Mild fluctuating elevation of unconjugated bilirubin (maximum 8 mg/dL) often with onset in adolescence
  - • Mild constitutional symptoms
  - • Transaminases and liver biopsy always normal. Mild increase in resting bilirubin with fasting. Genetic testing available but not necessary

- ■ Differential Diagnosis
  - • Hemolytic diseases
  - • Some drugs
  - • Hypothyroidism
  - • Infants with prolonged physiologic jaundice may later prove to have Gilbert syndrome

- ■ Treatment
  - • Specific treatment rarely needed
  - • Low-dose phenobarbital improves hepatic conjugation and excretion of bilirubin
  - • Avoid prolonged fasting

- ■ Pearl

New-onset fluctuating mild jaundice in a healthy teenaged boy with normal transaminases is Gilbert syndrome until proven otherwise.

Crigler-Najjar Syndrome

- ■ Essentials of Diagnosis
  - Autosomal recessive deficiency of uridine diphosphate-glucuronyl transferase-1
  - Consanguinity often present
  - Severe elevation of unconjugated bilirubin in neonate (>30 mg/dL)
  - Kernicterus occurs without adequate therapy
  - Milder Crigler-Najjar type 2 has both autosomal dominant and recessive inheritance. Is less severe with rare neurologic sequelae
  - Liver biopsy and liver function tests are normal
  - Duodenal fluid aspirate is colorless and contains minimal conjugated bilirubin

- ■ Differential Diagnosis
  - Other hemolytic disorders—Rh incompatibility, ABO incompatibility
  - Drug effect
  - Hypothyroid
  - Other infections—intra- and extrahepatic cholestatic do not have such severe elevation of total bilirubin and unconjugated bilirubin

- ■ Treatment
  - Phenobarbital ineffective
  - Exchange transfusion temporarily reduces bilirubin
  - Chronic phototherapy and cholestyramine helpful in type 2
  - Tin protoporphyrin is experimental
  - Liver transplant usually necessary in type 1

- ■ Pearl

Symptom onset in Crigler-Najjar type 1 may be delayed until adolescence when severe hyperbilirubinemia may develop suddenly with poor outcome.

Hepatitis A

4

- ■ Essentials of Diagnosis
  - • Subacute onset of anorexia, vomiting, diarrhea, and jaundice. Two-thirds of children asymptomatic
  - • Liver tenderness and hepatomegaly
  - • Usually self-limited with lifelong subsequent immunity. Fulminant hepatitis <1%
  - • May be a history of community epidemic
  - • Increased serum transaminases and bilirubin
  - • Positive anti–hepatitis A immunoglobulin (IgM) antibody
  - • Aplastic anemia is a rare complication that occurs late in the infection or shortly after resolution of infection

- ■ Differential Diagnosis
  - • Nonspecific viral illness
  - • Pancreatitis, cholecystitis, cholelithiasis
  - • Epstein-Barr virus (EBV), leptospirosis, hepatitis B virus (HBV), hepatitis C virus (HCV), cytomegalovirus (CMV), and other hepatotropic viruses
  - • Drug-induced hepatitis
  - • Wilson disease, autoimmune hepatitis, hepatic abscess, hepatic infiltration especially leukemia

- ■ Treatment
  - • Supportive therapy with fluids, rest, low fat diet are standard
  - • Prevention by immunization should be performed in endemic areas
  - • Isolation to prevent fecal oral spread. Passive immunization of contacts with immunoglobulin
  - • Avoid unnecessary medications or surgery during acute phase

- ■ Pearl

Edema of the gall bladder wall frequently seen on US of the abdomen.

Hepatitis B (HB)

- ■ Essentials of Diagnosis
  - Gradual onset of anorexia, vomiting, diarrhea, jaundice, and tender hepatomegaly. Macular rash, urticaria, arthritis, and nephritis may result from Ag-Ab complexes
  - History of sexual or household exposure, maternal HBV carriage, travel to endemic areas
  - Transfusion-acquired HBV has been eradicated with adequate screening of blood donors
  - Elevated serum transaminases and bilirubin
  - Positive HB surface antigen, HB core antibody, and (some cases) HB e antigen

- ■ Differential Diagnosis
  - Bacterial infections indirectly involving the liver (pneumococcal pneumonia, gonococcal perihepatitis)
  - Pancreatitis, cholecystitis, cholelithiasis
  - EBV, leptospirosis, HAV, HCV, CMV, and other hepatotropic viruses
  - Drug-induced hepatitis
  - Wilson disease, autoimmune hepatitis, hepatic abscess, hepatic infiltration especially leukemia

- ■ Treatment
  - Acquired infection is usually self-limited requiring supportive therapy only
  - Without treatment, 70–90% of neonatally acquired HB infection becomes persistent
  - Screening pregnant women for HB status allows for prevention of infection in newborns
  - Prevent transmission of HB from infected/carrier mothers to newborns by immediate administration of HB immune globulin and first dose of HB vaccine
  - In chronic infection, α-interferon or nucleoside analogues may eradicate infection
  - Liver transplantation is successful in fulminant HBV infection

- ■ Pearl

Chronic HB infection with or without symptoms or hepatic dysfunction is associated with late development of hepatocellular carcinoma. Screen chronic carriers by routine hepatic ultrasonography and serum α-fetoprotein.

Hepatitis C

4

- **Essentials of Diagnosis**
  - Most common cause of chronic hepatitis after HBV. Cirrhosis occurs after 10–30 years in 20% of patients with chronic infection
  - Risk factors are illicit IV drugs use (40%), occupational or sexual exposure (10%), transfusion (10%), unknown (30%)
  - Most acute infections are asymptomatic or with mild flu symptoms. Jaundice in <25%
  - Chronic infection follows 70–80% of acute infections associated with mild fluctuating transaminase elevation
  - Diagnosis by anti-HCV antibodies or HCV RNA. Liver biopsy indicated in chronic infection

- **Differential Diagnosis**
  - Must be differentiated from other hepatotrophic viral infections
  - Drug toxicity
  - Hepatic infiltrating tumor, especially leukemia
  - Wilson disease, α_1-antitrypsin deficiency, or other metabolic diseases

- **Treatment**
  - Supportive therapy
  - Treatment of chronic infection with α-interferon produces cure in <15%
  - Long-acting interferon with or without ribavirin is more effective in adults
  - Liver transplant indicated for end-stage liver disease
  - Immunoglobulin administration does not prevent disease in newborns

- **Pearl**

In infants <4 months, transplacentally acquired maternal antibodies will be present. Wait to test for HCV until maternal antibodies have disappeared unless there is obvious biochemical hepatitis. Alternatively, test by HCV RNA, which is not affected by maternal status.

Fulminant Hepatic Failure

- ■ Essentials of Diagnosis
  - A clinical description for acute hepatic damage severe enough to cause failure of critical liver functions
  - Laboratory tests usually show extreme elevation of serum transaminases, prolonged prothrombin time, international normalized ratio (INR), hypoglycemia, and hyperammonemia
  - Clinical findings—bleeding tendency, asterixis, fetor hepaticus, encephalopathy, cerebral edema, uncal herniation
  - Liver biopsy should be done if possible to assist in diagnosis and prognosis

- ■ Causes of Fulminant Hepatic Failure
  - Infectious hepatitis
  - Metabolic liver diseases—infantile tyrosinemia, Wilson disease
  - Drug toxicity (acetaminophen, aspirin, some herbal remedies, amanita mushrooms)
  - Reye-like syndrome and urea cycle abnormalities are usually anicteric at onset of hepatic failure
  - Autoimmune hepatitis, acute leukemia, cardiomyopathy, portal vein thrombosis, multisystem organ failure may all cause severe hepatic dysfunction
  - Veno-occlusive disease

- ■ Treatment
  - Intensive supportive care—maintain blood glucose, treat bleeding diathesis, decrease intracranial pressure, and maintain cerebral perfusion
  - Exchange transfusion for hyperammonemia
  - Extracorporeal hepatic support devices may help maintain life until liver transplant
  - Treat acetaminophen overdose with N-acetyl cysteine and avoid hepatotoxic drugs
  - Treat infections

- ■ Pearl

Mortality from all causes of fulminant hepatic failure is 60–80%. The higher the levels of clotting factors V, VII, and α-fetoprotein, the better the prognosis.

Autoimmune Hepatitis

- **Essentials of Diagnosis**
  - Acute or chronic hepatitis mainly in adolescent girls
  - Weight loss, fever, malaise, arthralgia, acne, amenorrhea, gynecomastia (in males), pleurisy, pericarditis, diarrhea, erythema nodosum, digital clubbing are all seen
  - Hypergammaglobulinemia, positive antinuclear antibody (ANA), anti–smooth muscle or anti–liver/kidney microsomal antibodies, elevated serum transaminases and bilirubin
  - Rarely evolves from drug-induced hepatitis. Associated with ulcerative colitis, Sjögren syndrome, autoimmune hemolytic anemia
  - Liver biopsy is essential to diagnosis

- **Differential Diagnosis**
  - Infection with hepatotropic viruses or bacteria
  - Wilson disease
  - α_1-Antitrypsin deficiency
  - Primary sclerosing cholangitis
  - Inflammatory bowel disease, especially ulcerative colitis
  - Drug toxicity—isoniazid (INH), methyldopa, pemoline
  - Tumor

- **Treatment**
  - Corticosteroids especially effective at time of diagnosis
  - Azathioprine used as sole maintenance if possible
  - Ursodeoxycholic acid, cyclosporine, tacrolimus, methotrexate used in resistant cases
  - Liver transplant may be required to treat progressive liver failure

- **Pearl**

Not every teenaged girl with weight loss and amenorrhea has anorexia nervosa. Look for palmar erythema, digital clubbing, spider telangiectasias, and macrocytosis in such patients as keys to chronic liver disease.

Nonalcoholic Fatty Liver Disease (NAFLD)

- ■ Essentials of Diagnosis
  - 10% of overweight teenagers have NAFLD
  - Usual presentation—overweight anicteric adolescent with asymptomatic hepatomegaly ± type 2 diabetes. In severe cases, steatohepatitis is present with mild aminotransferase elevation
  - Alanine aminotransferase (ALT) is usually higher than AST
  - Liver biopsy shows micro and macro vesicular fatty change with more severe cases showing portal inflammation, Mallory bodies, and variable fibrosis or even cirrhosis
  - US shows increased fat density

- ■ Differential Diagnosis
  - Other diseases with fatty liver—Wilson disease, hereditary fructose intolerance, tyrosinemia, HCV hepatitis, cystic fibrosis, kwashiorkor, fatty acid oxidation and respiratory chain defects, toxic hepatopathy from ethanol

- ■ Treatment
  - Weight reduction by diet and exercise
  - Diabetic control
  - Possibly vitamin E or oral hypoglycemics

- ■ Pearl

As the incidence of obesity increases above 30% American children, NAFLD is the most common pediatric liver disease. Obesity is hard to treat but the consequences may be a huge population of adults with cirrhosis.

α_1-Antitrypsin Deficiency

- **Essentials of Diagnosis**
  - Autosomal recessive mutation in protease inhibitor gene with numerous phenotypes. Liver disease affects ~20% of individuals with homozygous α_1-antitrypsin deficiency
  - Presents in neonates with hepatitis-like picture
  - Older children may present with insidious-onset cirrhosis
  - Serum α_1-antitrypsin level <50–80 mg/dL
  - Family history of early-onset pulmonary disease or liver disease
  - Protease inhibitor (Pi) phenotype ZZ or SZ most commonly have liver disease
  - Diastase-resistant glycoprotein deposits in periportal hepatocytes with variable fibrosis and inflammation

- **Differential Diagnosis**
  - In newborns, all other causes of neonatal cholestasis must be considered
  - In children—chronic HBV or HBC, autoimmune hepatitis, Wilson disease, cystic fibrosis, hemochromatosis, glycogen storage disease Type IV, tyrosinemia, cirrhosis from other causes

- **Treatment**
  - No specific therapy
  - Use bile acid binders, diet high in MCT, fat-soluble vitamin supplements in infants with cholestasis
  - Ursodeoxycholate use reduces transaminases and γ-glutamyltransferase (GGT) but long-term impact on outcome unknown
  - Reduce risk of pulmonary disease by avoiding smoking

- **Pearl**

Although only 20% of infants with Pi type ZZ will develop liver disease, all such patients are at risk for early-onset pulmonary emphysema, especially smokers.

Wilson Disease

- ■ Essentials of Diagnosis
  - Autosomal recessive condition with mutation of *ATP7B* gene that directs synthesis of protein needed in copper transport
  - Usual presentation in children—hepatomegaly and liver dysfunction in child >4 years. Liver disease at presentation may be fulminant hepatitis, chronic hepatitis, or silent cirrhosis
  - Occasional children present with severe hemolytic crisis followed by fulminant liver failure
  - 25% of childhood cases identified by screening after an affected sibling has been diagnosed
  - Kayser-Fleischer rings, neurologic deterioration and psychiatric symptoms occur late
  - Elevated liver, serum and urine copper with (usually) low and serum ceruloplasmin, low-alkaline phosphatase and uric acid

- ■ Differential Diagnosis
  - Acute hepatic presentation mimics viral hepatitis
  - α_1-Antitrypsin deficiency
  - Autoimmune hepatitis
  - Indian childhood cirrhosis
  - Drug-induced hepatitis
  - Other causes of cirrhosis
  - Degenerative neurologic conditions or psychiatric disease

- ■ Treatment
  - Copper chelation with D-penicillamine or trientine hydrochloride
  - Strict dietary restriction of copper
  - Vitamin B_6 prevents optic neuritis
  - Long-term copper chelation with D-penicillamine, trientine, or zinc salts
  - Liver transplant may be required when presentation is fulminant hepatitis

- ■ Pearl

The low-alkaline phosphatase with elevated transaminases is a very good clue that your patient with acute or chronic liver disease has Wilson disease.

Portal Hypertension

4

- ■ Essentials of Diagnosis
  - • Splenomegaly, ascites
  - • Variceal hemorrhage
  - • Hypersplenism with anemia, leucopenia, and thrombocytopenia
  - • Causes are prehepatic and suprahepatic vascular disease and intra-hepatic disease
  - • Abdominal US, wedge hepatic vein pressure, liver biopsy, and disease specific testing are indicated

- ■ Differential Diagnosis
  - • *Prehepatic obstruction of portal or splenic veins*—omphalitis, sepsis, dehydration, umbilical vein catheterization, hypercoagulable states, pancreatitis, congenital portal vein malformation
  - • *Suprahepatic obstruction (Budd-Chiari syndrome)*—vasculitis, tumor, trauma, hyperthermia, previous omphalocele/gastroschisis, hepatic vein malformation, oral contraceptives, hypercoagulable state. Usually no cause is found
  - • *Intrahepatic*—any disease-causing hepatic cirrhosis, veno-occlusive disease, congenital hepatic fibrosis, noncirrhotic portal fibrosis or nodular transformation, schistosoma infection
  - • *Other* conditions causing splenomegaly and ascites should be ruled out—tumor, infection

- ■ Treatment
  - • Prompt therapy of variceal hemorrhage and reduction of ascites
  - • Splenic rupture is a risk. Avoid contact sports
  - • Portosystemic vascular shunt indicated in some conditions
  - • Spontaneous resolution of prehepatic portal hypertension occurs in 50% over time but is rare in suprahepatic and intrahepatic portal hypertension
  - • Endoscopic ligation of varices is effective in reducing rebleeding

- ■ Pearl
  When a healthy 12-month-old suddenly vomits blood and has splenomegaly and thrombocytopenia, he probably has leukemia. However, cavernous malformation of the portal vein can produce the same symptoms and signs. Do an abdominal US.

Cholelithiasis

- **Essentials of Diagnosis**
  - Episodic right upper quadrant abdominal pain. Risk factors include hemolysis, females with prior pregnancy, obesity, rapid weight loss, portal vein thrombosis, Native Americans and Hispanics, ileal disease or resection, cystic fibrosis, Wilson disease, and prolonged IV nutrition
  - Elevated bilirubin, alkaline phosphatase, and GGT
  - Stones or sludge seen in gall bladder by US
  - Pigment stones most common up to 10 years; cholesterol stones most common in adolescents
  - US is the best diagnostic test

- **Differential Diagnosis**
  - Parenchymal liver disease
  - Peptic disease
  - Cardiac disease
  - Pancreatitis
  - Renal stones
  - Subcapsular liver lesions—abscess, tumor hematoma
  - Right lower lobe pneumonia

- **Treatment**
  - Cholecystectomy for symptomatic patients
  - Guidelines unclear for children with asymptomatic gall stones but surgery required in <20% of cases
  - Ursodeoxycholate and lithotripsy not approved for this indication

- **Pearl**

Gallstones are common harmless findings on prenatal ultrasound examinations. They resolve within several months of birth.

Hepatic Cancer

- **Essentials of Diagnosis**
  - Third most common intra-abdominal cancer of children
  - Abdominal enlargement, hepatomegaly, pain, weight loss, anemia, mass detected by abdominal computed tomography (CT) or US
  - Hepatoblastoma more common in male infants and associated with Beckwith Wiedemann syndrome, hemihypertrophy, familial adenomatous polyposis, prematurity
  - Hepatocellular carcinoma more common after 3 years of age. Associated with chronic HBV, HCV, cirrhosis, glycogen storage disease type I, tyrosinemia, α_1-antitrypsin deficiency, anabolic steroids
  - US and CT examination required. Laparotomy for tissue biopsy required

- **Differential Diagnosis**
  - Other conditions causing hepatomegaly—storage disease, cirrhosis, vascular tumors, malnutrition, heart failure, veno-occlusive disease, hepatic vein thrombosis
  - Infection or abscess
  - Pancreatic tumors or cysts
  - Inflammatory pseudotumor or mesenteric cysts

- **Treatment**
  - Aggressive surgical resection with resection of isolated lung metastases
  - Radiotherapy and chemotherapy are disappointing but may be used for tumor size reduction
  - Liver transplantation an option for hepatoblastoma only
  - Outcome of hepatocellular carcinoma may be better when tumor is associated with another of the disorders listed

- **Pearl**

Suspect hepatoblastoma in a male infant who develops galactorrhea.

Acute Pancreatitis

- ■ Essentials of Diagnosis
  - • Epigastric pain radiating to the back
  - • Nausea and vomiting
  - • Caused by drugs, infection, severe systemic disease (multiorgan system failure), abdominal trauma, hyperlipidemic states, pancreatic duct obstruction (gall stones, cyst, pancreas divisum, extrinsic tumors, ascariasis)
  - • Elevated serum amylase and lipase. Monitor for hypocalcemia, electrolyte abnormalities, acidosis
  - • CT scan or US showing pancreatic inflammation

- ■ Differential Diagnosis
  - • Acute gastroenteritis
  - • Atypical appendicitis
  - • Cholelithiasis
  - • Duodenal or gastric ulcer
  - • Intussusception
  - • Pneumonia
  - • Nonaccidental trauma

- ■ Treatment
  - • Intensive care may be needed for treatment of shock, fluid and electrolyte abnormalities, ileus, respiratory distress, hypocalcemia
  - • Pain management
  - • Acid suppression
  - • Parenteral or jejunal nutrition
  - • Surgery for stone obstruction or ruptured pancreas
  - • Antibiotics only useful for identified infection or in necrotizing pancreatitis
  - • Up to 20% of patients develop pseudocysts, but 2/3 of these resolve spontaneously

- ■ Pearl

Newborn infants are relatively amylase deficient. Thus, when they have pancreatitis they may not have an elevated serum amylase.

Exocrine Pancreatic Insufficiency

- **Essentials of Diagnosis**
    - Maldigestion, steatorrhea, diarrhea, poor weight gain, hyperphagia
    - Most common cause is cystic fibrosis
    - Distant second cause is Shwachman-Diamond syndrome—exocrine insufficiency, neutropenia secondary to granulocyte maturation arrest, metaphysical dysostosis, and fatty replacement of the pancreas with short stature
    - Pancreatic stimulation with secretin and cholecystokinin (CCK) results in low or absent pancreatic enzyme secretion
    - Fecal fat excretion is >10% in children over 12 months, >15% in children under 12 months

- **Differential Diagnosis**
    - Other rare causes of pancreatic insufficiency—Pearson bone marrow pancreas syndrome, congenital absence of the pancreas, duodenal atresia, or stenosis
    - Isolated trypsin deficiency usually caused by enterokinase deficiency
    - Malnutrition can cause temporary pancreatic insufficiency
    - Chronic and repeated pancreatitis cause exocrine deficiency

- **Treatment**
    - Exogenous pancreatic enzyme replacement
    - In infants, formulas with hydrolyzed fats, proteins, and starches may be used
    - Supplemental fat-soluble vitamins
    - Maldigestion improves with age in Shwachman-Diamond syndrome

- **Pearl**

Newborn infants are relatively amylase deficient. Giving a young infant too much cereal (complex carbohydrate) may cause diarrhea because of amylase deficiency.

5

Kidney and Urinary Tract

Polycystic Kidney Disease (PKD)

- ■ Essentials of Diagnosis
  - • Cystic dilation of renal tubules—caused by tubular cell hyperplasia, excess tubular fluid secretion, and abnormal tubular extracellular matrix
  - • 90% are autosomal dominant (AD). May present in childhood but most present at 30–40 years with pain, hypertension, infection, hematuria, enlarged kidneys, and renal failure
  - • Autosomal recessive (AR) PKD—often diagnosed by prenatal ultrasound. Newborns may have abdominal mass, Potter facies, club foot, and other findings of oligohydramnios caused by in utero renal failure
  - • Older infants with AR-PKD may present with congenital hepatic fibrosis, splenomegaly, portal hypertension, and variceal hemorrhage
  - • Diagnosis made by finding renal cysts on ultrasound in patients with suggestive signs and symptoms

- ■ Differential Diagnosis
  - • Other abdominal masses
  - • Other causes of hypertension
  - • Other structural urinary tract disorders with hematuria, proteinuria, and infection
  - • Acquired renal cysts secondary to isolated duct ectasia or chronic renal disease
  - • Medullary cystic disease—variable cysts in the medulla with Fanconi syndrome and renal failure

- ■ Treatment
  - • 50% of patients with AD-PKD require dialysis or renal transplant. Much less likely in AR-PKD
  - • Medical management of chronic renal insufficiency—decreased protein and sodium intake, calorie supplementation, vitamin D supplementation, antihypertensive medication (see section Chronic Renal Failure)
  - • Portosystemic shunt and/or variceal banding to treat variceal hemorrhage in patients with congenital hepatic fibrosis

- ■ Pearl

The major genes associated with AD-PKD are on chromosome 16 (85%) and chromosome 4 (15%). These genes code for the proteins polycystin 1 and 2. Abnormal proteins appear to produce renal ciliary dysfunction leading to tubular fluid accumulation and cyst formation.

Glomerulonephritis (GN)

- **Essentials of Diagnosis**
  - Most common form is poststreptococcal GN after infection with group A β-hemolytic *Streptococcus* serotypes 12 (pharyngitis) and 49 (impetigo)
  - Antigen-antibody complexes form after infection and are deposited in glomeruli causing inflammation and complement consumption
  - Usual presentation—hematuria, oliguria, proteinuria, edema, sodium and water retention, hypertension, headache, flank pain
  - Diagnosis requires proof of recent group A β-hemolytic streptococcus (GAS) infection (tonsils or skin), high-titer antistreptolysin O or other antistreptococcal antibodies, evidence of complement consumption
  - Other bacterial, viral, parasitic, and fungal infections may cause immune complex deposition and GN
  - Other conditions producing GN—immunoglobulin (IgA) nephropathy, HS purpura, membranoproliferative GN, systemic lupus erythematosus (SLE), hereditary GN (Alport syndrome), polyarteritis nodosa, Goodpasture syndrome, Berger disease

- **Differential Diagnosis**
  - Nephrotic syndrome
  - Renal stones, renal vein thrombosis, infection, PKD
  - Drug hypersensitivity nephritis usually has associated tubulointerstitial component
  - Angioedema
  - Hypertension
  - Idiopathic hematuria
  - Renal tumor

- **Treatment**
  - Most cases of poststreptococcal GN resolve without treatment
  - Antibiotics are given for persistent infection but do not change the course of disease
  - Treat hypertension—sodium and fluid restriction, diuretics and antihypertensives, corticosteroids (in severe cases)
  - Dialysis occasionally required

- **Pearl**

Although microscopic hematuria may persist for as long as a year, 85% of children with poststreptococcal GN recover completely. Severe proteinuria, atypical presentation, progressive renal insufficiency, or persistent hypocomplementemia suggest another entity.

Interstitial Nephritis

- **Essentials of Diagnosis**
  - Diffuse or focal inflammation of renal interstitium with secondary involvement of the tubules
  - Most often related to drug sensitivity—antibiotics (often β-lactams), anticonvulsants, nonsteroidal anti-inflammatory drugs (NSAIDs), thiazides, cimetidine, ranitidine. May be postinfectious
  - Fever, rigors, abdominal/flank pain, skin rash, hypertension. May present with acute renal failure. Eosinophilia often but not always present
  - Urinalysis shows white blood cells (WBCs) with eosinophils, hematuria, sometimes glucosuria, and low specific gravity because of tubular dysfunction
  - Biopsy may be needed if history and urinalysis are not diagnostic

- **Differential Diagnosis**
  - Lead toxicity causes chronic interstitial nephritis
  - Acute urinary tract infection (UTI)
  - Lupus, Goodpasture syndrome
  - Renal transplant rejection

- **Treatment**
  - Remove offending drug. Treat infection if present. Treat hypertension
  - Corticosteroids helpful
  - Dialysis for acute renal failure
  - Outcome generally good in drug-related nephritis. Progression to nephrotic syndrome or chronic renal failure may occur

- **Pearl**

The child with vesicoureteral reflux and recurrent infection is more likely to develop interstitial nephritis after infection that the child with a normal urinary tract.

Idiopathic Nephrotic Syndrome

5

- ■ Essentials of Diagnosis
  - • Proteinuria, hypoproteinemia, edema, and hyperlipidemia
  - • Most common form of nephrotic syndrome in childhood is idiopathic (nil disease, lipoid nephrosis, minimal change disease)
  - • Generally affects children <6 years. Often postinfectious
  - • Periorbital edema, peripheral edema, oliguria, malaise, abdominal pain, ascites, pulmonary edema, pleural effusion, dyspnea
  - • Urinary sediment often normal or with only microscopic hematuria. Significant proteinuria. Low serum albumin. High serum cholesterol and triglycerides
  - • Biopsy findings minor—mesangial foot process fusion, no immune deposits, occasional mesangial proliferation, or focal glomerular sclerosis

- ■ Differential Diagnosis
  - • Any glomerular disease can produce the findings of nephrotic syndrome
  - • Focal glomerular sclerosis
  - • Mesangial nephropathy
  - • Membranous nephropathy
  - • Renal vein thrombosis may be the cause of nephrotic syndrome or may be caused by it
  - • Congenital nephrosis—low birth weight, large placenta, widened cranial sutures, delayed ossification, edema, renal failure

- ■ Treatment
  - • Daily prednisone (2 mg/kg/day; maximum 60 mg/day) for 6 weeks. Same dose every other day for 6 weeks. Gradual taper over 2–4 months as proteinuria resolves
  - • Induce diuresis if necessary with intravenous (IV) albumin replacement followed by diuretics
  - • Administer pneumococcal vaccine to children with ascites to reduce risk of bacterial peritonitis
  - • Renal biopsy to rule out other disorders in patients with poor response to medications or relapse
  - • Patients unresponsive or relapsing on corticosteroid—use chlorambucil, cyclophosphamide, tacrolimus, or cyclosporine A as adjuncts

- ■ Pearl
  The cause of idiopathic nephrotic syndrome is unknown. There appears to be increased risk in individuals with HLA type B8 DR3, DR7, and DQ2. Relapsing disease associated with oligoclonal expansion of T-cell subsets, especially $CD8^+$ cells.

Renal Vein Thrombosis

- **Essentials of Diagnosis**
  - Most common in newborns—sepsis/dehydration, infant of diabetic mother, umbilical vein catheter, hypercoagulable state
  - Less common in children—trauma, nephrotic syndrome (possibly because of renal loss of antithrombotic proteins), membranoproliferative GN, hypercoagulable states (SLE, pregnancy, malignancy, Behçet disease), idiopathic
  - Sudden-onset abdominal mass, flank pain, oliguria (with bilateral thrombi), hematuria
  - Extension of clot into vena cava causes lower limb edema or pulmonary embolus
  - Diagnosis confirmed by ultrasound with Doppler flow study

- **Differential Diagnosis**
  - Acute papillary necrosis
  - Renal infarct
  - Renal cell cancer may invade and obstruct the renal veins
  - Extrinsic pressure from retroperitoneal fibrosis, tumor, lymph nodes
  - Renal colic from stones mimics some symptoms of renal vein thrombosis

- **Treatment**
  - Anticoagulation with heparin
  - Treat underlying problem
  - Recurrent thrombus may occur years after the original episode. Some patients require chronic anticoagulation
  - If there is underlying nephrotic syndrome, kidney biopsy should be performed to determine appropriate therapy

- **Pearl**

Children with renal vein thrombosis should be evaluated for hypercoagulable states. Factor V Leiden is found with increased frequency. Patients with nephrotic syndrome may also become hypercoagulable because of urinary loss of antithrombin III.

Hemolytic Uremic Syndrome (HUS)

- ■ Essentials of Diagnosis
  - Clinical triad of microangiopathic hemolytic anemia, thrombotic thrombocytopenia, and renal failure due to glomerular vascular injury
  - Usually preceded by infection with Shiga toxin (vero toxin) producing strains of *Shigella* or *Escherichia coli 0157:H7* which causes an initial bloody diarrhea bloody diarrhea
  - Absorbed toxin causes endothelial damage resulting in platelet deposition and microvascular occlusion
  - Other precipitants include cyclosporine A, human immunodeficiency virus (HIV), pneumococcal infection, genetic C3 complement or factor H deficiency
  - High index of suspicion in any child with recent history of acute bloody diarrhea. The history of oliguria is easy to miss
  - Laboratory testing—profound anemia, blood smear with microangiopathiced red blood cells (RBC) fragmentation, increased blood urea nitrogen (BUN) and creatine

- ■ Differential Diagnosis
  - Other causes of acute hemolytic anemia
  - Acute gastroenteritis with shock and oliguria
  - Sepsis with disseminated intravascular coagulation (DIC)
  - Ulcerative colitis, pseudomembranous enterocolitis
  - Intussusception
  - Lupus
  - Thrombotic thrombocytopenic purpura
  - Acute tubular necrosis or other causes of sudden renal failure

- ■ Treatment
  - Spontaneous recovery in 55%. Some residual renal disease and hypertension in 30%. End-stage renal failure in 15%
  - Meticulous management of fluid and electrolyte status
  - Antimotility agents and antibiotics may worsen HUS
  - Timely dialysis improves prognosis
  - Plasma infusion/plasmapheresis may increase plasma prostacyclin stimulating factor and prevent platelet aggregation
  - Platelet inhibitors early in the disease may improve prognosis
  - Erythropoietin may decrease the need for red cell transfusion

- ■ Pearl

The most common sources of E coli O157:H7 infection in the United States are undercooked ground beef or unpasteurized fruits, vegetables, or other food products contaminated with bovine feces. Notify your local health department of any case of HUS.

Acute Renal Failure

- ■ Essentials of Diagnosis
  - Sudden inability to excrete urine of adequate quantity or quality to maintain body fluid homeostasis
  - Most common cause in children is dehydration
  - Other causes—impaired renal perfusion, ischemia, acute renal disease, renal vascular compromise, acute tubular necrosis, obstructive uropathy
  - Major symptom is oliguria
  - Urine findings in prerenal failure—U_{Osm} 50 mOsm/kg >P_{Osm}; U_{Na} <10 mEq/L; U_{Cr}:P_{Cr} >14:1; urine SG >1.020
  - Urine findings acute tubular necrosis—U_{Osm} <P_{Osm}; U_{Na} > 20 mEq/L; U_{Cr}:P_{Cr} <13:1; urine SG 1.012–1.018

- ■ Differential Diagnosis
  - Postrenal obstruction preventing normal urine flow—anatomic anomalies of the urinary tract, bladder malignancy, severe fecal impaction, phimosis, balanitis
  - Drugs may cause urinary retention—antihistamines, narcotics, tricyclic antidepressants, atropines
  - Elevated BUN associated with gastrointestinal (GI) bleed may be high enough to suggest acute renal failure

- ■ Treatment
  - Ascertain intravascular volume, perfusion adequacy, and urine output with indwelling bladder catheter. Monitor intake
  - Specific treatment for prerenal disorders or postrenal obstruction
  - Re-establish normal plasma volume
  - Attempt to produce diuresis >.5 mL/kg/h with diuretics—furosemide, metolazone
  - If diuresis does not occur with a short trial of medication, dialysis may be needed
  - If severe oliguria lasts >3 weeks, acute tubular necrosis is unlikely. Consider vascular injury, ischemia, GN, or obstruction

- ■ Pearl

In patients suspected of acute renal failure, it is important to adjust both the amount of fluid and medication administered to the degree of renal failure to avoid fluid overload or drug toxicity.

Chronic Renal Failure

- **Essentials of Diagnosis**
  - In infants, most common causes are structural anomalies of kidneys or urinary tract—renal dysgenesis, obstructive uropathy, severe vesicoureteral reflux
  - In older children, chronic glomerulonephritides, irreversible nephrotoxic injury, and HUS are most common causes
  - Complications—growth failure, polyuria/oliguria, salt wasting/retention, metabolic bone disease, hypertension
  - Symptoms of uremia—anorexia, nausea, electrolyte abnormalities, confusion, apathy, seizures, anemia, bleeding tendency, pericarditis, colitis, pulmonary edema, and hypertension

- **Classification of Renal Failure**
  - *Prerenal*—dehydration, hemorrhage, diabetic acidosis, hypovolemia, shock, heart failure
  - *Renal*—HUS, acute GN, nephrotoxins, acute tubular necrosis (ATN), renal cortical necrosis, renal vascular disease, severe infection, fresh water drowning, hyperuricacidemia during cancer therapy, hepatorenal syndrome
  - *Postrenal*—obstruction (tumor, hematoma, posterior urethral valves, UP junction stricture ureterocele), stones, trauma, renal vein thrombosis

- **Treatment**
  - Control hypertension—diuretics, antihypertensives, Na, and fluid restriction
  - Control hyperkalemia—dietary restriction
  - Control hyperphosphatemia—dietary restriction, dietary phosphate binders (Ca carbonate), vitamin D supplementation
  - Control uremia—protein restriction
  - Promote growth—supplemental calories, growth hormone sometimes used
  - Control anemia—erythropoietin
  - Reassess need for dialysis or renal transplant regularly

- **Pearl**

1-year graft survival rate in living related kidney transplantation is 90% overall. 5-year overall survival is 75%. Mortality and morbidity of renal transplantation are significantly increased in infants <1 year or <15 kg.

Hypertension

- **Essentials of Diagnosis**
  - Diagnosis is age dependent—patient is normotensive if the average systolic and diastolic blood pressures are <90% for age and sex
  - Renal disease is most common cause—congenital anomaly of kidney or renal vasculature, renal obstruction, renal vein or artery thrombosis, volume overload, loss of one kidney, diabetic or SLE-related renal disease
  - Other causes—cardiac (coarctation of aorta), drugs (cocaine, amphetamines, steroids, ephedrine, estrogens, EPO, cyclosporine A), endocrine (hyperthyroidism, pheochromocytoma, Wilms tumor, neuroblastoma, Cushing syndrome, hyperaldosteronism), increased intracranial pressure
  - Essential hypertension—risk factors include obesity and family history
  - Symptoms often not present. Headache, signs of intracranial hypertension, cardiac failure may indicate a hypertensive crisis

- **Differential Diagnosis**
  - Measuring blood pressure with a cuff too small for the patient is the most common cause of hypertension
  - Anxiety causes increase in systolic pressure

- **Treatment**
  - Acute hypertensive emergency may require diuretic (furosemide), α- or β-blockers, angiotensin-converting enzyme inhibitors, calcium channel blockers (nifedipine), vasodilators (sodium nitroprusside, hydralazine) in an intensive care setting
  - Sustained hypertension of renal origin—angiotensin-converting enzyme inhibitor
  - Sustained essential hypertension treated with vasodilators usually requires concomitant diuretic and β-blockade

- **Pearl**

The most common organic cause of hypertension in infants is congenital renal/renovascular or cardiac disease. In adolescence, essential hypertension becomes the most common diagnosis.

Renal Tubular Acidosis (RTA)

- **Essentials of Diagnosis**
  - *Type 1 (distal RTA)*—hereditary disorder with failure to thrive, anorexia, vomiting, and dehydration. Metabolic acidosis, hyperchloremia, hypokalemia, urinary pH >6.5
  - Type 1 RTA usually permanent. Differentiated from type 2 RTA by the large amount of bicarbonate required to normalize plasma level (>10 mEq/kg/24 h)
  - *Type 2 (proximal RTA)*—most common RTA of childhood. Mildly low serum bicarbonate, excess bicarbonate in urine with low renal threshold for loss. Normal distal tubular function allows for acidification of urine at bicarbonate concentrations below threshold
  - Type 2 RTA may be a developmental immaturity of renal function. Dose of alkali required to achieve normal plasma bicarbonate is low (2–3 mEq/kg/24 h)
  - Both types 1 and 2 may be associated with hypercalciuria, stones, or nephrocalcinosis

- **Differential Diagnosis**
  - Fanconi syndrome
  - Other conditions with tubular defects—Hartnup disease, Lowe syndrome, cystinosis, Wilson disease, hereditary tyrosinemia
  - Secondary RTA may result from chronic reflux

- **Treatment**
  - Treat distal RTA with bicarbonate. Doses greater than 3 mEq/day are rarely required
  - Prognosis good in uncomplicated distal RTA in the absence of complications
  - Treat proximal RTA with at least 3 mEq/day of bicarbonate or citrate. Doses over 10 mEq/kg/day may be required. Concomitant potassium supplementation may be needed
  - Prognosis good in proximal RTA. Therapy usually discontinued by 2 years

- **Pearl**

Young infants don't like the taste of bicarbonate, citrate, or potassium solutions. They may develop food refusal behavior and diarrhea (from the osmotic load of the solutions), which aggravates failure to thrive.

Urinary Tract Infection (UTI)

- ■ Essentials of Diagnosis
  - 8% of girls and 2% of boys will have $\geq$1 UTI during childhood
  - Most UTIs are ascending infections—risk factors are chronic constipation, uncircumcised males, dysfunctional voiding in girls, poor perineal hygiene, instrumentation of the urethra, sexual activity
  - Infants—congenital anomalies of kidneys and collecting system are risk factors for UTI
  - Usal organisms—*E coli* (>85%), *Klebsiella, Proteus,* other gram negatives, *Enterococcus,* coagulase negative staphylococcus
  - Infant symptoms are fever, vomiting, irritability and sepsis. Childhood symptoms are frequency dysuria, urgency, enuresis and flank pain
  - Catheterized urine required for culture and antibiotic choice. Urine analysis shows WBCs, protein, blood and sometimes bacteria
  - Leukocyte esterase test often false positive. Urinary nitrite most sensitive in older children with less frequent voiding

- ■ Differential Diagnosis
  - In infants and children with pyelonephritis differential is wide—sepsis, appendicitis, abdominal surgical condition, heart or lung disease, child abuse, neurologic disease, metabolic disease, gastrointestinal (GI) disease (especially gastroesophageal [GE] reflux
  - In children with dysuria—orchitis, prostatitis, urethritis, epididymitis, gonorrhea, phimosis, balanitis
  - Prostatic tumor, tumors of other pelvic organs, fecal impaction may obstruct bladder neck and produce symptoms of UTI
  - Spine injury or spinal cord tumor or infection

- ■ Treatment
  - IV antibiotics in infants <3 months and patients with toxicity
  - Uncomplicated cystitis use oral amoxicillin, trimethoprim-sulfamethoxazole, or first-generation cephalosporin
  - Cystitis in sexually mature teenagers use 3 days of fluoroquinolone
  - Acute pyelonephritis treated for 10 days
  - Prophylactic antibiotics for high-grade vesicoureteral reflux, recurrent UTI, spastic or atonic bladder, anatomic abnormalities

- ■ Pearl

Voiding cystourethrogram (VCUG) is indicated in boys with first UTI. Posterior urethral valve is the most common anatomic abnormality discovered in infant boys with UTI.

Henoch-Schönlein Purpura (HSP)

- **Essentials of Diagnosis**
  - Postinfectious leukocytoclastic vasculitis of children <20 years, affecting many organ systems
  - Males affected more often than females for unknown reasons
  - Usual clinical constellation is purpuric rash on dorsa of lower extremities and buttocks (often more extensive), abdominal pain, bloody diarrhea, joint pain. Cerebritis, intussusception, duodenitis, pancreatitis cholecystitis, scrotal edema, DIC also occur
  - Renal involvement in 20–100% of cases ranges from mild GN with microscopic hematuria, hypertension to end-stage renal failure
  - Diagnosis is clinical. High platelet count common. Hyper- or hypo-IgA often seen
  - IgA deposits seen in blood vessels of kidney, skin, and GI tract biopsies

- **Differential Diagnosis**
  - GI symptoms (vomiting, pain, bloody diarrhea) suggesting surgical emergency
  - Headache may predominate suggesting brain tumor or meningitis
  - Nephritis may predominate suggesting other glomerular nephritides
  - Septicemia with DIC, meningococcemia, Rocky Mountain spotted fever

- **Treatment**
  - No specific therapy. Self-limited in most cases
  - Patients with severe abdominal pain at risk for intussusception with intramural bowel hemorrhages as lead point and may require surgery
  - Renal failure may develop in those with severe hematuria, proteinuria many months after resolution of acute symptoms
  - Corticosteroids often used for severe abdominal pain and for renal disease

- **Pearl**

Respiratory infections are the most likely trigger (strep throat, Mycoplasma, adenovirus, and others) but odd things like bug bites and stress have been blamed.

Renal Stones

- ■ Essentials of Diagnosis
  - Kidney stones may occur in certain metabolic diseases—cystinosis (cystine), hyperglycinuria (glycine), Lesch-Nyhan syndrome (urate), oxalosis (oxalate)
  - Stones may be caused by hypercalciuria—distal RTA, immobilization syndrome, spina bifida or spinal injury, corticosteroid use
  - Chronic urinary infection with or without obstruction increases the risk of struvite stones (magnesium and ammonia)
  - Underlying anatomic anomaly often found in children
  - Symptoms are pain, hematuria, obstruction
  - Diagnosis by ultrasound and other imaging studies

- ■ Differential diagnosis
  - Hematuria from infection, obstruction, trauma, tumor, nephritis
  - Flank pain from trauma, cholecystitis, urinary infection or obstruction, tumor, spinal injury

- ■ Treatment
  - Treat the underlying cause
  - Increase fluid intake, decrease sodium intake to decrease calciuria
  - Most small stones pass spontaneously
  - Extracorporeal shockwave lithotripsy is sometimes used in children
  - Surgical removal may be required for very large stones, obstruction, intractable pain, chronic infection

- ■ Pearl

The incidence of kidney stones in children is increasing and is blamed on increasing prevalence of obesity and type 2 diabetes. Risk factors may be high dietary sodium intake and physical inactivity in obese children.

Neurological and Neuromuscular Disorders

Brain Death

- **Essentials of Diagnosis**
  - Stage IV coma, no spontaneous respiration after 3 minutes with P_{CO_2} >60 mm Hg, no brainstem functions, normal blood pressure and body temperature, flaccid muscle tone, no spontaneous movements
  - Consistent findings in 2 examinations over 24 hours (children > 1 year)
  - Cerebral angiography, radionuclide scanning, and transcranial ultrasound useful to confirm clinical diagnosis
  - Testing needed in neonates in whom clinical diagnosis is difficult
  - Electroencephalogram (EEG) silence for 30 minutes in absence of suppressing drugs or hypothermia also confirms clinical diagnosis, especially in neonates

- **Differential Diagnosis**
  - Deep coma may simulate brain death—hypothermia, paralytic agents; sedative—hypnotic drug overdose, toxins, trauma
  - Stroke, hypoxic-ischemic injury, massive bleed
  - Vegetative state

- **Treatment**
  - By definition, brain death is irreversible
  - Recommended observation period to confirm clinical diagnosis of brain death is 48 hours in neonates and 24 hours in others
  - Withdrawal of life-sustaining medical therapy requires sensitive education and support of family

- **Pearl**

The Task Force on Brain Death in Children published the most widely used criteria for brain death in Pediatrics 1987;80:298–300. The criteria are regularly reviewed and updated by the American Academy of Pediatrics.

Febrile Seizures

- **Essentials of Diagnosis**
  - Occur in 2–3% of children between 3 months and 5 years
  - >90% of are generalized, lasting <5 minutes and occurring early in an infectious illness causing fever
  - Acute viral respiratory infection is the most common associated illness
  - Other infections associated with febrile seizure—gastroenteritis (Shigella, Campylobacter), urinary tract infection, roseola infantum
  - Only 1–2.4% of children with a febrile seizure have subsequent epilepsy
  - Risk factors for later epilepsy—fever <38.8°C, seizure lasting >15 minutes, >1 seizure in the same day, focal seizure, abnormal baseline neurologic status, age <1 year, family history of epilepsy
  - Check serum glucose, electrolytes, calcium
  - Investigate nontypical seizure with immediate spinal tap and brain imaging and EEG at least 1 week after seizure

- **Differential Diagnosis**
  - Electrolyte (especially sodium and calcium) and blood glucose abnormalities
  - Seizures associated with breath-holding spells or syncope
  - Head trauma
  - Central nervous system (CNS) infection
  - New-onset epilepsy

- **Treatment**
  - Control fever
  - Stop ongoing seizure. Drugs rarely needed as seizures are usually brief
  - Diagnostic evaluation for unusual seizures or risk factors
  - Educate parents about future fever control
  - Anticonvulsant prophylaxis can reduce recurrent febrile seizures and may be appropriate after the second febrile seizure
    - Use diazepam at onset and for duration of febrile illness
    - Use a regular bedtime dose phenobarbital
    - Phenytoin and carbamazepines are ineffective

- **Pearl**

Simple febrile seizures do not have any long-term adverse consequences. Minor EEG abnormalities seen in ~20% of children after a febrile seizure have little value in predicting risk of recurrence or long-term prognosis.

Epilepsy

- ■ Essentials of Diagnosis
  - Recurrent nonfebrile seizures with interictal EEG abnormalities
  - *Benign idiopathic neonatal seizures* account for 6% of neonatal seizures. Onset at 3–7 days, multifocal, brief, with spontaneous resolution
  - *Infantile spasms*—onset 3–18 months, violent contractions of muscle groups, hypsarrhythmia on EEG, 90% have mental/ motor retardation
  - *Generalized tonic-clonic (GTCS)*—onset 3–11 years, family or personal history of febrile seizures, 3/s spike wave EEG in 50%
  - *Absence seizures (petit mal)*—onset 10–12 years, more frequent in boys, 3–4/s spike wave EEG, most also have GTCS, may remit spontaneously
  - *Myoclonic epilepsy*—onset 12–18 years, myoclonic jerks of upper limbs, 4–6/s general spike wave EEG, 90% also have GTCS if not treated
  - *Rolandic epilepsy*—autosomal dominant, onset 3–13 years, brief 2–5/min simple partial seizures during sleep, bilateral spikes on EEG
  - *Complex partial seizures*—preseizure aura, stereotypic movements and vocalizations lasting 15–90 seconds, followed by confusion

- ■ Differential Diagnosis
  - Secondary seizures—trauma, bleed/stroke, infection, drugs, toxins, hypoglycemia, hypocalcemia, hyponatremia, febrile seizure
  - Breath-holding spells, especially pallid spells
  - Tourette syndrome tics
  - Night terrors
  - Migraine
  - Benign nocturnal myoclonus
  - Gastroesophageal (GE) reflux with Sandifer posturing
  - Masturbation
  - Conversion reaction
  - Benign paroxysmal vertigo
  - Staring spells

- ■ Treatment
  - Status epilepticus occurs in all seizure types; most common in GTCS
  - Status epilepticus is a medical emergency requiring airway and circulation support, administration of glucose and calcium, diagnostic search for primary cause, and intravenous medications (diazepam, phenytoin, phenobarbital, midazolam, valproate, pentobarbital)
  - Phenytoin, phenobarbital, valproate, carbamazepine are used for maintenance in most types of childhood epilepsy
  - Adjunctive medications include—Diamox, levetiracetam, oxcarbazepine, Felbatol, Neurontin, topiramate, Gabitril, lamotrigine

- ■ Pearl

The key to the clinical diagnosis of a seizure disorder is obtaining an accurate description of the spell.

Syncope and Fainting

■ Essentials of Diagnosis

- Transient loss of consciousness and postural tone due to cerebral ischemia—vasovagal/vasodepressive/neurocardiogenic etiology
- 20–50% of children will faint at some point before age 20 years
- Prodromal symptoms—dizziness, light-headedness, nausea, gray-out, sweating, pallor
- Brief tonic-clonic seizure occurs in many cases
- Family history often positive
- EEG and cardiac evaluation normal except for occasional evidence of autonomic dysfunction (tilt table test) with exaggerated orthostatic hypotension

■ Differential Diagnosis

- Prolonged QT_c interval, ventricular tachycardia or fibrillation, or other arrhythmia, mitral valve prolapse, hypertrophic cardiomyopathy
- Hypercyanotic spell—tetralogy of Fallot
- Seizures
- Migraine
- Hypoglycemia
- Hysteria, hyperventilation, vertigo
- Pallid breath-holding spell

■ Treatment

- Search for a primary cause indicated in recurrent syncope—complete blood count (CBC), glucose, electrolytes, Holter monitor, and possible cardiology or neurology evaluation
- Protect patient from self-injury during spell—bite, fall
- Education and avoidance of precipitating situations
- Lie down during prodrome. Adequate fluid and salt intake
- Rarely β-blockers and fludrocortisone may be used

■ Pearl

Common precipitants for fainting include watching or undergoing venipuncture, prolonged standing, overheating, fatigue, poor fluid and salt intake (especially in thin teenaged girls), athleticism with baseline bradycardia.

Headaches

- **Essentials of Diagnosis**
  - 3 types of headaches—tension, vascular, traction/inflammatory—account for 25% of all neurology referrals
  - 15% of children have had a *vascular headache (migraine)* by age 14 years—recurrent, paroxysmal, pulsatile, often unilateral, located in forehead or eye, nausea, emesis, occasional paralysis/seizure. Prodromal aura rare in children
  - *Traction/inflammatory headaches*—chronic with gradually increasing frequency and severity, signs of increased intracranial pressure (ICP), papilledema, nausea, and emesis especially with position change
  - *Tension headaches*—chronic recurrent, band-like or diffuse, source of psychic stress often identified at home or school
  - Careful history is the first diagnostic test. Imaging of head indicated with signs of increased ICP

- **Differential Diagnosis**
  - Drug abuse/overuse, depression, sleep disorders may present as tension headache
  - Sinusitis often gives unilateral headache
  - Refractive error
  - Emesis may be such a prominent symptom of vascular headache that gastrointestinal (GI) obstruction is suggested

- **Treatment**
  - *Tension headache*—Tylenol or ibuprofen ± biofeedback usually suffice. Trial of amitriptyline in teenagers with severe/frequent attacks
  - *Migraine* usually responds to prompt administration of ibuprofen. With/without addition of caffeine, caffeine-ergotamine, isometheptene
  - Sumatriptan, rizatriptan, naratriptan effective for *migraine* in teenagers
  - *Severe migraine* may require prophylaxis with propranolol, amitriptyline, cyproheptadine, valproate, calcium channel blockers
  - CNS disease must be ruled out if signs of increased ICP are present

- **Pearl**

The cyclic vomiting syndrome causes episodic attacks of intractable emesis and abdominal pain with/without headache. It may be a form of migraine. Family history of migraine is often present and attacks can be treated/prevented with migraine therapy.

Cerebrovascular Disease—Stroke, Hemorrhage, Vasculitis

- **Essentials of Diagnosis**
  - Stroke affects 2–8 in 100,000 children. 10% cause death, 60–80% cause permanent neurologic deficit or seizures, 20–35% of affected children have recurrent strokes
  - Etiologies—infection (Varicella, Mycoplasma HIV, bacterial endocarditis), minor head and neck trauma, hematologic disorders (coagulopathies, sickle cell disease, polycythemia, hypercoagulable states), neoplastic disorders, congenital heart disease, neurocutaneous disorders, intracranial vascular anomalies, vascular occlusive disorders, vasculitis, or combinations of several factors
  - Symptoms depend on distribution of clot or hemorrhage. Multifocal symptoms are common. Hemiplegia, unilateral weakness, sensory disturbance, dysarthria, dysphagia, depressed level of consciousness, and mood disturbance in bilateral stroke
  - Evaluation—clotting studies, inflammatory markers, examination of cerebrospinal fluid (CSF), electrocardiogram (ECG), and echocardiography. Cranial computed tomography (CT), magnetic resonance imaging (MRI), magnetic resonance angiography (MRA), magnetic resonance venography (MRV), and diffusion-weighted imaging are helpful

- **Differential Diagnosis**
  - Hypoglycemia
  - Prolonged focal seizure or postictal paresis
  - Encephalomyelitis, meningitis, encephalitis, brain abscess
  - Migraine with focal neurologic deficit
  - Neurodegenerative disorders
  - Drug abuse or toxin

- **Treatment**
  - Initial supportive treatment of cardiac, pulmonary, and renal function
  - Determine underlying cause if possible
  - Blood pressure management, fluid management, anticoagulation, thrombolysis, and anti-inflammatory therapy depend on underlying diagnosis
  - Anticoagulation in nonhemorrhagic stroke—both heparin and aspirin
  - In adults, thrombolytic agents (tissue plasminogen activator) are used within hours of stroke. No controlled studies available in childhood

- **Pearl**

Delay in the diagnosis of stroke is a major cause of morbidity. Delayed diagnosis is more common in children than in adults because initial caregivers may not consider the diagnosis.

Congenital Malformations

- **Essentials of Diagnosis**
  - *Neural tube defects*—spina bifida with meningomyelocele, anencephaly, encephalocele. Prenatal diagnosis by ultrasound
  - Depending on extent, spina bifida is associated with hydrocephaly, bowel and bladder dysfunction, distal motor and sensory defects, orthopedic abnormalities of spine and sacrum
  - *Cellular proliferation and migration defects* produce lissencephaly, agenesis of corpus callosum, pachygyria, agyria, Dandy-Walker syndrome
  - *Craniosynostosis*—premature closure of cranial sutures, usually sporadic and idiopathic. Genetic forms include Crouzon (calvarial, cranial base sutures) and Apert's syndromes (coronal suture)
  - *Hydrocephalus*—increased CSF volume causes ventricular dilation and macrocephaly. Noncommunicating forms (hemorrhage, infection, tumor, congenital malformations) cause obstruction to CSF flow in the ventricular system. Communicating hydrocephaly is caused by abnormal reabsorption of CSF

- **Differential Diagnosis**
  - Skull molding and deformity due to intrauterine pressure
  - Hydrocephalus "ex-vacuo" is enlargement of ventricles in a normal-sized head caused by brain atrophy (alcoholism, hypoxic injury)
  - Macrocephaly with normal brain growth may be familial
  - Megalencephaly (large brain) from neurofibromatosis (NF), tuberous sclerosis, Soto syndrome, achondroplasia, storage diseases (mucopolysaccharidoses, mucolipidosis, leukodystrophy) causes macrocephaly

- **Treatment**
  - Adequate folic acid before and during pregnancy reduces the risk of neural tube defects
  - If spina bifida is diagnosed by prenatal ultrasound, delivery is by Caesarian section with immediate surgical skin closure over defect to prevent infection
  - Most children with spina bifida will develop hydrocephaly. These children and others with noncommunicating hydrocephaly have shunts placed to relieve intraventricular pressure
  - Craniosynostosis treated surgically if cranial nerves, eye, or brain growth and function are impacted or if cosmetic effects are severe

- **Pearl**

Malformations of the nervous system occur in 1–3% of neonates and are present in 40% of neonates who die in the first 30 days of life.

Neurofibromatosis (NF)

- ■ Essentials of Diagnosis
  - Type 1 NF is a genetic neuroectodermal disorder with 1:4000 prevalence. 50% of cases are due to new mutations in *NF1* gene
  - Learning disabilities (40%), mental retardation (8%); strabismus or amblyopia (optic glioma), unexplained skin masses, macrocephaly, neurologic symptoms of spine or brain tumor, hypertension
  - Many asymptomatic patients are identified after a first-degree relative is diagnosed
  - Diagnostic criteria—>6 café au lait spots of >5 mm diameter (prepuberty) or >15 mm (postpuberty); ≥2 neurofibromas of any type or 1 plexiform neurofibroma; axillary or inguinal freckles; optic glioma; ≥2 Lisch nodules (iris hamartoma), osseous lesions (pseudarthroses, thinning of long bones)

- ■ Differential Diagnosis
  - McCune-Albright syndrome patients have larger café au lait spots
  - Normal children frequently have 1 or 2 café au lait spots. A large single café au lait spot is usually innocent
  - Café au lait spots occasionally seen in tuberous sclerosis

- ■ Treatment
  - Genetic counseling of parents and screening examination of siblings
  - Lifelong regular monitoring for brain and spinal tumors, hypertension, scoliosis and other orthopedic problems, optic glioma, acoustic neuroma, disfiguring skin masses, delayed puberty, emotional and psychiatric problems
  - Cognitive and psychological testing should be done early to maximize effectiveness of interventions

- ■ Pearl

Although patients with NF type 1 may have brain, spinal cord, and optic nerve tumors, auditory nerve tumors (acoustic neuromas) only occur in NF type 2, a rare autosomal dominant form of NF.

Tuberous Sclerosis

- **Essentials of Diagnosis**
    - Autosomal dominant. Deletions in tumor suppressor genes on chromosome 9 (*TSC1* gene, hamartin) or 16 (*TSC2*, tuberin) allow tumors to develop in CNS, renal, skin, cardiac, lungs, and other tissues
    - Facial angiofibromas, subungual and gingival fibromas, hypomelanotic macules (ash leaf spots in 96% of patients), retinal hamartoma, cortical tubers, subependymal glial nodules (often calcified), giant cell astrocytoma, renal angiomyolipoma
    - Rarer findings—cystic lung disease, cardiac rhabdomyoma, cystic rarefaction of bones of fingers and toes
    - Seizures of all types, mental retardation, autism

- **Differential Diagnosis**
    - Facial rash may be confused with acne, acne rosacea, cystic acne
    - Intrauterine infection may cause intracranial calcification and seizures
    - 3 or fewer ash leaf spots is normal
    - When café au lait spots are present, there may be some consideration of NF
    - Trauma may cause subungual fibroma

- **Treatment**
    - Regular monitoring for complications
    - Control seizures
    - Skin lesions may require laser or dermabrasion
    - Tumors must be treated
    - Genetic counseling. Heterozygotes have a 50% chance of passing the condition to offspring

- **Pearl**

Of babies presenting with infantile spasms, 5% will be found to have tuberous sclerosis. The cranial CT scan and family history are key as other signs and symptoms confirming the clinical diagnosis may be absent in infancy.

Ataxia

- **Essentials of Diagnosis**
  - *Acute cerebellar ataxia*—post-infectious syndrome of children 2–6 years old (varicella, rubeola, mumps, rubella, echovirus, polio, EBV, and influenza) involving trunk and extremities. Normal CSF and head imaging
  - *Polymyoclonus-opsoclonus*—lightning-like jerking of extremities, truncal ataxia, jerking irregular eye movements, irritability, emesis, occurs after infection (often β-hemolytic streptococcus) and with neural crest tumors (usually benign ganglioneuroblastoma)
  - *Friedreich ataxia*—autosomal recessive, gait ataxia develops before puberty. Diminished reflexes, position sense and light touch, dysarthria, cardiomyopathy, diabetes mellitus, pes cavus, and scoliosis develop over time
  - *Dominant ataxia*—autosomal dominant disorder of CAG repeats. 10% of patients present in childhood. Ataxia progresses to ophthalmoplegia, extrapyramidal symptoms, polyneuropathy, and dementia

- **Differential Diagnosis**
  - Mimickers of acute cerebellar ataxia—drug effect (phenytoin, phenobarbital, primidone) lead intoxication, infection, corticosteroid withdrawal, CNS vasculitides (polyarteritis nodosa)
  - Polymyoclonus-opsoclonus may look like acute cerebellar ataxia until the eye movements are recognized
  - Ataxia is a feature of untreated Wilson disease, ataxia telangiectasia, Refsum disease, Rett syndrome, abetalipoproteinemia (vitamin E deficiency), gangliosidoses, Chediak-Higashi, Charcot-Marie-Tooth disease

- **Treatment**
  - Acute cerebellar ataxia improves spontaneously, sometimes leaving permanent learning disability, abnormal eye movements, and dysarthria. Corticosteroids do not help. IVIg has been used but no controlled studies
  - Polymyoclonus-opsoclonus responds variably to adrenocorticotropic hormone (ACTH), IVIg, and plasmapheresis. Look for tumor in every case with urinary catecholamines, head and abdominal CT
  - Patients with Friedreich ataxia may need surgery for scoliosis, medical treatment of heart disease and diabetes. Antioxidants may slow cardiomyopathy
  - Dominant ataxia sometimes responds to levadopa

- **Pearl**

Differentiating ataxia from motor weakness caused by CNS disease, infection, myopathy, and trauma may be surprisingly difficult in children, especially in frightened toddlers.

Extrapyramidal Disorders

- **Essentials of Diagnosis**
  - Major symptoms are dyskinesia, athetosis, ballismus, tremor, rigidity, dystonia
  - *Sydenham chorea*—autoimmune disorder associated with β-hemolytic streptococcal infection. Choreiform movements, psychological disturbance (see Cardiovascular Disorders: Rheumatic fever)
  - *Paroxysmal dyskinesias*—short episodes of choreoathetosis/dystonia occurring spontaneously or set off by movement (rising from a chair) or sustained exercise. Genetic disorder possibly related to ion channel function
  - *Tremor*—essential tremor is most common. Dominant inheritance. Worsened by anxiety, fatigue, stress, activity, caffeine. Comorbidities are attention deficit-hyperactivity disorder (ADHD), dystonia, Tourette syndrome. Most often affects hands and arms

- **Differential Diagnosis**
  - Tourette syndrome is not clearly extrapyramidal in origin, but motor tics sometimes resemble ballismus or athetosis
  - Cerebral palsy may have prominent extrapyramidal symptoms
  - Hyperthyroidism
  - Hypocalcemia
  - Wilson disease
  - Parkinson disease, Huntington chorea rarely start in childhood
  - Ataxia syndromes
  - Systemic lupus erythematous (SLE)

- **Treatment**
  - Sydenham chorea usually resolves spontaneously with occasional reappearance of chorea. Dopaminergic blockers (haloperidol, pimozide), corticosteroids, valproate occasionally used
  - Carbamazepine used in paroxysmal dyskinesias. Spontaneous resolution sometimes occurs. Ion channel disorders are as yet untreatable
  - Tremor—avoid stimulating factors. Alcohol gives only temporary relief and should not be considered a therapy because of side effects

- **Pearl**

"Shuddering spells" in infancy may be a forerunner of essential tremor in children and adults.

Acute Flaccid Paralysis

- **Essentials of Diagnosis**
  - *Anterior horn cells* of the spinal cord may be damaged by infection (polio), immune-mediated inflammation (acute transverse myelitis)
  - *Spinal nerve trunks* may be damaged by immune-mediated polyneuritis (Guillain-Barré syndrome) or toxins (diphtheria, porphyria)
  - *Encephalitis of spinal cord and brain stem*—enterovirus 71, HIV, West Nile virus
  - *Neuromotor junctions* may be blocked toxin (tick, botulinum), metabolic disease (periodic paralysis)
  - *Muscles* may be affected directly (myositis)
  - Diagnostic information from spinal fluid, nerve conduction studies, spinal and brain MRI, viral studies, careful neurologic examination help differentiate causes

- **Differential Diagnosis**
  - Polyneuritis syndromes may present with flaccid paralysis
  - Epidural spinal abscess or tumor causing external spinal cord pressure
  - Intravenous (IV) drug abuse may lead to myelitis and paralysis

- **Treatment**
  - Intensive care unit support of respiratory function and nutrition may be required
  - Treat causative infectious agents (abscess, encephalomyelitis) if possible
  - Corticosteroids are of little benefit
  - Plasmapheresis or IV immunoglobulin (IgG) sometimes beneficial in Guillain-Barré
  - Always look for ticks even without a history of exposure
  - Toxicology screen

- **Pearl**

Ascending symmetric paralysis is characteristic of Guillain-Barré syndrome. Asymmetric paralysis is typical of poliomyelitis. Infant botulism causes generalized weakness with constipation. Tick bite paralysis is generalized and symmetric. Transverse myelitis causes paraplegia with early areflexia below the motor level.

Myasthenia Gravis

- **Essentials of diagnosis**
  - Weakness and easy fatigability, especially of muscles innervated by brainstem—extraocular, mastication, deglutition, respiration
  - *Neonatal form*—occurs in 12% of infants of myasthenic mothers due to placental transfer of maternal acetylcholine receptor antibodies
  - *Congenital*—not due to acetyl choline receptor antibodies. Genetic abnormality of acetylcholine receptor protein, postsynaptic membrane structure, or other myoneural transmission defects
  - *Juvenile form*—female predominant, autoimmune disorder with acetylcholine receptor antibodies. May be acute fulminant, but usually slowly progressive. Thyrotoxicosis occurs in 10% of female patients
  - Electromyogram (EMG) and nerve conduction studies demonstrate decremental response to repetitive stimuli. Anticholinesterase antibodies present in patients with neonatal form and those with juvenile form. Neostigmine improves symptoms briefly as does edrophonium.

- **Differential Diagnosis**
  - Acute fulminant form is mistaken for Guillain-Barré or bulbar polio
  - Neonatal and congenital forms must be distinguished from other causes of "floppy baby" syndrome
  - Thyrotoxicosis, SLE, rheumatoid arthritis, thymoma occur with increased frequency in myasthenia gravis but may also occur in its absence
  - Polyneuropathy
  - Drug-related neuromotor blockade—aminoglycosides

- **Treatment**
  - Newborns may urgently require neostigmine, mechanical ventilation, oral suctioning, gastrostomy insertion, and intensive supportive care until symptoms resolve spontaneously (usually 2–3 weeks)
  - Patients with myasthenic crisis require anticholinesterase therapy and intensive supportive care
  - Prednisone, mycophenolate mofetil, plasmapheresis sometimes used in crises to eliminate anticholinesterase and muscle-specific receptor tyrosine kinase antibodies
  - Patients with juvenile form respond to oral pyridostigmine
  - Thymectomy beneficial in patients with symptoms not restricted to ocular muscles

- **Pearl**

Given the fluctuating and unpredictable nature of weakness in juvenile myasthenia gravis, patients are often evaluated first by a psychiatrist for nonspecific symptoms and fatigue.

Multiple Sclerosis (MS)

- **Essentials of Diagnosis**
  - Degenerative inflammatory condition of brain, spinal cord, and optic nerves. Rarely presents before adolescence. Female predominance
  - Variable presentation. Recurrent remissions and relapses. Slow progression
  - Paresthesias, weakness, fatiguability, slurred speech, diplopia, sphincter control problems, emotional and concentration problems
  - Multiple sclerotic foci demonstrated on brain MRI. Slight CSF pleocytosis, elevated CSF protein and γ-globulin with oligoclonal bands
  - Auditory, visual, and somatosensory evoked responses often abnormal

- **Differential Diagnosis**
  - CNS vasculitis—SLE, polyarteritis nodosa
  - Acute demyelinating encephalomyelitis, Devic disease
  - Small vessel infarcts
  - Neurosyphilis
  - Optic neuritis due to other causes
  - Cerebellar ataxia of other causes
  - Metastatic or primary brain tumor, spinal cord injury, tethered cord, transverse myelitis, or spinal syrinx
  - Emotional/psychiatric problems

- **Treatment**
  - Suggested medical therapies are based on adult experience
  - Corticosteroids reduce inflammation and limit duration of relapse
  - β-Interferon reduces relapse rate but side effects are significant
  - Immunomodulators have been tried but little controlled data
  - Medications for muscle spasticity, depression, constipation, incontinence, and bladder spasticity may be needed
  - Physical therapy

- **Pearl**

A single focus of CNS disease rarely explains the numerous signs and symptoms of MS. Recognition of this fact is often the key to diagnosis of this multifocal disorder.

Facial Nerve Palsy (Bell's Palsy)

- ■ Essentials of Diagnosis
  - Unilateral nuclear or peripheral facial nerve (VII) injury causes sagging of the mouth, inability to close the eye, inability to wrinkle the forehead, loss of taste on the anterior two-thirds of the tongue
  - Neonatal VII nerve palsy now less frequent with decreasing number of forceps deliveries, but still occurs due to chronic intrauterine pressure. Bilateral facial palsy in neonate suggests agenesis of the VII nerve nuclei (Möbius syndrome)
  - Acquired peripheral VII palsy is sudden, usually unilateral, often postviral (respiratory infection, Lyme disease, EBV, Herpes simplex)
  - VII nerve palsy may result from brain stem tumor or thrombosis/hemorrhage in the carotid distribution

- ■ Differential Diagnosis
  - Syndromes with VII nerve palsy plus other findings—neonatal myasthenia gravis, Miller Fisher syndrome (infantile polyneuropathy)
  - Myotonic dystrophy may look like VII nerve palsy
  - Autosomal dominant absence of the depressor anguli oris—lower lip on the affected side fails to depress with crying. Occasionally other anomalies associated (cardiac septal defects)

- ■ Treatment
  - Postviral or intrauterine pressure-associated VII nerve palsies improve with time
  - Genetic absence of depressor anguli oris becomes less obvious with time
  - Protect the cornea with 1% methylcellulose drops and night-time eye patching until eyelid function improves
  - Prednisone probably ineffective in postviral Bell's palsy
  - Plastic surgery and cranial nerve reattachment may help disfiguring facial weakness

- ■ Pearl

The most common antecedent event in a child with Bell's palsy is otitis media or herpes infection. The condition is almost always unilateral, onset is rapid (within 24–38 hours), and spontaneous resolution is the rule within 2–4 weeks.

The Floppy Infant

- **Essentials of Diagnosis**
  - Clinical term to describe neonates with abnormal motor tone. The differential is broad and very important
  - Abnormal motor tone in infancy is reflected in decreased motor activity (both voluntary and in response to stimulation), abnormal deglutition, cough, and defecation, chronic assumption of frog leg or other abnormal body positions, delay in motor milestones
  - Physical examination shows abnormal neck and back muscle strength during ventral suspension (infant supported supine with a hand under the chest), and excessive head lag
  - Older infants come to medical attention because of poor endurance and delays in walking and climbing

- **Differential Diagnosis**
  - *Paralytic*—spinal muscular atrophy, infantile neuropathy, birth injury to brain or spine
  - *Myopathic*—neonatal and congenital myasthenia gravis, myotonic dystrophy, genetic myopathy (nemaline, central core, mitochondrial myopathy
  - *CNS degenerative disease*—Tay-Sachs disease, metachromatic leukodystrophy
  - *Syndromes with hypotonia*—trisomy 21, Prader-Willi, Marfan syndrome, dysautonomia, Turner syndrome, Ehlers-Danlos syndrome
  - *Systemic disease*—malnutrition, chronic illness (especially cardiac and pulmonary), metabolic disease, endocrinopathy (hypothyroid)
  - *Muscular glycogen storage*—Pompe disease (II) and McArdle disease (VII)
  - *Drug toxicity*—antihistamines, narcotics, antiepileptic medications

- **Treatment**
  - Treatment of the floppy infant depends upon the diagnosis reached by thorough evaluation

- **Pearl**

Benign hypotonia *is a term used to describe a weak, otherwise normal child with no obvious cause for weakness. It is a diagnosis of exclusion. As tests of muscle and nerve function improve, this diagnosis is likely to disappear altogether.*

Chronic Polyneuropathy

- **Essentials of Diagnosis**
  - Clinical description—insidious-onset gait disturbance, fatigability, weakness, clumsiness of hands, pain, paresthesias
  - Muscle weakness worse distally, ↓deep tendon reflexes, occasional cranial nerve signs, glove and stocking sensory deficits, muscle pain, trophic skin changes, thickened ulnar and peroneal nerves, ↓sensitivity to pain
  - Sensory and motor nerve conduction studies, nerve biopsy (identifies inflammation, degeneration, demyelination, storage), muscle biopsy (identifies denervation) will direct further investigation
  - Spinal fluid may show increased protein in inflammatory disease

- **Differential diagnosis**
  - *Chronic neuropathy of insidious onset*—idiopathic, inflammatory demyelinating neuropathy
  - *Toxins*—lead, arsenic, mercurials, vincristine, benzene
  - *Systemic disorders*—diabetes mellitus, uremia, recurrent hypoglycemia, porphyria, polyarteritis nodosa, SLE
  - *Inflammatory states*—Guillain-Barré, chronic, inflammatory demyelinating neuropathy, mumps, diphtheria
  - *Hereditary*—storage diseases, leukodystrophies, spinocerebellar degeneration, familial dysautonomia (Riley-Day syndrome), Charcot-Marie-Tooth disease, and other hereditary motor and sensory neuropathies
  - *Polyneuropathy* of malignancy, beriberi, excess vitamin B_6 very rare

- **Treatment**
  - Treat the specific disorder when possible
  - With bulbar involvement, tracheostomy and respiratory assistance may be required
  - Corticosteroids often tried in cases of unknown or apparent inflammatory origin (except for Guillain-Barre or acute inflammatory demyelinating neuropathy)
  - Steroid sparing regimens for chronic disease include IVIG, plasmapheresis, mycophenolate mofetil and rituximab

- **Pearl**

In some hereditary neuropathies, ataxia may be such a prominent symptom that polyneuropathy is overshadowed. Examples are Friedreich ataxia, dominant cerebellar ataxia, Marinesco-Sjögren syndrome.

Cerebral Palsy

- **Essentials of Diagnosis**
  - Descriptive term describing chronic and static impairment of muscle tone, strength, coordination, or movement of CNS origin
  - In infants, other neurologic deficits often coexist—seizures (50%), mild (26%), or severe (27%) mental retardation; disorders of language, speech, vision, hearing, and sensory perception
  - In infancy, 75% have predominance of spasticity, 15% ataxia, 5% choreoathetosis, 1% hypotonia without spasticity
  - Causes include anoxic/ischemic brain injury (before, during, or after birth), intrauterine viral infection, small for gestational age (SGA) and severe prematurity, congenital malformations, kernicterus, hypoglycemia, metabolic disorders. No etiology obvious in 25% of infants

- **Differential Diagnosis**
  - Primary motor and neurologic disorders with neonatal onset (see Floppy Infant)
  - Drugs producing athetosis—metoclopramide, Compazine, antihistamines
  - Progressive neurologic symptoms suggest a careful search for brain tumor, inflammatory, infectious, degenerative neurologic diseases at any age

- **Treatment**
  - In spastic cerebral palsy, treatment is directed at helping child to attain maximal physical and developmental potential
  - Physical, occupational, speech therapy
  - Orthopedic monitoring and intervention
  - Special educational assistance
  - Medications to reduce spasticity may improve overall motor function—botulinum toxin injection, baclofen
  - Adequate seizure control

- **Pearl**

In the child with mild cerebral palsy, there may be significant improvement in motor and cognitive function with age and maturity. In severely affected children, morbidity is higher. Aspiration pneumonia and intercurrent infection are the most common causes of death.

7

Hematologic Disorders

Constitutional Aplastic Anemia (Fanconi Anemia)

- ■ Essentials of Diagnosis
  - • Caused by several autosomal recessive mutations involved in DNA repair
  - • Presents at 2–10 years with gradual-onset pancytopenia and high mean cell volume (MCV)
  - • Complications—bleeding, infection, growth retardation, hypothyroidism, diabetes, malignancies (nonlymphocytic leukemia, solid head, neck and genital tumors, myelodysplastic syndromes)
  - • Diagnosis—macrocytosis, anisocytosis, chromosome breakage in peripheral lymphocytes. Bone marrow hypoplasia or aplasia
  - • Associated congenital anomalies in 50%—hyper- or hypopigmentation, short stature, delicate features, abnormal radii or thumbs, aplastic kidneys, horseshoe kidney, microcephaly, microphthalmia, strabismus, ear anomalies, hypogonadism

- ■ Differential Diagnosis
  - • Postinfectious aplastic anemia—viral hepatitis (usually non-A, non-B, non-C), Epstein-Barr virus (EBV), human immunodeficiency virus (HIV), parvovirus B19 (in immunocompromised patients)
  - • Drug reactions—phenylbutazone, sulfonamides, chloramphenicol, nonsteroidal anti-inflammatory drugs (NSAIDs), anticonvulsants
  - • Toxin exposure—benzene, insecticides, heavy metals, antineoplastic drugs, radiation
  - • Osteopetrosis, acute leukemia, and other malignancies may depress all 3 blood cell lines. Differentiated by bone marrow examination

- ■ Treatment
  - • Supportive care for bleeding, anemia, and infections
  - • 50% of patients respond partially to oxymetholone, but side effects include masculinization, hepatotoxicity, hepatic adenoma
  - • Avoid blood transfusions from human leukocyte antigen (HLA)–matched family members. They decrease the success of bone marrow transplantation from these donors
  - • Bone marrow transplantation cures aplastic anemia but probably does not reduce malignancy risk

- ■ Pearl

Exposure of lymphocytes to diepoxybutane stimulates chromosome breaks and rearrangements. This is a sensitive test for Fanconi anemia even before symptoms occur and is important in screening potential sibling bone marrow donors.

Transient Erythroblastopenia of Childhood

- **Essentials of Diagnosis**
  - Acquired anemia of children 6 months to 4 years with gradual onset
  - Normocytic anemia with low reticulocyte count, no hemolysis, no hepatosplenomegaly or lymphadenopathy, Coombs test negative
  - Most common presentation is pallor in a relatively well child
  - Bone marrow shows isolated absence of red blood cell (RBC) precursors and rules out other disorders

- **Differential Diagnosis**
  - Diamond-Blackfan anemia
  - Hemolytic anemia in aplastic crisis
  - Malignancy (especially acute leukemia)
  - Iron, folate, or vitamin B_{12} deficiency
  - Anemia of chronic disease—inflammatory bowel disease, autoimmune hepatitis, collagen vascular diseases

- **Treatment**
  - Monitor patient for signs of cardiac decompensation, infection, or bleeding
  - Resolution is usually spontaneous in 4–8 weeks
  - Transfusion occasionally needed for anemia causing cardiac decompensation
  - Monitor routine complete blood count (CBC). Recovery preceded by dramatic increase in reticulocyte count

- **Pearl**

The autoimmune nature of the disorder is suggested by the fact that immunoglobulin (IgG) from some patients has been shown to suppress erythropoiesis in vitro.

Diamond-Blackfan Anemia

- ■ Essentials of Diagnosis
  - Mechanism unknown but may be in utero stem cell injury. Autosomal dominant and recessive cases are seen
  - Presents in infancy with pallor, anemia, congestive heart failure. Short stature, congenital anomalies seen in one-third of patients (head, face, and thumbs)
  - Macrocytic anemia, reticulocytopenia, near-normal platelets and white cells. Increased fetal hemoglobin (Hb). Elevated erythrocyte adenosine deaminase
  - Bone marrow shows decreased or absent erythropoiesis

Differential Diagnosis
  - Transient erythroblastopenia of childhood (usually presents later)
  - Renal failure with low erythropoietin or erythropoietin antibodies
  - Anemia of chronic disease
  - Hypothyroidism
  - Thymoma, lymphoproliferative diseases, autoimmune disorders have been associated with pure red cell aplasia
  - Postinfectious—parvovirus B19 causes red cell aplasia especially in immunosuppressed patients or those with hemolytic disorders
  - Drug reactions—isoniazid, sulfa, chloramphenicol, azathioprine, antiepileptics

- ■ Treatment
  - Corticosteroids improve bone marrow erythropoiesis in two-thirds of patients
  - Chronic transfusion therapy for those unresponsive to corticosteroids
  - Iron chelation for transfusion-induced hemosiderosis
  - Bone marrow transplant
  - Hematopoietic growth factors have limited efficacy

- ■ Pearl

Although the dose of corticosteroid (prednisone) can be tapered in responsive patients, anemia recurs upon complete withdrawal. There may be significant long-term side effects of steroids—glaucoma, cataracts, diabetes, osteopenia, short stature, increased risk of infection.

Iron Deficiency Anemia

- **Essentials of Diagnosis**
  - Most common cause of childhood anemia
  - Nutritional deficiency presents at 6–12 months. Neonatal iron stores usually sufficient for the first 6 months of life
  - Nutritional deficiency occurs earlier in premature infants with smaller neonatal iron stores
  - Diet exclusively of whole cow's milk is most common cause of nutritional iron deficiency in older infants and toddlers
  - Symptoms vary with severity of anemia—irritability, poor feeding, pallor, fatigue, pica, cardiac decompensation
  - Testing—microcytosis, hypochromia (low MCV and mean corpuscular hemoglobin [MCH]), anisocytosis, poikilocytosis, high reticulocyte count, low serum iron, and high total iron binding capacity (TIBC)

- **Differential diagnosis**
  - Congenital microcytic anemias—α- and β-thalassemia, Hb E disease in patients of African, Mediterranean, or Asian ethnicity
  - Anemia of chronic disease—normo or microcytic anemia with low iron and low TIBC
  - Lead toxicity
  - Sideroblastic anemia
  - Chronic blood loss—milk allergy, polyps, ulcer disease, esophagitis, menorrhagia
  - Iron malabsorption—celiac disease, excessive liquid antacid use, excessive plant phytate ingestion

- **Treatment**
  - Oral elemental iron (6 mg/kg/day) in infants and toddlers
  - Reticulocyte count should begin to increase in 3–5 days
  - Continue treatment for several months to replenish iron stores
  - Nutritional evaluation to improve daily iron intake, especially in excessive milk drinkers

- **Pearl**

β-Thalassemia trait (Thalassemia minor) can be missed on Hb electrophoresis in the presence of concomitant iron deficiency.

Megaloblastic Anemia

- ## Essentials of Diagnosis
  - Macrocytic anemia caused by vitamin B_{12} and/or folic acid deficiency
  - Dietary deficiency in infants seen in breast-fed infants of strict vegans or infants of B_{12} deficient mothers with pernicious anemia
  - B_{12} deficiency in children—intestinal malabsorption, Crohn disease, exocrine pancreatic insufficiency, small bowel bacterial overgrowth, *Diphyllobothrium latum* infestation, ileal resection, intestinal bypass
  - Folate deficiency in children—inadequate intake, intestinal malabsorption (especially celiac disease), phenytoin, phenobarbital, methotrexate, liver disease
  - Blood smear shows macrocytic red cells and large neutrophils with hypersegmented nuclei (megaloblasts)
  - Check red cell folate, serum vitamin level, ↑serum methylmalonic acid (B_{12} deficiency), ↑serum homocystine (folate and B_{12} deficiency)

- ## Differential Diagnosis
  - Other macrocytic states without megaloblasts—Down syndrome, drugs (nucleoside analogues, anticonvulsants), hypothyroidism, liver disease
  - Fanconi and Diamond-Blackfan anemia
  - Inborn errors of B_{12} and folate synthesis—eg, methylmalonic aciduria, homocystinuria
  - Chronic hemolysis increases folic acid requirement. Deficiency state occurs despite normal folic acid intake
  - Intrinsic factor deficiency and pernicious anemia cause B_{12} deficiency. Rare in childhood

- ## Treatment
  - Oral supplements of B_{12} in nutritional deficiency states
  - Correct conditions causing intestinal malabsorption. If not correctable, give parenteral B_{12}
  - Intranasal gel, skin patches, and sublingual preparations are convenient vehicles for parenteral administration of vitamin B_{12}
  - Folic acid deficiency usually responds to oral therapy
  - Very high dose B_{12} may be required in metabolic disorders of synthesis

- ## Pearl

All women should receive extra folic acid during pregnancy. Folate supplementation reduces the risk of fetal neural tube defects even in women with normal levels and normal intake.

Red Cell Membrane Defects

- ■ Essentials of Diagnosis
  - *Hereditary spherocytosis* (HS)—autosomal dominant abnormality of spectrin synthesis causes abnormal RBC shape, increases splenic sequestration, and decreases RBC survival
  - HS—variable anemia, ↑indirect bilirubin, splenomegaly, chronic hemolysis with hemolytic and aplastic crises, microspherocytes on blood smear, ↑RBC osmotic fragility
  - *Hereditary elliptocytosis* (HE)—autosomal dominant disorder of RBC membrane skeletal proteins usually with mild symptoms
  - HE—most severe in neonates with jaundice, hemolysis, anemia, bizarre RBC morphology, low MCV
  - Direct (DAT) and indirect (IAT) antiglobulin tests negative

- ■ Differential Diagnosis
  - Immune hemolytic states—often have spherocytes on smear
  - ABO incompatibility—neonates show spherocytes
  - Cirrhosis with portal hypertension—hypersplenism, anemia, and bizarre RBC morphology with some spherocytes
  - Other hemolytic states with spherocytes and elliptocytes—disseminated intravascular coagulation (DIC) and hemolytic uremic syndrome (HUS)
  - Paroxysmal nocturnal hemoglobinuria. Defect in phosphatidylinositol-glycan of RBC membrane proteins causes hemolysis. Associated with thromboses, aplastic anemia, and malignancy and spherocytes on blood smear

- ■ Treatment
  - Erythroid hyperplasia in the bone marrow compensates for the anemia in mild HS and in most HE
  - Supplemental folic acid to support rapid red cell production
  - Severe HS may require regular transfusion
  - In HS, postinfectious hemolytic crises after parvovirus B19 may require transfusion
  - In HS, monitor for gall stones. Cholecystectomy often required
  - Neonates with elliptocytosis may require transfusion but hemolysis improves during first year
  - After age 5 years, splenectomy can be performed in HS to increase RBC survival. Rarely required in elliptocytosis

- ■ Pearl

Patients with autosomal dominant HS have better spectrin synthesis than the rarer individuals with homozygous recessive HS. Symptoms are therefore likely to be milder in children who have 1 obviously affected (dominant HS) parent.

α-Thalassemia

- **Essentials of Diagnosis**
  - α-Thalassemia caused by deletions of 1 or more of the 2 α-globin genes on each chromosome 16. Disease severity depends on the number and location of deletions
  - Abnormal genotypes are -α/αα (silent carrier), - -/-α (Hb H disease), - -/αα or -α/-α (α-thalassemia trait), - -/- - (α-thalassemia major)
  - *2 gene deletions* (α-thalassemia trait)—mild microcytic anemia looks like iron deficiency but normal iron binding capacity and high/normal serum iron
  - *3 gene deletions* (Hb H disease)—mild/moderate microcytic hemolytic anemia, hepatosplenomegaly, high reticulocyte count, hypochromia, poikilocytosis, basophilic stippling, 15–30% Bart's hemoglobin (4 β-chains)
  - *4 gene deletions* (α-thalassemia major)—severe hydrops fetalis or still birth. Incompatible with postnatal survival
  - Diagnosis by Hb electrophoresis. Bart's hemoglobin (γ-chain tetramer) or Hb H (β-globin chain tetramer) detected

- **Differential Diagnosis**
  - Iron deficiency and other conditions with microcytic anemia may resemble heterozygous forms of α-thalassemia

- **Treatment**
  - Occasional blood transfusions needed in Hb H disease especially during infections
  - Folate supplements for Hb H disease
  - Avoid oxidant drugs and foods in Hb H. They may cause hemolysis
  - Splenomegaly may produce hypersplenism and splenectomy may become necessary

- **Pearl**

The offspring of 2 persons of Asian decent with α-thalassemia trait are at higher risk of severe disease than the offspring of 2 persons of African descent. The explanation is that Asian carriers usually have deletions of 2 α-genes on the same chromosome while Africans carriers usually have deletions of 1 α-gene on each chromosome.

β-Thalassemia

■ Essentials of Diagnosis
- Recessive mutation in the single β-globin gene on chromosome 11
- *β-Thalassemia minor* (heterozygous)—mild hypochromic anemia, normal serum iron, increased red cell number. Ratio of mean red cell volume (MCV) to red cell count is <13. Increased HgA_2
- *β-Thalassemia major* (homozygous)—severe hypochromic anemia with microcytosis, anisocytosis, and poikilocytosis by 12 months. Mild ↑serum indirect bilirubin. Hb electrophoresis shows only Hb F and A_2
- β-Thalassemia minor patients—little morbidity beside mild anemia
- Without regular transfusion, children with β-thalassemia have growth failure, hepatosplenomegaly, enlarged medullary bone spaces, thin bony cortices, facial deformities, and pathologic fractures

■ Differential Diagnosis
- β-Thalassemia minor resembles iron deficiency states and α-thalassemia
- Double heterozygotes of β-thalassemia with other hemoglobino-pathy—Hb E/β-thalassemia may resemble β-thalassemia major

■ Treatment
- β-Thalassemia minor requires no therapy. Most common problem is overuse of iron because of mistaken diagnosis of iron deficiency
- In β-thalassemia major, chronic transfusion with iron chelation therapy prevents or improves most complications. Even with chelation therapy, iron overload may cause liver and heart disease
- 90% of β-thalassemia cases cured by bone marrow or umbilical cord blood transplantation from HLA identical sibling if transplant done before iron related liver or heart disease develops

■ Pearl
Individuals of Mediterranean, Middle Eastern, and Asian ancestry have a higher incidence of β-thalassemia major and minor.

Sickle Cell Disease

■ Essentials of Diagnosis

- Homozygotes for the sickle gene produce mostly Hb S. Deoxygenated Hb S polymerizes causing distorted red cell anatomy, ↑blood viscosity, ↓red cell survival, and a predisposition to vaso-occlusion
- In heterozygotes (sickle cell trait) there is enough Hb A in red cells to prevent polymerization of Hb S
- Prevalence increased in Central African, Sicilian, Italian, Greek, Turkish, Saudi Arabian, and Indian ethnicity
- Symptoms—gall stones, splenomegaly, functional asplenia, sepsis, osteomyelitis, meningitis, pain crises due to infarcts, stroke, acute chest syndrome, fat emboli, failure to thrive, priapism, aplastic crises

■ Differential Diagnosis

- Once sickle cells are seen on peripheral blood, the diagnosis of sickle cell disease, trait, or sickle syndrome (SC, Sthal) is likely
- Double heterozygotes with Hb C and β-thalassemia may have symptoms suggesting sickle cell syndrome

■ Treatment

- Neonatal screening has markedly reduced complications associated with delayed diagnosis
- Multispecialty clinics are the most efficient way to monitor and treat SS disease
- Prophylactic penicillin reduces infection from pneumococcus in double heterozygotes and homozygous SS with functional asplenia
- Red cell transfusion or exchange transfusion in pain crises, vaso-occlusive disease, stroke, acute chest syndrome, preoperatively or before angiograms with hypertonic contrast
- Bone marrow or cord blood transplant from a matched sibling is curative
- Oral hydroxyurea increases production of fetal Hb and decreases hemolysis and pain crises

■ Pearl

Dactylitis (hand-and-foot syndrome) is the most common initial symptom of SS disease and occurs in 50% of children before age 23 years.

Glucose-6-Phosphate Dehydrogenase Deficiency (G6PD)

7

- **Essentials of Diagnosis**
  - X-linked recessive congenital hemolytic anemia due to absence of red cell glucose-6-phosphate dehydrogenase. Many variants exist
  - Red cells with deficient G6PD don't contain enough nicotinamide adenine dinucleotide phosphate (NADP) to maintain normal levels of reduced glutathione and hemolyze during oxidant stress
  - Symptomatic newborns may need exchange transfusion for high bilirubin
  - Children are usually well. Hemolytic crises triggered by infection, drugs (sulfonamides, naphthalene, nitrofurantoin, furazolidone, primaquine, methylene blue), and some foods
  - Diagnosis made by enzyme assay in mature red cells. Direct antiglobulin test is negative

- **Differential Diagnosis**
  - Other disorders of red cell metabolism—pyruvate kinase deficiency
  - Red cell membrane defects—HS, HE, paroxysmal nocturnal hemoglobinuria
  - Hemoglobinopathies
  - Autoimmune hemolytic anemia—postinfectious systemic lupus erythematosus (SLE), or other autoimmune syndromes, immunodeficiency states or malignancy
  - Nonimmune hemolytic anemia—associated with liver disease, renal disease, splenomegaly HUS, DIC, giant hemangioma (Kasabach-Merritt syndrome), mechanical heart valves
  - Paroxysmal nocturnal hemoglobinuria—intravascular hemolysis due to complement activation

- **Treatment**
  - Avoid drugs that precipitate hemolysis
  - Avoid foods that precipitate hemolysis—fava beans
  - Treat infection promptly, using antibiotics when appropriate
  - Red cell transfusion may be required if sudden anemia precipitates cardiac decompensation
  - In rare G6PD patients with chronic anemia, monitor for gall stones and hypersplenism

- **Pearl**

  In G6PD patients of Mediterranean extraction, the most common food precipitant of hemolysis is the fava bean. Patients of African extraction are not as sensitive to this dietary trigger.

Acquired Hemolytic Anemia

- Essentials of Diagnosis
  - Acquired autoimmune hemolysis (AIHA) occurs in isolation or complicating infection, immunodeficiency, autoimmune conditions (SLE), malignancy. There are 3 major forms:
    - *Warm AIHA*—IgG with panagglutinin or Rh specificity binds to RBCs maximally at 37°C causing extravascular hemolysis and splenic consumption. Associated with immune disorders. May become chronic
    - Cold AIHA—complement with I/i antigen specificity binds to RBCs causing intravascular hemolysis. Maximal in vitro activity at 4°C
    - Paroxysmal cold hemoglobinuria—complement with P antigen specificity binds to RBCs causing intravascular hemolysis. Maximal in vitro activity at 4°C. Associated with *Mycoplasma,* EBV, and cytomegalovirus (CMV) infections
  - Acquired nonimmune hemolysis is associated with liver disease, renal disease (HUS), DIC, cavernous hemangioma (Kasabach-Merritt syndrome), hypersplenism, artificial heart valves, other intravascular foreign bodies, drug and toxin exposure
  - Reticulocyte count, indirect bilirubin, serum lactate dehydrogenase (LDH) and urine urobilinogen are increased. Direct and indirect antiglobulin tests (DAT and IAT) positive in autoimmune hemolysis, negative in nonimmune hemolysis

- Differential Diagnosis
  - Other hemolytic anemias (see Differential Diagnosis of G6PD)

- Treatment
  - Diagnosis and treatment of underlying disease important for all acquired hemolytic anemias
  - Warm AIHA often responds to corticosteroid or IVIG. In severe chronic AIHA, use cyclophosphamide, azathioprine, busulfan, cyclosporine, rituximab. Splenectomy may be of benefit
  - Cold and paroxysmal AIHA usually self-limited. Poor response to corticosteroids. Plasma exchange may be effective to remove IgM
  - RBC transfusion may be needed, but cross-matching may be difficult to impossible in warm AIHA

- Pearl

Some patients with severe AIHA may have associated DIC and may require therapy with heparin.

Methemoglobinemia

- **Essentials of diagnosis**
  - Methemoglobin is hemoglobin with iron trapped in the ferric state. Met Hb is unable to transport oxygen. Cyanosis visible with >15% Met Hb
  - *Congenital methemoglobinemia* caused by autosomal recessive diaphorase I deficiency. Patients usually asymptomatic with compensatory polycythemia
  - *Hemoglobin M* (HbM)—abnormal hemoglobins with amino acid substitutions on either α- or β-globin chains that form Met Hb. Patients mildly cyanotic but otherwise well
  - *Drug induced*—lidocaine, benzocaine, aniline dyes, nitrates, nitrites, sulfonamides, phenacetin, bismuth subnitrate, potassium chlorate, dapsone, pyridium
  - Drugs can induce very high Met Hb levels causing oxygen unresponsive deep cyanosis, dyspnea, cardiac failure, and death
  - Hb M diagnosed by isoelectric focusing of Hb. Met Hb is detected by co-oximetry.

- **Differential Diagnosis**
  - Hypoxia and ischemia from underventilation (neurologic injury or drugs), lung disease, heart disease
  - Raynaud phenomenon and acrocyanosis sometimes suggest methemoglobinemia
  - Sulfhemoglobinemia
  - Exposure to blue dyes and silver compounds producing skin discoloration

- **Treatment**
  - Identify and discontinue offending drug. In acute exposure with very high Met Hb, try to remove remaining drug by gastric lavage
  - Acute methemoglobinemia usually responds quickly to methylene blue 1–1.5 mg/kg IV
  - Ascorbic acid is effective but response is slower
  - Congenital diaphorase I deficiency rarely requires therapy but responds to methylene blue and ascorbic acid
  - Hyperbaric oxygen has been used in life-threatening situations

- **Pearl**

Newborns and infants are more susceptible to acquired methemoglobinemia because their red cells contain less NADH Met Hb reductase. Acidosis caused by diarrhea and dehydration also increases susceptibility.

Neutrophil Function Defects

■ Essentials of Diagnosis

- *Chédiak-Higashi syndrome*—abnormal neutrophil membrane fusion processes with giant granules, abnormal chemotaxis, reduced bactericidal power and degranulation causes recurrent skin and respiratory infection. Late development of lymphoproliferative disease

- *Leukocyte adhesion deficiency*—2 genetic deficits of cell surface adhesive glycoproteins producing neutrophils with deficient adherence, abnormal chemotaxis, deficient rolling interaction with endothelium and recurrent infections

- *Chronic granulomatous disease* (CGD)—most forms are X-linked recessive with defects in oxidase components. Recurrent purulent infections of skin, mucous membranes, lymph nodes, lung, liver, and bones with catalase-positive bacteria and fungi

- *Myeloperoxidase deficiency*—post-translational defect in processing of myeloperoxidase causes poor neutrophil microbicidal activity. Affected patients with systemic disease (eg, diabetes) have recurrent infections

■ Differential Diagnosis

- Glycogen storage disease Ib, diabetes mellitus, renal disease, hypophosphatemia, viral infections all have associated neutrophil dysfunction

- Drug-induced neutrophil dysfunction

- Abnormal neutrophil motility and bactericidal activity are characteristic of newborns and patients with burn injury, trauma, and severe infection

■ Treatment

- In all disorders, anticipate infection, aggressively identify focus and causative agent, treat with antibiotics

- In all disorders, prophylactic antibiotics occasionally indicated

- Ascorbic acid improves neutrophil function in Chédiak-Higashi

- Trimethoprim-sulfa enhances bactericidal activity of neutrophils in CGD

- Recombinant γ-interferon decreases number and severity of infections in CGD

- Bone marrow transplantation has been used in these conditions

■ Pearl

Patients with Chédiak-Higashi syndrome also display oculocutaneous albinism, photophobia, nystagmus, and ataxia. Many die during the lymphoproliferative phase, which may be an EBV-related hemophagocytic syndrome. Older patients may develop degenerative central nervous system (CNS) disease.

Idiopathic Thrombocytopenic Purpura (ITP)

- **Essentials of Diagnosis**
  - Most common bleeding disorder of childhood. Usual age 2–5 years
  - Occurs after viral infections—rubella varicella, measles, influenza, EBV, CMV, and other common viruses
  - Sudden petechiae, bruises, epistaxis. Splenomegaly, lymphadenopathy, and hepatomegaly after EBV or CMV infections
  - Severe hemorrhage into vital organs is rare but a serious complication
  - Platelet count <50,000/μL due to splenic consumption of antibody-coated platelets. Large platelets seen in peripheral smear
  - Bone marrow normal with increased megakaryocytes. Other cell lines normal

- **Differential Diagnosis**
  - Antibody-mediated platelet destruction—idiopathic thrombocytic purpura, infection, immunologic disorders
  - Platelet consumption and destruction—DIC, sepsis, thrombosis, cavernous hemangioma, HUS, thrombotic thrombocytopenic purpura (TTP), hypersplenism
  - Decreased production of platelets—aplastic anemia, osteopetrosis, Wiskott-Aldrich syndrome, Fanconi's anemia, leukemia
  - Vitamin B_{12} and folate deficiency
  - Infants of mothers with ITP and infants with platelet alloimmunization have thrombocytopenia

- **Treatment**
  - ITP is self-limited. Most children require no therapy
  - Protective helmet and avoidance of trauma while platelet count is low
  - Platelet transfusion is only used for life-threatening bleeding or in preparation for surgery
  - Short-course prednisone or IVIG usually helpful when platelet count <10,000/μL
  - Rituximab useful in reducing antibody production
  - Splenectomy is a last resort in life-threatening or chronic thrombocytopenia

- **Pearl**

In Rh+ patients with ITP, administration of polyclonal Ig against the Rho-D antigen coats the red cells. While the spleen works to clear these coated red cells, it does a poorer job at clearing platelets and the platelet count rises! This therapy may cause severe RBC hemolysis, but 80% of children respond favorably.

Inherited Bleeding Disorders of Procoagulants

- Essentials of Diagnosis
  - *Factor VIII deficiency* (hemophilia A)—X-linked recessive. Factor VIII activity <1% causes spontaneous bleeding in skin, joints, muscles, and viscera. Mild disease with 5–40% activity has bleeding only with trauma. Prothrombin time (PT) normal. Prolonged activated partial thromboplastin time (aPTT)
  - *Factor IX deficiency* (hemophilia B)—genetics and presentation similar to factor VIII. PT normal. aPTT variably prolonged
  - *Factor XI deficiency* (hemophilia C)—autosomal recessive with mild symptoms. Bleeding after surgery or trauma. Severity of bleeding does not correlate well with factor activity level
  - *von Willebrand disease*—autosomal dominant or recessive. von Willebrand factor binds factor VIII and is a cofactor in endothelial adhesion of platelets. Mild symptoms. Menorrhagia may be the first manifestation
  - *Rare genetic deficiencies* of other factors in the clotting cascade have been described and are detected by specific factor analysis

- Differential Diagnosis
  - Severe liver disease causes decreased synthesis of prothrombin; fibrinogen; factors V, VII, IX, X, XII, and XIII; plasminogen; antithrombin III (AT III); protein C; and protein S. There may be both bleeding and thrombotic tendencies
  - Vitamin K deficiency. Vitamin K is a cofactor in synthesis of factors II, VII, IX, and X. Newborn infants and children with poor intake or fat malabsorption are at risk
  - DIC

- Treatment
  - In mild factor VIII deficiency, factor VIII and vWF released from endothelium after desmopressin administration are adequate to prevent bleeding
  - Most factor VIII deficient patients require exogenous factor VIII to treat hemorrhage. Some require prophylactic factor VIII to prevent progressive arthropathy
  - Exogenous factor IX used for factor IX deficiency
  - Peri-operative or peripartum treatment with fresh frozen plasma (FFP) and platelets for factor XI deficiency. Desmopressin also used
  - Intravenous or intranasal desmopressin used for bleeding in von Willebrand disease

- Pearl

Acquired von Willebrand disease can develop in association with Wilm tumor, hypothyroidism, cardiac disease, renal disease, SLE, and valproic acid therapy.

Disseminated Intravascular Coagulation (DIC)

- ■ Essentials of Diagnosis
  - • Acquired consumptive coagulopathy precipitated by release of tissue factors results in excess thrombin generation, intravascular fibrin deposition, consumption or inactivation of platelets, consumption of procoagulant factors, and activation of fibrinolysis
  - • Precipitants are endothelial damage (virus, bacterial endotoxin), tissue necrosis (burns, crush injury), ischemia (shock, hypoxia, acidosis), release of tissue procoagulants (some cancers, placental abruption, septic abortion)
  - • Clinical signs are shock, diffuse bleeding, and thrombotic lesions in multiple sites
  - • Tests—prolonged PT and aPTT; decreased platelet count; variable decreases in plasma fibrinogen, AT III, and protein C; increased plasma fibrin split products and D-dimer

- ■ Differential Diagnosis
  - • Synthetic coagulopathy of liver disease occurs in patients with multisystem organ failure especially when there is portal hypertension, splenomegaly, and consumptive thrombocytopenia

- ■ Treatment
  - • Identify and treat the triggering event
  - • Replace procoagulant factors with FFP and platelets
  - • Cryoprecipitate is a rich source of fibrinogen and factor VIII
  - • Cautious anticoagulation with unfractionated heparin decreases coagulation activation and thrombosis
  - • Some positive experience with use of AT III concentrate and protein C concentrate in coagulopathy associated with meningococcemia and purpura fulminans
  - • Use of anticytokines not effective in established DIC

- ■ Pearl
  Hepatic coagulopathy can be distinguished from DIC by factor VII levels (low in liver disease; near normal in DIC) and factor VIII levels (normal or high in liver disease; low in DIC).

Inherited Thrombotic Disorders

- ■ Essentials of Diagnosis
  - • *Protein C deficiency*—protein C normally inactivates factor V procoagulant. Autosomal heterozygotes present with venous thromboembolic events (VTE). Homozygotes or compound heterozygotes present at birth with purpura fulminans or VTE
  - • *Protein S deficiency*—since protein S is a cofactor for protein C, deficiency of protein S has presentation similar to protein C deficiency
  - • *Factor V Leiden*—mutant factor V protein is resistant inactivation by protein C and promotes thrombosis
  - • *Antithrombin III deficiency* (AT III)—AT III inhibits activated factors IX, X, XI, and XII. Patients with AT III deficiency present in adolescence or early adulthood with venous thrombotic events
  - • Inherited dysfibrinogenemias occasionally develop venous or arterial thromboses. Some have bleeding tendencies and most are asymptomatic

- ■ Differential Diagnosis
  - • DIC
  - • Venous thrombosis associated with vascular surgery or foreign body, cardiac disease, malignancy, infection, trauma, immobilization, chronic inflammatory disease, renal disease, sickle cell anemia
  - • Hyperhomocysteinemia increases risk of venous and arterial thrombosis
  - • Acquired disorders—antiphospholipid antibodies, deficiency of proteins C, S, and AT III during sepsis, veno-occlusive disease following bone marrow transplant
  - • Acute phase elevations of procoagulants during infections may promote venous thrombosis (especially fibrinogen, factor VIII, and ↑platelets)

- ■ Treatment
  - • Thrombolytic therapy with tissue plasminogen activator (tPA) may be warranted in life-threatening venous thrombosis
  - • After first non–life-threatening thrombotic event, anticoagulate for 3 months
  - • Lifelong anticoagulation with warfarin may be required for recurrent thrombotic episodes

- ■ Pearl

Factor V Leiden is present in ~5% of Caucasians. However, the abnormal protein is found in 20% of Caucasians with deep vein thrombosis (DVT) and 40–60% of those with a family history of venous thrombotic events. Female heterozygotes for factor V Leiden have a 35-fold risk of VTE. Estrogen-containing oral contraceptives are contraindicated in these women.

8

Oncology

Acute Lymphoblastic Leukemia (ALL)

- ■ Essentials of Diagnosis
  - Most common malignancy of childhood (25% of all cancers)
  - Pallor, fatigue, bruising, petechiae (50%), bone pain (25%), unexplained fever, hepatosplenomegaly (60%), lymphadenopathy (50%)
  - Rare findings include mediastinal mass, cranial nerve palsies, leukemic exudates in optic fundi, congestive failure, and hemorrhage
  - Decrease in mature peripheral leukocytes, platelets, and red cells with leucocytosis (50%) secondary to immature lymphoblasts
  - Diagnosis by bone marrow aspirate or biopsy with >25% lymphoblasts

- ■ Differential Diagnosis
  - Children with Down syndrome have 14-fold increase in rate of leukemia
  - Chronic infection, especially Epstein-Barr virus (EBV) and cytomegalovirus (CMV)
  - Immune thrombocytopenia or anemia
  - Juvenile rheumatoid arthritis
  - Lymphocytosis is typical of pertussis

- ■ Treatment
  - Induction of remission commonly by prednisone, vincristine, daunorubicin, asparaginase, intrathecal methotrexate, cyclophosphamide (in T-cell leukemia)
  - Consolidation therapy—intrathecal and continued intensive systemic chemotherapy
  - Intensification therapy—prednisone, vincristine, doxorubicin, cytoxan, cytarabine, 6-thioguanine
  - Maintenance—daily oral 6-MP, monthly vincristine, oral prednisone, and intermittent intrathecal methotrexate ± cytarabine and hydrocortisone

- ■ Pearl

A child 1–9 years old with initial WBC <50,000 and with normal chromosomes is at "standard" risk. Patients >10 years old with initial WBC >50,000 or with chromosomal translocations (9;22 or 4;11) are at "high" risk and require more intensive chemotherapy regimens.

Acute Myeloid Leukemia (AML)

- **Essentials of Diagnosis**
  - Bone marrow aspirate or biopsy with >20% leukemic blasts
  - Neutropenia (69%), anemia (44%), thrombocytopenia (33%)
  - 8 subtypes (M0–M7) based on histopathology and maturation of leukocyte precursors and cytogenetic associations
  - Fatigue, bleeding (M3–M5), infection, adenopathy, hepatosplenomegaly, skin nodules (M4–M5)
  - Venous sludging and infarction (lung and central nervous system) occur with WBC >100,000/μL

- **Differential Diagnosis**
  - Increased AML risk in Diamond-Blackfan anemia, neurofibromatosis, Down syndrome, Wiskott-Aldrich syndrome, Kostmann syndrome, Li-Fraumeni syndrome, chromosomal instability syndromes (Fanconi anemia)
  - Acquired risk factors—ionizing radiation, cytotoxic chemotherapy, benzenes

- **Treatment**
  - Less responsive to therapy than ALL. Medication side effects common
  - Induction usually with anthracyclines, cytarabine, and etoposide followed by allogeneic stem cell transplant or additional aggressive chemotherapy
  - M3 subtype treated with transretinoic acid, cytarabine, and daunorubicin
  - M7 (megakaryocytic AML) in Down syndrome responds well to less intensive treatment

- **Pearl**

Recognition of genetic subtypes of AML has led to development of antibody-targeted cytotoxic agents such as Mylotarg, a humanized anti-CD33 monoclonal antibody conjugated with calicheamicin. This and similar drugs under investigation may improve the generally poor outcome of AML.

Myeloproliferative Disorders

- **Essentials of Diagnosis**
  - Leukocytosis with predominant immature cells
  - Indolent fever, bone pain, respiratory symptoms, anemia, hepatosplenomegaly, bleeding problems
  - Three types of myeloproliferative disorder
    - Chronic myeloid leukemia (CML)—translocation of chromosomes 9 and 22 (Philadelphia chromosome) causes production of a novel fusion protein tyrosine kinase that disregulates cell proliferation, decreases cell adherence and apoptosis
    - Juvenile myelomonocytic leukemia (JMML)—there is 7 monosomy or 7q deletion in 20% of cases
    - Transient myeloproliferative disorder—mutations in *GATA1* gene on chromosome 21 may be responsible

- **Differential Diagnosis**
  - Neurofibromatosis type 1 increases risk of JMML
  - Transient myeloproliferative disorder is unique to patients with trisomy 21 or mosaicism of chromosome 21
  - ALL, AML both mimic myeloproliferative disorders but are differentiated by bone marrow findings
  - Chronic infection with leukemoid reactions

- **Treatment**
  - CML—hydroxyurea or busulfan to reduce Philadelphia chromosome-positive cells followed by stem cell transplantation
  - CML—targeted molecular therapy with tyrosine kinase inhibitor (imatinib mesylate; trade name Gleevec) produces dramatic but short-lived remission
  - Transient myeloproliferative disorder—usually resolves with no or minimal chemotherapy
  - JMML—response to chemotherapy disappointing. Stem cell transplant is the only current therapy

- **Pearl**

The durability of remission produced by tyrosine kinase inhibitors in children with CML is unclear. This drug is now accepted first-line therapy in this disorder.

Brain Tumors

- ■ Essentials of Diagnosis
  - • Most common solid tumor of childhood
  - • Classic symptom triad (morning headache, vomiting, papilledema) found at presentation in <30%
  - • Increasing head circumference (in infants), cranial nerve palsies, dysarthria, ataxia, hemiplegia, hyperreflexia, cracked pot sign
  - • Seizures, personality change, blurred vision, diplopia, weakness, decreased coordination, precocious puberty
  - • Computed tomography/Magnetic resonance imaging (CT/MRI) of neuraxis, spinal fluid examination, and sometimes brain biopsy used in diagnosis

- ■ Differential Diagnosis
  - • Posterior fossa—medulloblastoma, cerebellar astrocytoma, brainstem glioma, ependymoma account for 49%
  - • Hemispheric—low- or high-grade astrocytoma and others account for 37%
  - • Midline—craniopharyngioma, chiasmal glioma, pineal tumors account for 14%
  - • Diagnosis often delayed by focus on these alternative diagnoses—failure to thrive, infant gastroesophageal reflux, emotional problems, endocrine disease, eye problems

- ■ Treatment
  - • Recent surgical developments allow more complete tumor resection—operating microscope, ultrasonic tissue aspirator, computed stereotactic resection, electrocorticography, CO_2 laser, better intraoperative monitoring
  - • Radiation used mainly for tumors with high risk of neuraxis dissemination
  - • Dexamethasone prior to surgery
  - • Anticonvulsants for preoperative or anticipated postoperative seizures
  - • High-intensity systemic chemotherapy may be followed by autologous stem cell or homologous bone marrow transplantation

- ■ Pearl

Major challenges remain in devising effective treatment brain tumors not amenable to surgical resection, especially in children <3 years of age. Quality of life after high-intensity therapies is a crucial concern.

Lymphoma

- ■ Essentials of Diagnosis
  - Common signs and symptoms include adenopathy (especially cervical and supraclavicular), fever, mediastinal mass, cough, dyspnea, orthopnea, pleural effusion
  - Hodgkin lymphoma divided into 4 groups—lymphocyte predominant, nodular sclerosing, mixed cellular, and lymphocyte depleted. Reed-Sternberg cells (malignant germinal center B cells) essential to diagnosis in all
  - Non-Hodgkin disease divided into 4 groups—lymphoblastic lymphoma, small non-cleaved-cell lymphoma, large B-cell lymphoma, and anaplastic large cell lymphoma
  - Non-Hodgkin disease—more common in males, often have abdominal tumors, associated with immunodeficiency, EBV infection (Burkitt), and other viral infections

- ■ Differential Diagnosis
  - Other malignancies (neuroblastoma, rhabdomyosarcoma), infection, autoimmune diseases, storage diseases
  - Lymphoproliferative disease (LPD) after solid organ or bone marrow transplant
  - Spontaneous LPD in immunodeficiency syndromes—Bloom syndrome, Chédiak-Higashi syndrome, X-linked lymphoproliferative syndrome, congenital T-cell immunodeficiencies, human immunodeficiency virus (HIV) infection

- ■ Treatment
  - Staging of Hodgkin disease by areas of involvement determines treatment. Most often treated by chemotherapy alone—cyclophosphamide, vincristine, procarbazine, prednisone or adriamycin, bleomycin, vinblastine, dacarbazine
  - Standard therapy for non-Hodgkin's disease includes systemic chemotherapy and prophylactic CNS chemotherapy. Anti-CD20 monoclonal antibodies are in trial in children
  - Post-transplant LPD treated with chemotherapy, reduced immunosuppression, and anti-CD20 monoclonal antibody

- ■ Pearl

Stage I and II Hodgkin lymphoma has 90% disease-free 5-year survival. Non-Hodgkin disease has a better prognosis in children than adults. Localized non-Hodgkin lymphoma has 90% disease-free survival.

Neuroblastoma

■ Essentials of Diagnosis

- Tumor arise from neural crest tissue of the sympathetic chain or adrenal medulla
- Biologically diverse tumor that may resolve spontaneously or progress despite intensive chemotherapy
- Bone pain, abdominal pain, anorexia, weight loss, fatigue, fever, irritability. 90% in children <5 years
- Abdominal mass (65%), adenopathy, proptosis, periorbital ecchymosis, skull masses, subcutaneous nodules, hepatomegaly, spinal cord compression
- Opsoclonus-myoclonus is a paraneoplastic symptom that suggests neuroblastoma
- Watery diarrhea due to tumor production of secretory proteins (vasoactive intestinal peptide [VIP]) may predominate
- Metastasizes to skeletal and skull bones, bone marrow, lymph nodes, liver, and subcutaneous tissue
- Urinary catecholamines are elevated in 90% of patients

■ Differential Diagnosis

- Histology must differentiate neuroblastoma cells from similar small round blue cell malignancies—Ewing sarcoma, rhabdomyosarcoma, peripheral neuroectodermal tumor, lymphoma
- Neck masses often misdiagnosed as infected lymphadenitis
- Behavioral changes may suggest psychiatric disease

■ Treatment

- Outcome based on location and histologic characteristics. Aggressive disease is associated with amplification of the MYCN proto-oncogene
- The goal of therapy is complete surgical resection coupled with chemotherapy (curative in stage I and II disease). High-risk disease requires surgery, chemotherapy, radiation, and occasionally stem cell transplantation
- *Cis*-retinoic acid promotes tumor cell differentiation and prolongs disease-free survival in patients with residual tumor after aggressive therapy

■ Pearl

A child with peri-orbital ecchymoses and proptosis requires evaluation for neuroblastoma with metastases to the sphenoid bone.

Wilms Tumor (Nephroblastoma)

- **Essentials of Diagnosis**
  - Asymptomatic abdominal distension or mass (83%)
  - Fever (23%), hematuria, (21%), hypertension (25%), genitourinary malformations (6%), aniridia, hemihypertrophy
  - Usually sporadic but may be associated with other malformations—aniridia, hemihypertrophy, cryptorchidism, hypospadias, gonadal dysgenesis, pseudohermaphroditism, horseshoe kidney
  - Mean age at diagnosis 4 years
  - Surgical exploration required for potential removal and for staging of tumor

- **Differential Diagnosis**
  - Bone and brain metastases are uncommon and suggest other renal tumors such as clear cell sarcoma or rhabdoid tumor
  - Increased risk of Wilms tumor in Beckwith-Wiedemann syndrome, Denys-Drash syndrome, and WAGR syndrome (Wilms, aniridia, ambiguous genitalia, mental retardation)

- **Treatment**
  - Initial surgical exploration with en bloc removal of tumor, evaluation of contralateral kidney, excision, and/or biopsy of affected nodes or liver masses
  - Prognosis depends upon localization, extent of histologic dedifferentiation, loss of heterozygosity of chromosomes 1p and 16q
  - Survival rates improved by intensifying the initial therapy. Chemotherapy should start directly postoperative and radiation of the tumor bed within 10 days
  - Bilateral involvement (stage V) requires intensive chemotherapy and second-look kidney sparing surgery to remove tumor

- **Pearl**

The contralateral kidney may be affected. The vena cava is a common site of local extension. The lungs and liver are the most common metastatic sites.

Rhabdomyosarcoma

■ **Essentials of Diagnosis**

- Most common soft tissue sarcoma of childhood. Peak incidence 2–5 years
- Painless enlarging mass; proptosis; chronic drainage from nose, ear, sinus, or vagina; cranial nerve palsies; urinary obstruction; constipation; hematuria
- 5 subtypes—embryonal and botryoid (60–80%), alveolar (15–20%), undifferentiated (8%), pleomorphic (1%), other (11%) with differing locations and metastatic potential
- Genetic predisposition in Li-Fraumeni syndrome (mutation of p53 tumor suppressor gene), chromosome translocations (2;13) and (1;13)
- 35% involve the head and neck; 22% involve bladder, prostate, vagina, uterus or testicles; 18% involve the extremities
- Therapy depends on location, tissue type, and presence of metastases

■ **Differential Diagnosis**

- Inflammatory swellings
- Other bony or soft tissue malignancies or benign masses (cysts, nasal polyps)
- Urinary obstruction from stone

■ **Treatment**

- Surgical excision if possible. Debulking may improve prognosis
- Chemotherapy may convert an inoperable tumor to a resectable one. Radiation used for local tumor control and residual tumor
- Chemotherapy usually includes vincristine, dactinomycin, and cyclophosphamide
- Second-look surgery after initial debulking and chemotherapy and/or radiation to remove residual tumor
- Patients receiving intensive chemotherapy and radiation may require stem cell transplantation

■ **Pearl**

Children with localized disease at diagnosis have a 70–75% 3-year disease-free survival. Children with metastatic disease at presentation have a 39% 3-year disease-free survival.

Retinoblastoma

- **Essentials of Diagnosis**
    - Neuroectodermal malignancy arising in embryonic retinal cells
    - Causes 5% of childhood blindness in the United States
    - Probably present from birth. 90% diagnosed before age 5 years
    - Bilateral in 20–30%
    - Some patients are homozygous for a mutation of the retinoblastoma gene *RB1*, a tumor suppressor gene on chromosome 13q14
    - Leukocoria, often seen best in photographs, is the most common sign (60%). Other symptoms are strabismus (if macula involved), glaucoma, eye pain, hyphema, proptosis

- **Differential diagnosis**
    - Leukocoria is also caused by *Toxocara canis* granuloma, astrocytic hamartoma, retinopathy of prematurity, Coats' disease, hyperplastic primary vitreous

- **Treatment**
    - Treatment determined by the potential for useful vision, size, location, and number of intraocular lesions
    - Indications for enucleation are no vision, neovascular glaucoma, inability to control tumor growth
    - External beam irradiation is the mainstay of therapy.
    - Chemotherapy sometimes used for tumors confined to the globe and always for metastatic disease

- **Pearl**

5-year survival is 90% in retinoblastoma confined to the retina. Mortality is high with optic nerve involvement, orbital extension, choroid invasion, meningeal or metastatic spread.

Bone Tumors

- **Essentials of Diagnosis**
  - Osteosarcoma accounts for 60% of bone tumors in children
  - Osteosarcoma incidence peaks during adolescence and is most frequent in the fastest growing, longest tubular bones (distal femur most common)
  - Pain is the most common symptom, systemic symptoms rare, mass sometimes present
  - Ewing sarcoma is the second most common tumor. Found in white postadolescent males usually in the diaphyses of long bones and central axial skeleton
  - 85–90% of Ewing tumors have a consistent cytogenetic abnormality with transposition between chromosome 11 and 22
  - X-ray and biopsy are diagnostic. Serum alkaline phosphatase and lactate dehydrogenase elevated

- **Differential Diagnosis**
  - Benign cysts, osteomyelitis, Langerhans cell histiocytosis, leukemia, lymphoma all may present with lytic bone lesions
  - The differential of Ewing sarcoma includes the other small round blue cell malignancies—rhabdomyosarcoma, lymphoma, and neuroblastoma
  - *C-myc* proto-oncogene is expressed in Ewing tumor cells but not in neuroblastoma
  - Peripheral neuroectodermal tumor is an extraosseous form of Ewing sarcoma

- **Treatment**
  - With surgery alone, 50% of osteosarcoma patients will develop pulmonary metastases. Adjuvant chemotherapy improves disease-free survival even in apparently completely resected tumors
  - Radiation therapy is useless in osteosarcoma, but is sometimes used in Ewing sarcoma
  - Surgery, radiation, and subsequent chemotherapy with combinations of dactinomycin, vincristine, doxorubicin, cyclophosphamide, etoposide, and ifosfamide are used for Ewing sarcoma
  - Stem cell transplantation may be lifesaving in advanced bony tumors

- **Pearl**

Whenever a child has a fracture, be on the alert for bony abnormalities—cyst, benign or malignant primary tumors, or metastatic disease.

Immunodeficiency Disorders

Complement Defects

■ Essentials of Diagnosis

- The classical complement factors (C1, 2, and 4); the alternative pathway factors (BD and properdin); and the terminal pathway factors (C3–9) are innate immunity proteins facilitating opsonization/lysis of bacteria, phagocyte recruitment, and antibody-mediated immunity
- Mannose binding lectin (MBL) is also an innate immunity protein, facilitating nonspecific opsonization of bacteria
- C1, 2, or 4 deficiency associated with systemic lupus erythematous (SLE) and other autoimmune diseases.
- C3 deficiency associated with pyogenic infections *Neisseria* species, *Streptococcus pneumoniae, Staphylococcus aureus, Pseudomonas aeruginosa, Haemophilus influenzae, Ureaplasma urealyticum*
- C5–9 and properdin deficiency associated with *Neisseria* infections
- MBL deficiency permits frequent bacterial infections
- C1 esterase inhibitor deficiency produces hereditary angioedema
- Deficiency of the modulatory proteins decay accelerating factor (DAF) and CD59 causes paroxysmal nocturnal hemoglobinuria
- Complement factor deficiency is excluded if total hemolytic complement (CH50) and alternative pathway screens (AH50) are normal. Individual factor assays confirm specific deficiency

■ Differential Diagnosis

- Leukocyte function and immunoglobulin deficiency disorders
- Generalized ↓in serum complement protein concentrations can occur in liver disease (↓synthesis), renal disease, and burns (↑loss) with partial loss of complement functions

■ Treatment

- MBL and terminal pathway deficiencies—treat infections aggressively. Fresh frozen plasma (FFP) containing complement proteins may augment antibiotic therapy
- C1 esterase inhibitor deficiency—danazol increases C1 esterase levels and prevents angioedema attacks. C1 inhibitor replacement is useful in emergencies (airway edema) or when steroids are contraindicated (pregnancy)
- Terminal pathway deficiencies—immunize against *Neisseria* species, *S pneumoniae.* FFP may be useful in severe infections

■ Pearl

Cystic fibrosis (CF) patients with chronic pseudomonas infections who carry MBL variant alleles seem to have poorer lung function and greater risk of Burkholderia cepacia *lung infections than other CF patients.*

Neutrophil Defects

- **Essentials of Diagnosis**
  - *Neutropenia*—usually acquired but also seen in bone marrow disorders, Shwachman syndrome, Kostmann syndrome, Chédiak-Higashi syndrome, Griscelli syndrome, X-linked a-γ-globulinemia (XLA), and others
  - *Chronic granulomatous disease* (CGD)—↓white blood cell (WBC) superoxide generation prevents normal killing of catalase positive organisms causing recurrent *S aureus, B cepacia, Serratia* species*, Nocardia* and *Aspergillus* infections. 65% are X-linked recessive
  - *Leukocyte adhesion deficiency I* (LAD I)—defective or absent β_2-integrin impairs neutrophil migration and adherence at sites of infection. Variable presentation includes recurrent infection, absence of pus (cold abscesses), poor wound healing, periodontal disease
  - *Glucose-6-phosphate dehydrogenase deficiency* (G6PD)—severe forms of X-linked recessive disorder affect neutrophil respiratory function and increase the risk of malaria infection
  - *Myeloperoxidase deficiency*—autosomal recessive defect causing poor intracellular killing of *Candida albicans.*

- **Diagnostic Evaluation**
  - Neutropenia—search for secondary causes (infection, leukemia, drug toxicity, alloimmune disease), bone marrow aspiration
  - CGD—ability of neutrophils to reduce nitroblue tetrazolium (NBT) is helpful. Dihydrorhodamine flow cytometry differentiates X-linked from autosomal recessive CGD and identifies carriers
  - LAD I—peripheral blood leucocytosis often striking. Flow cytometry analysis for β_2-integrin (CD18) is diagnostic
  - G6PD—red blood cell (RBC) or WBC enzyme activity
  - Myeloperoxidase deficiency—WBC enzyme activity

- **Treatment**
  - CGD—prophylactic and symptomatic antibiotic and antifungal agents combined with interferon-γ. Bone marrow transplant has been used
  - LAD I—aggressive antibiotic therapy during infections. Meticulous oral hygiene and wound care
  - G6PD—malaria prophylaxis in endemic areas. Avoid drugs and foods precipitating hemolysis
  - Myeloperoxidase deficiency—most patients do not have systemic candida infections. Some require antifungal prophylaxis

- **Pearl**

Neonates with LAD deficiency are sometimes recognized when the umbilical cord fails to separate. This process requires neutrophil function. Omphalitis may occur.

Hypo-γ-globulinemia

- Essentials of Diagnosis
  - *X-linked agammaglobulinemia* (XLA)—life-threatening infections with *S aureus, S pneumoniae, Ureaplasma* species, and vaccine strains of poliovirus; clinical onset in males in about 4 months of age as transplacental maternal IgG declines.
  - *Common variable immunodeficiency* (CVID)—exclusionary diagnosis in child with recurrent infections (especially sinus, pulmonary, gastrointestinal) and no other cause of ↓serum IgG and IgA. At risk for autoimmune diseases, gastric carcinoma, and lymphoma
  - *Transient hypo-γ-globulinemia of infancy*—delayed-onset immunoglobulin synthesis in infants causes recurrent otitis and upper respiratory infections (URI)
  - *IgA deficiency*—common disorder (1:700). Mostly asymptomatic but may have ↑URI, GI infections, later autoimmune disorders
  - *IgG subclass deficiency*—decrease in 1 of the 4 major subclasses of IgG. Associated consistent pattern of disease is not established. Possibly associated with recurrent URI

- Diagnostic Testing
  - XLA—scant lymphoid tissue, poor growth, low or absent serum immunoglobulins, low or absent B cells, molecular analysis shows B lymphocyte tyrosine kinase (blk) gene mutation
  - CVID—low serum IgG and IgA, poor antibody response to vaccines, low or absent isohemagglutinins, normal B cell count but reduced memory B cells by flow cytometry
  - Transient hypo-γ-globulinemia—IgG and IgA levels low for age; normal IgM and B cell count; normal specific antibody responses; normal T-cell function
  - IgA deficiency—serum IgA <7 mg/dL with normal serum IgM, IgG, specific antibody formation, T and B cells

- Treatment
  - XLA—lifelong replacement of IgG, aggressive prevention and treatment of infection. Bone marrow transplant has been used
  - CVID—prognosis often good. IgG replacement if needed; monitor for bronchiectasis, autoimmune disease, malignancy, gastric achlorhydria, and vitamin B_{12} deficiency
  - Transient hypo-γ-globulinemia—spontaneous recovery at 18–30 months. Antibiotics and intravenous immunoglobulin (IVIG) if needed
  - IgA deficiency—replacement therapy not feasible because of short half-life and anaphylaxis. Treat infections and monitor for autoimmune complications

- Pearl

When measuring serum immunoglobulin levels, age-related normal values should be used as standards to avoid overdiagnosis of deficiency states.

Severe Combined Immunodeficiency Diseases (SCID)

- **Essentials of Diagnosis**
  - Neonates present with recurrent infection (bacterial, viral, fungal, and opportunistic), chronic diarrhea, failure to thrive, oral or diaper candidiasis. Some present with cough, tachypnea, hypoxia (*Pneumocystis carinii*)
  - Physical examination—poor growth, lack of tonsils, lymph nodes, and thymus. Skin, pulmonary, GI infections, jaundice, and hepatosplenomegaly
  - Most infants are lymphopenic. Some have normal lymphocyte counts due to maternal lymphocyte engraftment at birth
  - Poor lymphocyte response to mitogens. No specific antibody formation

- **Major SCID Subtypes**
  - *X-linked SCID*—most common form. Mutation in IL-2 receptor gene encoding γ-globulin chain that is part of many cell surface cytokine receptors. Low T-cell count, normal B-cell count but no functional antibody production, absent NK cells
  - *Adenosine deaminase deficiency*—autosomal recessive; homozygotes have absence of adenosine deaminase (ADA) which removes toxic cell metabolites. T-cell death with total absence of T-cell function
  - *Janus kinase 3 deficiency*—homozygous mutations interrupt intracellular signaling through the common γ-chain. Resembles X-linked SCID
  - *IL-7 receptor α-chain deficiency*—homozygous mutations cause abnormal T-cell maturation, ↓T-cell count and dysfunctional B and NK cells
  - *Recombinase activating gene deficiency*—homozygous mutations in these genes (RAG1 and RAG2) encoding proteins critical for assembling antigen receptor genes in T and B cells cause ↓T- and B-cell count with normal NK count
  - *CD3 δ-chain deficiency*—homozygous mutations halt normal T-cell maturation. Presentation similar to IL-7 receptor α-chain deficiency. Thymus normal on x-ray

- **Treatment**
  - Aggressive treatment of infection and care to avoid unnecessary exposure to infection
  - Bone marrow transplant with human leukocyte antigen (HLA)-matched sibling donor, T-cell depleted HLA haploidentical donor or umbilical cord stem cells

- **Pearl**

Gene therapy, using viral vectors to carry and insert missing genes, has been tried in ADA deficiency, but many problems have prevented widespread use.

Wiskott-Aldrich Syndrome (WAS)

- ■ **Essentials of Diagnosis**
  - X-linked recessive disorder with immune deficiency and recurrent infections (especially lung and sinuses), microplatelet thrombocytopenia and eczema
  - Mutation in the WASP gene directing synthesis of proteins regulating actin rearrangements essential to the cross-talk between T cell and antigen presenting cell
  - Presents with bloody diarrhea, cerebral bleeding, severe infections with polysaccharide-encapsulated bacteria, eczema. Milder mutations produce only X-linked thrombocytopenia (XLT)
  - High mortality from bleeding and infection. Increased incidence of hematologic malignancy and autoimmune diseases with age
  - Laboratory findings—↓platelet count, ↓isohemagglutinins, ↓production of antibodies to polysaccharide antigens of *S pneumoniae and H influenzae*, ↓serum IgM, ↑serum IgA and IgE, ↓CD8 T cells

- ■ **Differential Diagnosis**
  - Other disorders causing thrombocytopenia
  - Severe exematoid disorders
  - Other immune deficiency disorders

- ■ **Treatment**
  - Prophylaxis with antibiotics including trimethoprim sulfamethoxazole for *P carinii*
  - IVIG for patients with poor antibody responses
  - Splenectomy may be helpful for patients with XLT
  - Avoid platelet transfusions except for life-threatening hemorrhage
  - Monitor for malignancy
  - HLA-matched bone marrow transplant may be curative

- ■ **Pearl**

Only about one-fourth of patients have the classic triad of sinopulmonary infection, platelet abnormalities, and eczema.

Ataxia-Telangiectasia (A-T)

- **Essentials of Diagnosis**
  - Autosomal recessive defect in synthesis of protein kinase on chromosome 11 required in cell cycle regulation and DNA repair
  - Cerebellar ataxia secondary to Purkinje cell degeneration develops by age 5 years with progressive loss of motor coordination and weakness
  - Telangiectasias of conjunctivae and exposed skin develop later
  - Respiratory infections and malignancy are major causes of death
  - ↑ serum α-fetoprotein, thymic hypoplasia, lymphopenia, ↓IgA, E, and/or G, defect in ability to repair DNA damage caused by ionizing radiation

- **Differential Diagnosis**
  - Nijmegen breakage syndrome is a variant of A-T with more severe features, microcephaly, and bird-like facies. No telangiectases
  - Cerebellar tumor
  - Friedreich ataxia, cerebral palsy, spinocerebellar ataxia, multiple sclerosis, Charcot-Marie-Tooth
  - Vitamin E deficiency
  - Acute cerebellar ataxia

- **Treatment**
  - No specific therapy available
  - Antibiotics and IVIG have been used with limited success

- **Pearl**

Prior to the development of pathognomonic conjunctival telangiectases, ataxia may be the only symptom of A-T. An elevated α-fetoprotein in an ataxic child makes A-T a likely diagnosis.

Chronic Mucocutaneous Candidiasis (CMC)

- **Essentials of Diagnosis**
  - Autosomal dominant disorder with *C albicans* infection of skin, nails, and mucous membranes. Rarely associated with endocrine or autoimmune disorders
  - Rare complications of autosomal dominant CMC include mycotic central nervous system (CNS) aneurysm, thymoma, oral, and GI cancers
  - Autosomal recessive form—autoimmune polyendocrinopathy, abnormal T-cell response to Candida antigen, and ectodermal dysplasia
  - APECED syndrome caused by mutations in genes promoting synthesis of transcription regulator protein necessary for normal thymocyte development
  - Anergy to candida prick test. Candida extracts fail to produce lymphocyte proliferation in vitro testing

- **Differential Diagnosis**
  - SCID
  - DiGeorge syndrome
  - Hyper-IgE syndrome (Job syndrome)
  - Human immunodeficiency virus (HIV) infection and other acquired or inherited T-cell disorders
  - Candida overgrowth associated with antibiotic use, drug-induced immunosuppression, intravascular foreign bodies
  - Biotin deficiency

- **Treatment**
  - Autoimmune endocrinopathies (thyroiditis, Addison disease, type 1 diabetes) if present require specific therapy
  - Cutaneous fungal infections may require systemic therapy and relapse off therapy is common
  - There is some interest in adjunctive use of T-cell transfer factor from Candida immune donors to treat severe infection
  - Ectodermal dysplasia is treated symptomatically with attention to prevention of skin injury, hyperthermia, dehydration and electrolyte loss, careful scalp and dental care

- **Pearl**

Not every recalcitrant Candida diaper dermatitis is a result of poor hygiene. Consider CMC here and in infants with severe oral thrush.

X-Linked Lymphoproliferative Syndrome

- **Essentials of Diagnosis**
  - Affected males appear normal until they develop fulminant, usually fatal infectious mononucleosis with their first Epstein-Barr virus (EBV) infection usually by age 5 years
  - Fulminant mononucleosis is characterized by hemophagocytic syndrome, liver failure, disseminated intravascular coagulation (DIC), multiple organ system failure, bone marrow aplasia
  - Mutation is in genes on X chromosome encoding the SLAM-adapter protein, a signaling protein used by T cells and NK cells
  - Boys who do not encounter EBV or who survive a first infection are at risk for recurrent EBV infection, lymphoma (especially B cell non-Hodgkin type), vasculitis, CVID, or hypo-γ-globulinemia with elevated IgM

- **Differential Diagnosis**
  - Severe mononucleosis infection can occur in the absence of XLPD
  - Hemophagocytic syndrome (hemophagocytic lymphohistiocytosis; macrophage activation syndrome) can be familial or can occur with other infections. Appears to be stimulated by a massive release of cytokines, especially IFN-γ with macrophage activation
  - X-linked hyper-IgM syndrome
  - Late-stage Chédiak-Higashi syndrome has a terminal lymphohistiocytic phase

- **Treatment**
  - Antenatal diagnosis is possible
  - Use of antiviral agents (ganciclovir, acyclovir) rarely effective
  - Intensive supportive care may permit survival of initial infection, but ultimate outcome usually fatal
  - Isolated reports of successful treatment by bone marrow transplantation

- **Pearl**

Hemophagocytosis occurs when macrophages are strongly activated. In many patients with severe infections, occasional phagocytosed red cells can be seen in liver or bone marrow without full-blown hemophagocytic syndrome.

Graft-Versus-Host Disease (GVHD)

- Essentials of Diagnosis
  - GVHD occurs when immunologically competent donor T cells are grafted into a host who cannot reject them
  - GVHD occurs most frequently after allogeneic bone marrow transplant but also after blood transfusion to an immuno-incompetent host, maternal-to-fetal transfusion and (rarely) via T cells contained in a solid organ transplant
  - Engrafted T cells attack host tissues causing rash, enteritis with diarrhea, hepatitis, nephritis, pneumonitis, fever, and bone marrow injury
  - Peripheral eosinophilia and leukocytosis. Early skin biopsy shows changes at the epidermal basement membrane (vacuolation, cell necrosis, lymphocyte infiltration). GI biopsies may show lymphocytic infiltrate and gland destruction
  - Chronic GVHD skin biopsy shows hyperkeratosis, acanthosis, and thick granular layer

- Differential Diagnosis
  - GVHD must be differentiated from specific organ infections and autoimmune disorders, eg, viral hepatitis, tuberculous enteritis, Crohn disease, chronic glomerulonephritis
  - Drug eruption, viral exanthem may mimic acute GVHD skin rash
  - Scleroderma may resemble chronic GVHD skin rash

- Treatment
  - Prevention is the best option in high-risk situations. Prophylactic immunosuppressant regimens include methotrexate, cyclosporine, mycophenolate mofetil
  - Treatment regimens include drugs used in prevention plus additional agents such as antithymocyte globulin, corticosteroids, and monoclonal antibodies against activated T cells (daclizumab) and cytokines (infliximab, etanercept)

- Pearl

Syngeneic bone marrow and cord blood stem cell transplant are less likely to cause GVHD. T-cell depletion of donor hemopoietic tissue carries reduced risk of GVHD but higher risk of graft failure.

10

Endocrine Disorders

10

Growth Hormone (GH) Deficiency

- **Essentials of Diagnosis**
  - Major symptoms—decreased growth velocity, delayed skeletal maturation, truncal adiposity, other pituitary-related hormone deficiencies
  - *Congenital*—septo-optic dysplasia, interrupted pituitary stalk syndrome, empty sella
  - *Genetic*—mutations in genes for GH, GH-releasing hormone (GHRH), or GH receptor
  - *Acquired*—craniopharyngioma, germinoma, histiocytosis, cranial irradiation
  - *Idiopathic*—most common
  - Newborns with GH deficiency have normal birth weight, hypoglycemia, cholestatic jaundice, micropenis, adrenal and thyroid deficiency
  - Diagnosis by noting ↓GH response to insulin, arginine, levodopa, clonidine, or glucagon
  - Serum insulin-like growth factor (IGF-1) and IGF binding protein are reduced in GH deficiency

10

- **Differential Diagnosis**
  - Constitutional growth delay
  - Hypothyroidism
  - Syndrome associated—Down, Turner, Prader-Willi, Russel-Silver dwarfism, skeletal dysplasia syndromes, many others
  - Psychosocial short stature—emotional deprivation
  - Chronic systemic disease—inflammatory bowel and liver disease, celiac disease, glycogen storage disease, cardiac and renal insufficiency
  - Malnutrition

- **Treatment**
  - Exogenous GH approved for GH deficiency, Turner syndrome, renal insufficiency prior to transplant, Prader-Willi syndrome, small for gestational age (SGA) babies with failure of catch-up growth
  - Exogenous GH for constitutional growth delay is Food and Drug Administration (FDA)-approved but still controversial
  - Rare side effects of GH therapy—intracranial hypertension, slipped capital femoral epiphysis

- **Pearl**

Consider Turner syndrome (XO genotype) in any short girl even those without typical Turner phenotype. Early diagnosis is critical to appropriate therapy. GH therapy starts at a young age and estrogen and progesterone at the time of puberty.

Diabetes Insipidus (DI)

- **Essentials of Diagnosis**
  - *Central DI*
    - Genetic—mutations in vasopressin gene and *WFS1* gene (Wolfram syndrome)
    - Midline brain defects—septo-optic dysplasia, holoprosencephaly
    - Brain injury, infection, or surgical resection
    - Hypothalamic or pituitary tumors—craniopharyngioma, germinoma, histiocytosis, lymphocytic hypophysitis
  - *Nephrogenic DI*—chronic renal disease with failure to concentrate urine
  - Polydipsia, polyuria (>2 L/m^2/day), nocturia
  - Patients unable to produce concentrated urine during fluid restriction. Urine SG remains <1.010 with urine osmolality <600 mOsm/kg even with plasma osmolality > 300 mOsm/kg
  - Hypernatremia and dehydration with serum sodium as high as 180 mEq/L. Serum vasopressin level is low

- **Differential Diagnosis**
  - Psychogenic polydipsia
  - Diabetes mellitus
  - Hypertonic dehydration secondary to diarrhea
  - Exogenous salt administration

- **Treatment**
  - Identify treatable causes of DI
  - Treat children with desmopressin acetate (DDAVP) orally or intranasally
  - Do not use DDAVP in young infants. With their normally large fluid intake (formula and breast milk), DDAVP use may cause water intoxication
  - Use extra free water as needed in infants
  - Chlorothiazides may be helpful in infants with central DI

- **Pearl**

Measuring glucose, sodium, and osmolality in urine and serum can quickly distinguish diabetes mellitus, hypertonic dehydration, psychogenic polydipsia, and exogenous salt intake from DI.

Hypothyroidism

- **Essentials of Diagnosis**
  - *Congenital causes*—thyroid aplasia/hypoplasia, dyshormono-genesis, iodine transport defects, maternal iodine deficiency, pituitary hypoplasia
  - *Acquired causes*—thyroiditis, surgical removal of thyroid or pituitary, radiation injury, chronic excess or deficient iodide intake, lithium, amiodarone
  - Symptoms in children—growth retardation, delayed puberty, decreased energy, goiter, hypothermia, dry skin, weight gain, constipation, bradycardia, dull affect
  - Symptoms in infants—prolonged neonatal jaundice, constipation, hypotonia, ↓deep tendon reflexes, hoarse cry, big tongue, hypotonia, umbilical hernia, developmental delay
  - Thyroid-stimulating hormone (TSH) is elevated in primary thyroid disease and low or normal in pituitary or hypothalamic disease
  - Low to low normal total T_4, free T_3, and T_3 resin uptake

- **Differential Diagnosis**
  - Pituitary and hypothalamic disease with central hypothyroidism
  - Thyroxine-binding globulin (TBG) deficiency (low total T_4 with normal TSH and free T_4)
  - Depression
  - Transient postpartum hypothyroidism or postpartum pituitary insufficiency
  - Sick euthyroid syndrome caused by severe illness and anorexia nervosa

- **Treatment**
  - Levothyroxine is the drug of choice
  - Medication and monitoring are lifelong in most cases
  - Identify and treat acquired forms

- **Pearl**

Symptoms are often absent in hypothyroid neonates. Newborn screening and early treatment are the keys to preventing mental retardation from congenital hypothyroidism.

10

Chronic Lymphocytic (Autoimmune) Thyroiditis

- **Essentials of Diagnosis**
  - Most common cause of goiter and hypothyroidism in children. Female/Male ratio 4:1
  - Autoimmune-mediated disorder
  - Usual presentation—hypothyroid symptoms, goiter, positive antithyroid peroxidase antibodies. May present with hyperthyroid symptoms
  - TSH generally normal. TSH low during hashitoxicosis. TSH high during hypothyroid phase of thyroiditis
  - Associated with autoimmune polyglandular syndrome type 2 (adrenal failure, autoimmune thyroid disease, type 1 diabetes mellitus, vitiligo, celiac disease, atrophic gastritis, gonadal failure)

- **Differential diagnosis**
  - Idiopathic goiter
  - Graves disease
  - Viral thyroiditis
  - Iodine deficiency
  - Goitrogen ingestion
  - Congenital hypothyroidism

- **Treatment**
  - Ideal treatment has not been established
  - Exogenous thyroid hormone—decreases goiter size but does not prevent progression of disease
  - Regular monitoring for the development of hypothyroidism or Graves disease

- **Pearl**

Hypothyroidism and Graves disease can develop at any time in patients with autoimmune thyroiditis. Be on the alert for the insidious development of thyroid dysfunction in patients with autoimmune thyroiditis.

Hyperthyroidism

- ■ Essentials of Diagnosis
  - Graves disease is the most common cause of childhood hyperthyroidism. Increased incidence in adolescent females
  - Symptoms—nervousness, emotional lability, fatigue, tremor, palpitations, hyperphagia, weight loss, sweating, heat intolerance, moist skin, insomnia, inability to concentrate, school failure, polyuria
  - Physical examination—goiter, thyroid bruit, exophthalmos, tachycardia, widened pulse pressure, systolic hypertension, proximal muscle weakness
  - Serum T_4 and T_3 concentrations elevated; TSH suppressed; TSH receptor antibody detected
  - Neonatal Graves disease—transient hyperthyroidism caused by transplacental transfer of TSH receptor antibodies from mother with Graves disease to fetus

10

- ■ Differential Diagnosis
  - Acute, subacute, or chronic thyroiditis
  - Autonomously functioning thyroid nodule
  - TSH-producing tumor
  - McCune-Albright syndrome
  - Hypermetabolic states may resemble hyperthyroidism—anemia, chronic infection, carcinoid, pheochromocytoma, muscle-wasting diseases
  - Panic attacks and anxiety disorder
  - Exogenous thyroid hormone overdose
  - Iodine overdose

- ■ Treatment
  - β_1-Adrenergic blockers for symptom relief
  - Propylthiouracil and methimazole interfere with hormone synthesis
  - Radio-iodine ablation or surgical thyroidectomy in resistant cases
  - Large-dose iodide sometimes used in hyperthyroid crisis
  - Treat neonatal Graves disease with β_1-adrenergic blockers to relieve cardiac symptoms
  - Monitor for Graves ophthalmopathy

- ■ Pearl

Neonatal Graves disease occurs in 1% of babies born to mothers with Graves disease. Severe cases may result in arrhythmia, cardiac failure, and death.

Thyroid Cancer

- **Essentials of Diagnosis**
  - Rare disorder presents in childhood with thyroid nodule or neck mass
  - Thyroid functions tests usually normal
  - Fine needle aspiration for histological evaluation key to diagnosis
  - Papillary thyroid carcinoma most common, followed by follicular carcinoma, medullary carcinoma, anaplastic carcinoma, lymphoma, and sarcoma
  - Papillary carcinoma may be metastatic at presentation but responds well to therapy
  - Medullary carcinoma is highly malignant and associated with autosomal dominant *RET* gene mutations (multiple endocrine neoplasia type II)

10

- **Differential Diagnosis**
  - Other causes of thyroid enlargement—hypothyroidism, hyperthyroidism
  - Branchial cleft cysts
  - Cervical lymphadenopathy

- **Treatment**
  - Treat papillary carcinoma by total or subtotal surgical thyroidectomy, removal of metastases, and radioiodine ablation of thyroid remnants followed by chronic thyroid hormone therapy to suppress regrowth
  - Other cancers usually treated surgically
  - Outcome poor in medullary carcinoma

- **Pearl**

All family members of patients with medullary thyroid carcinoma should be screened for the RET mutation and those with the mutation should have prophylactic thyroidectomy.

Hypoparathyroidism

- ■ Essentials of Diagnosis
  - • Hypocalcemia causes tetany, facial and extremity numbness, tingling, carpopedal spasm, positive Trousseau and Chvostek signs, diarrhea, laryngospasm, loss of consciousness, and convulsions
  - • Prolongation of electrical systole (QT interval) on electrocardiogram (ECG)
  - • Defective nails and teeth, cataracts, ectopic calcification of subcutaneous tissues and basal ganglia

- ■ Differential Diagnosis
  - • Pseudo-hypoparathyroidism
  - • Transient tetany in newborns is a relative parathyroid hormone (PTH) deficiency associated with high phosphate diet (whole cow's milk), infant of diabetic mother, fetal alcohol syndrome
  - • Severe vitamin D deficiency
  - • Gastrointestinal (GI) malabsorption syndromes, chronic renal disease, tumor lysis syndrome, rhabdomyolysis
  - • DiGeorge syndrome—congenital absence of parathyroid gland
  - • Autoimmune polyendocrine syndrome type 1
  - • Autosomal dominant hypocalcemia—gain of function mutation in extracellular calcium receptor. Causes low serum PTH despite calcium loss and hypocalcemia
  - • Postoperative or postradiation for thyroid disease
  - • Iron or copper overload—hemochromatosis, thalassemia, Wilson disease
  - • Other syndromes—velocardiofacial syndrome (Shprintzen), Zellweger syndrome, mitochondrial abnormalities, hyper- and hypomagnesemia

10

- ■ Treatment
  - • Establish and maintain normocalcemia and normophosphatemia
  - • During intravenous (IV) calcium infusion, monitor ECG
  - • High calcium diet and dietary calcium supplements
  - • Vitamin D supplementation with calcitriol
  - • Treat underlying cause if possible
  - • PTH is not generally used

- ■ Pearl

The only FDA-sanctioned use of exogenous PTH at present is adult osteoporosis. Diet, vitamin D, and treatment of underlying causes are the mainstays of therapy in pediatric hypocalcemia syndromes.

Pseudo-hypoparathyroidism

- **Essentials of Diagnosis**
  - Heterozygous inactivation of stimulatory G protein subunit of PTH receptor causes impaired signaling and PTH resistance in renal tubule and/or bone
  - Several phenotypes with hypocalcemia, hyperphosphatemia, and elevated PTH levels
  - Albright hereditary osteodystrophy—common phenotype with short stature, round facies, short fourth and fifth metacarpals and metatarsals, delayed and defective dentition, mild mental retardation, corneal and lens opacity, calcified basal ganglia
  - Pseudo-pseudo-hypoparathyroidism—patients have Albright phenotype but normal calcium homeostasis

- **Differential Diagnosis**
  - There are many causes of hypocalcemia (see section Hypoparathyroidism)
  - Typical body appearance makes diagnosis relatively straightforward

- **Treatment**
  - Same as for hypoparathyroidism
  - Specific remediation for ocular, mental, and physical disabilities

- **Pearl**

Genomic imprinting is thought to be responsible for different phenotypic expressions. Heterozygous loss of the maternal allele results in pseudo-hypoparathyroidism while heterozygous loss of the paternal allele results in pseudo-pseudo-hypoparathyroidism.

Hypercalcemia

- ■ Essentials of Diagnosis
  - • Symptoms—abdominal pain, hypertension, failure to thrive, constipation, impaired concentration, altered mental status, mood swings, coma
  - • Peptic ulcer and pancreatitis more commonly seen in adults
  - • Bone changes—bone pain, pathologic fractures, osteitis fibrosa cystica, subperiosteal bone resorption
  - • Renal disease—kidney stones, parenchymal calcification, antidiuretic hormone unresponsiveness causing polyuria, polydipsia
  - • 80% of children with serum Ca >12 mg/dL have either malignancy or hyperparathyroidism. Milder elevations suggest Williams syndrome or benign familial hypocalciuric hypercalcemia

10

- ■ Causes of Hypercalcemia
  - • Primary hyperparathyroidism—adenoma, familial ectopic PTH secretion, parathyroid hyperplasia
  - • Increased intestinal or renal absorption of calcium—hypervitaminosis D, familial hypocalciuric hypercalcemia, lithium, sarcoidosis, phosphate depletion, aluminum toxicity
  - • Increased mobilization of bone calcium—hyperthyroidism, immobilization, thiazides, vitamin A intoxication, malignancy (myeloma, PTH-secreting tumors, prostaglandin secreting tumors, cancers metastatic to bone)

- ■ Treatment
  - • Vigorous hydration
  - • Forced calcium diuresis with furosemide
  - • Glucocorticoids or calcitonin may be helpful
  - • Biphosphonates are being used cautiously in pediatric patients
  - • Diagnose and treat underlying causes

- ■ Pearl

Because of albumin binding, every gram decrease in serum albumin produces a 0.8 mg/dL decrease in total calcium. Thus in a hypoalbuminemic child, total serum calcium may not be a good indicator of hypercalcemia. Add 0.8 mg/dL to the total serum calcium for every gram decrease in albumin. Better yet, measure ionized calcium which is independent of serum albumin.

Familial Hypocalciuric Hypercalcemia

- **Essentials of Diagnosis**
  - Increased PTH secretion causes decreased renal calcium excretion and high renal calcium reabsorption
  - "Inactivating" mutation in the membrane-bound calcium-sensing receptor in parathyroid and renal tubule cells
  - Autosomal dominant with high penetrance
  - Heterozygous patients usually symptom free with normal or mildly elevated PTH
  - Homozygous infants have severe neonatal hyperparathyroidism (NSHP), a metabolic emergency

- **Differential Diagnosis**
  - Other forms of hyperparathyroidism with increased renal absorption of calcium—hypervitaminosis D, lithium, sarcoidosis, phosphate depletion, aluminum intoxication
  - Primary hyperparathyroidism
  - Williams syndrome

- **Treatment**
  - Usually not needed
  - In homozygous infants with NSHP, surgical removal of parathyroids may be required
  - Important to recognize this disorder in mildly affected patients to avoid unnecessary therapy or parathyroid removal

- **Pearl**

Often discovered by accident, these are healthy individuals whose major long-term complication is gall stones. Leave them alone.

Hypervitaminosis D

- **Essentials of Diagnosis**
  - Accidental or intentional vitamin D overdose usually of long standing
  - Signs and symptoms in infants include emesis, constipation, irritability, fatigue, anorexia, hypertension, and hypercalcemia
  - More than 1000 IU vitamin D taken daily for several months will result in toxicity in childhood
  - Massive overdose may cause symptoms within 2–8 days
  - Excess vitamin D during pregnancy may cause fetal hypocalcemia from suppression of PTH
  - Excess vitamin D intake during lactation may cause infant hypercalcemia
  - Gall stones, renal stones may result
  - Measure vitamin D and vitamin D metabolites in serum

10

- **Differential Diagnosis**
  - Hypercalcemic states especially occult malignancy
  - Williams syndrome (neonatal hypercalcemia)—abnormal responsiveness to vitamin D with transient neonatal hypercalcemia, elfin facies, supravalvular aortic stenosis, failure to thrive, mental retardation, hypotonia, irritability, polyuria, polydipsia, and hypertension. Mutations in elastin gene on chromosome 7
  - Be alert for other vitamin toxicities in self-medicated patients

- **Treatment**
  - Corticosteroids to promote calcium excretion
  - Hydration
  - Low calcium diet (Calcilo in formula-fed infants)
  - Education of patient and caregiver

- **Pearl**

Vitamin D is stored in adipose tissue. Elimination of excess body stores of vitamin D and return of normocalcemia in overdosed patients may take several months.

Rickets

- ■ Essentials of Diagnosis
  - • Inadequate vitamin D causes reduced calcification of osteoid matrix, failure of calcification of cartilage
  - • Symptoms—weakness, bone pain, anorexia, refusal to walk, irritability
  - • Physical findings—wide tender epiphyses at ankles and wrists, enlarged costochondral junctions (rachitic rosary), bow legs, craniotabes, scoliosis, kyphosis, fractures
  - • Risk factors—vitamin D-deficient breast-feeding mother, limited sun exposure, inadequate vitamin D intake or absorption
  - • Laboratory testing—low serum phosphate, normal-to-low serum calcium, low serum 25-OH vitamin D, increased serum alkaline phosphatase, elevated PTH (in nutritional vitamin D deficiency)
  - • X-ray findings—cupping, widening, and fraying of long bone metaphyses

- ■ Differential Diagnosis
  - • Hypophosphatemic rickets due to abnormal renal phosphorus loss
  - • Hypophosphatasia—rickets-like skeletal abnormality with very low serum alkaline phosphatase and hypercalcemia
  - • Vitamin D and calcium malabsorption—untreated celiac disease, short bowel syndrome, liver disease, pancreatic disease
  - • Failure of 25-hydroxylation in advanced liver disease

- ■ Treatment
  - • Biochemical vitamin D deficiency without signs or symptoms— oral vitamin D supplement
  - • Rickets—large-dose vitamin D until alkaline phosphatase normal then maintenance dose
  - • Hypophosphatemic rickets—lifelong therapy with oral phosphorus and calcitriol (to prevent secondary hyperparathyroidism due to phosphorus excess)

- ■ Pearl

Vitamin D deficiency is increasing due to the use of unfortified milk, extensive use of sunscreen, increasing religious diversity, and long-term survival of medically complicated children with liver and bowel disease who have malabsorption of fat-soluble vitamins.

Ambiguous Genitalia

- **Essentials of Diagnosis**
  - *Gonad differentiation defects*—gonadal dysgenesis with inadequate testicular differentiation, mosaicism of X or Y chromosome, idiopathic failure of the fetal testis, true hermaphroditism
  - *Defects in testosterone synthesis/action*—micropenis, genital ambiguity or absence of male external genitalia in an XY individual. Most common testosterone synthetic enzyme defects are 12-ketoreductase deficiency and 5α-reductase deficiency. Testosterone synthesis defects may be associated with cortisol and aldosterone deficiency with salt wasting.
  - *Adrenal androgen overproduction*—21-hydroxylase deficiency interferes with cortisol and aldosterone synthesis allowing excess adrenal androgen causing 95% of newborn female virilization (congenital adrenal hyperplasia). 11-Hydroxylase deficiency causes salt retention and hypertension with masculinization in girls. Rarer is 3β-hydroxysteroid dehydrogenase deficiency causing ambiguous genitalia in males
  - *Syndromic*—VATER syndrome, Wilms tumor/aniridia syndrome, Smith-Lemli-Opitz, Denys-Drash

- **Differential Diagnosis**
  - Maternal exposure to androgen or androgen antagonists may cause genital ambiguity
  - Mild clitoromegaly may be normal in female neonates
  - Vaginal bleeding (in females), breast hypertrophy, and galactorrhea (both sexes) are benign effects of in utero progesterone excess

- **Treatment**
  - Neonate with ambiguous genitalia—immediate consultation with pediatric endocrinologist for parent education, parent support, rapid diagnosis, and monitoring for complications of salt wasting
  - Chromosome analysis
  - Endocrine screening with serum steroid metabolites
  - Imaging to assess adrenal size and presence/type of gonads may include ultrasound (U/S), computed tomography (CT), and magnetic resonance imaging (MRI)
  - Gender assignment requires close collaboration with family and should not be made until results of evaluation are complete
  - In salt losers, fluid management and hormone replacement are indicated

- **Pearl**

There is substantial family distress at the birth of a child with ambiguous genitalia. However, experience teaches the importance of completing a thorough evaluation before gender assignment is made. Appropriate support will help the family weather the delay.

Precocious Puberty—Girls

- **Essentials of Diagnosis**
  - Secondary female sexual characteristics before age 8 years
  - *Central precocious puberty*—activation of hypothalamic gonadotropin-releasing hormone (GnRH) pulse generator increases luteinizing hormone (LH), follicle stimulating hormone (FSH) secretion and release of sex steroids with normal-sequence pubertal development
  - Central precocious puberty is usually idiopathic but may be caused by hypothalamic hamartoma, central nervous system (CNS) tumors, cranial irradiation or inflammation, hydrocephalus, head trauma
  - *Peripheral precocious puberty*—occurs independent of gonadotropin secretion
  - Peripheral precocity caused by ovarian or adrenal tumors, ovarian cyst, congenital adrenal hyperplasia, McCune-Albright syndrome, exogenous estrogen
  - Evaluation is indicated if bone age is advanced or growth velocity increased

- **Differential Diagnosis**
  - Benign premature thelarche—no associated acceleration of linear growth or bone age
  - Premature adrenarche—development of pubic/axillary hair, body odor, acne without acceleration of linear growth or bone age. Associated with polycystic ovarian syndrome during puberty

- **Treatment**
  - Central precocious puberty—GnRH analogs (leuprolide) down-regulate pituitary GnRH receptors and decrease gonadotropin secretion
  - McCune-Albright—antiestrogens (tamoxifen) or aromatase inhibitors may be effective
  - Attention to psychological issues important in all cases

- **Pearl**

Unilateral or bilateral premature thelarche usually occurs in girls <2 years or >6 years. In the absence of other signs of pubertal development, advanced bone age or accelerated height velocity, no evaluation is needed.

Delayed Puberty—Girls

- **Essentials of Diagnosis**
  - Absence of pubertal signs by 13 years or menarche by 16 years
  - Failure to complete puberty (Tanner stage V) within 4 years of onset
  - *Primary hypogonadism*—Turner syndrome or other gonadal dysgenesis, ovarian failure due to autoimmune disease, surgery, radiation, chemotherapy, galactosemia
  - *Central hypogonadism*—pituitary or hypothalamic tumors, congenital hypopituitarism, Kallmann syndrome, chronic illness, undernutrition, excess exercise, hyperprolactinemia
  - *Anatomic*—Mullerian agenesis, complete androgen resistance
  - Primary ovarian failure causes elevated FSH (Turner syndrome). Central hypogonadism causes low gonadotropin

10

- **Differential Diagnosis**
  - Constitutional growth delay
  - Secondary amenorrhea—weight loss, medication, chronic intercurrent illness
  - Hypothyroidism and GH deficiency
  - Absence of the uterus—androgen insensitivity, Mayer-Rokitansky-Küster-Hauser syndrome
  - Polycystic ovarian syndrome—failure to menstruate with normal estrogen

- **Treatment**
  - Replacement therapy in girls with hypogonadism starts with estrogen followed in 12–18 months with cyclic estrogen-progesterone therapy
  - Treat primary cause

- **Pearl**

Be on the alert for anorexia nervosa in the underweight teenaged girl with secondary amenorrhea.

Precocious Puberty—Boys

- ■ Essentials of Diagnosis
  - • Secondary sexual characteristics before age 9 years
  - • Male precocious puberty less common than female
  - • *Central precocious puberty*—basal LH and FSH not in pubertal range. LH response to GnRH is pubertal. Bone age advanced. Growth velocity increased. Testicular size increased for age
  - • *Peripheral precocious puberty*—Premature secondary sexual characteristics with normal testicular size for age

- ■ Differential Diagnosis
  - • Central precocious puberty often associated with CNS tumor
  - • Peripheral precocious puberty
    - • McCune-Albright syndrome
    - • Familial Leydig cell hyperplasia (testotoxicosis)—abnormal Leydig cell LH receptor is autonomously activated causing increased testicular production of testosterone
    - • Human chorionic gonadotropin (HCG)-secreting tumor
    - • Congenital adrenal hyperplasia

- ■ Treatment
  - • Central precocious puberty treated with GnRH analog
  - • McCune-Albright or familial Leydig cell hyperplasia—steroid synthesis blockers (ketoconazole) or combination of antiandrogen and aromatase inhibitor

- ■ Pearl

Imaging of the brain is mandatory in evaluating boys with central precocious puberty. There is a high likelihood of finding a CNS lesion.

Delayed Puberty—Boys

- **Essentials of Diagnosis**
  - Lack of secondary sexual characteristics by age 14 years
  - *Primary testicular failure*—testicular absence or hypoplasia (Klinefelter), destruction of testes by irradiation, infection (mumps), autoimmune inflammation, trauma or tumor, enzyme defects
  - *Secondary failure*—pituitary or hypothalamic disease, isolated LH or FSH deficiency due to GnRH deficiency (Prader-Willi and Laurence-Moon syndrome), destructive brain tumors or infections, chronic debility, hypothyroidism
  - Primary testicular failure—low plasma testosterone with elevated LH and FSH
  - Secondary testicular failure—testosterone, LH, and FSH are below normal
  - Presence of testes and their ability to respond is measured by plasma testosterone after intramuscular HCG

- **Differential Diagnosis**
  - Constitutional growth delay—most common cause of delayed puberty. Normal growth velocity and delayed bone age
  - Masculinized female—check karyotype and look for adrenal hyperplasia
  - Cryptorchidism—isolated finding or associated with hypothalamic-pituitary-gonadal axis, androgen synthesis or receptor defects
  - Abdominal testes—plasma testosterone after HCG stimulation will be normal

- **Treatment**
  - Specific therapy depends on cause
  - Constitutional delay may respond to short course of low-dose Depo-testosterone
  - Permanent hypogonadism requires regular Depo-testosterone or testosterone gel

- **Pearl**

Klinefelter syndrome is the most common cause of primary hypogonadism in boys. Affected males have small testes but moderate virilization. They can usually attain Tanner stage IV pubic hair development.

Cryptorchidism

- **Essentials of Diagnosis**
  - 3% of term male newborns, higher in prematures
  - Unilateral or bilateral
  - 80% of undescended testes will be in scrotum by 1 year with further descent during puberty
  - Malignancy risk increased (22 times) in both the undescended and contralateral testis
  - Increased temperature in undescended testis reduces fertility

- **Differential Diagnosis**
  - Retractile testis
  - Absence of testis
  - Masculinized female—in the newborn, consider congenital adrenal hyperplasia
  - Abdominal testis—check plasma testosterone after HCG stimulation. It will be normal.

- **Treatment**
  - Surgical orchidopexy should be performed by 12 months
  - Short spermatic artery and poor testicular blood supply increases the risk of testicular loss during orchidopexy
  - HCG given twice weekly for 5 weeks causes descent of retractile testis but not helpful in true cryptorchidism
  - Androgen therapy at puberty if the testis is nonfunctional

- **Pearl**

Orchidopexy decreases but does not eliminate the risk of testicular malignancy. The undescended testis may be dysplastic and carry an inherent risk of malignant change. These boys should be educated and monitored.

Adrenocortical Insufficiency (Adrenal Crisis, Addison Disease)

- **Essentials of Diagnosis**
  - Leading causes—hereditary enzyme defects (congenital adrenal hyperplasia), autoimmune destruction (Addison disease), cranial irradiation or surgery, congenital midline defects (septo-optic dysplasia)
  - Low serum sodium and bicarbonate with high potassium and blood urea nitrogen. Urinary sodium inappropriately high for the degree of hyponatremia
  - Eosinophilia (Addison disease)
  - Serum adrenocorticotropic hormone (ACTH) high in end-organ insufficiency, low in central insufficiency
  - Decreased urinary free cortisol and 17-OH corticosteroid
  - Chronic insufficiency—fatigue, weakness, salt craving, vomiting, hyperpigmentation (melanocyte stimulation by ACTH), small heart on x-ray
  - Acute adrenal crisis—vomiting, diarrhea, dehydration, fever or hypothermia, weakness, hypotension, coma, death

- **Differential Diagnosis**
  - Congenital adrenal leukodystrophy
  - Polyglandular autoimmune syndromes
  - Adrenal tumor, calcification, and hemorrhage (Waterhouse-Friderichsen)
  - Adrenal tuberculous or fungal infections (especially in immunodeficiency)
  - Anterior pituitary tumor
  - Temporary salt losing due to mineralocorticoid deficiency or renal under-responsiveness (pseudo-hypoaldosteronism) in infants with pyelonephritis
  - Septic shock, diabetic coma, CNS diseases, and acute poisoning mimic adrenal crisis. Anorexia nervosa, myasthenia gravis, salt-losing nephritis, and chronic infections mimic chronic adrenal insufficiency.

- **Treatment**
  - Adrenal crisis requires IV hydrocortisone, fluid, and electrolyte resuscitation
  - Fludrocortisone given for chronic insufficiency
  - Inotropes (dopamine, dobutamine) may be needed during crisis

- **Pearl**

If your patient is taking prednisone chronically, sudden discontinuation of medication may leave him/her with adrenal suppression and therefore at risk for adrenal crisis during subsequent intercurrent illness.

10

Congenital Adrenal Hyperplasia (CAH)

- **Essentials of Diagnosis**
  - Leading cause (80%) is 21-hydroxylase deficiency
  - Low-serum sodium and bicarbonate. High-serum potassium. High-serum ACTH and rennin
  - In 21-hydroxylase deficiency, increased serum 17-OH progesterone and testosterone cause virilization of newborn females
  - Males with 21-hydroxylase deficiency look normal and present during the first months with salt-losing crisis or isosexual precocity
  - Increased linear growth. Advanced skeletal maturation
  - Diagnosis confirmed by failure of hormone response to ACTH stimulation

- **Differential Diagnosis**
  - Chromosome abnormalities
  - Polycystic ovarian syndrome
  - Mild enzyme defects may present later in life with virilization, precocious puberty, irregular menses, infertility
  - In 20,22-desmolase deficiency and 3β-ol dehydrogenase deficiency, decreased plasma androgens cause ambiguous genitalia in males

- **Treatment**
  - Salt-losing crises treated with IV hydrocortisone, fluid, and electrolyte replacement
  - Chronic therapy with oral hydrocortisone and fludrocortisone
  - Increased corticosteroids during stress
  - Maternal dexamethasone during pregnancy reduces virilization of female fetus

- **Pearl**

Hypertension occurs in 11-hydroxylase deficiency due to accumulation of 11-deoxycortisol.

Adrenocortical Hyperfunction (Cushing Syndrome)

- ### Essentials of Diagnosis
  - Adrenocortical hyperfunction occurs with adrenal tumor, adrenal hyperplasia, pituitary adenoma, ectopic ACTH producing tumors
  - Truncal adiposity, thin extremities, moon facies, muscle wasting, weakness, plethora, easy bruising, purple striae, decreased height gain, delayed skeletal maturation
  - Hypertension, osteoporosis, glycosuria, variable masculinization, menstrual irregularities, acne
  - Elevated plasma cortisol without diurnal variation, low serum potassium, high serum sodium and chloride, lymphopenia, eosinopenia, low ACTH in central disease, high ACTH in adrenal disease
  - Abnormal dexamethasone suppression test in adrenal disease
  - Pituitary imaging to demonstrate adenoma. Adrenal imaging to demonstrate hyperplasia or adenoma

10

- ### Differential Diagnosis
  - Exogenous administration of corticosteroid or ACTH
  - Exogenous obesity mimics adrenocortical hyperfunctional but stature and bone age are normal or mildly advanced. Striae are pink, not purple

- ### Treatment
  - Remove central or adrenal tumors if possible and supplement with corticosteroids if there is adrenal insufficiency postoperatively
  - Minotane (toxic to adrenal cortex) and aminoglutethimide (steroid synthesis inhibitor) have not been tested in children

- ### Pearl
  Measurement of midnight salivary cortisol is accurate. It is less invasive than venopuncture and allows for repeated measurements. Urinary free cortisol may be slightly elevated in obesity but the salivary cortisol measurement at midnight is normal.

Primary Hyperaldosteronism

- **Essentials of Diagnosis**
  - Most common cause is adrenal adenoma or adrenal hyperplasia secondary to familial hyperaldosteronism
  - Hypertension, paresthesias, tetany, weakness, polydipsia, enuresis, periodic paralysis
  - Hypokalemia, hypernatremia, metabolic alkalosis, abnormal glucose tolerance
  - Large-volume alkaline urine with inappropriately high potassium and low sodium
  - Elevated plasma and urine aldosterone with low plasma renin
  - Improved signs and symptoms after aldosterone antagonist (spironolactone)

- **Differential Diagnosis**
  - Renal disease or Bartter syndrome have associated hyperaldosteronism but the plasma renin is high

- **Treatment**
  - Surgery for tumors
  - Subtotal resection of adrenal gland for hyperplasia
  - Glucocorticoid therapy for hyperaldosteronism type 1
  - Spironolactone for familial hyperaldosteronism type 2

- **Pearl**

Glucocorticoid responsive familial hyperaldosteronism (type 1) is a rare autosomal dominant condition. Genetic screening is available and allows for early identification of asymptomatic family members before they develop severe hypertension or stroke.

Pheochromocytoma

- ■ Essentials of Diagnosis
  - • Uncommon tumor of chromaffin tissue (adrenal medulla, sympathetic ganglia, carotid body)
  - • Possibly due to disregulated (decreased) apoptosis of neural crest cells
  - • May be multiple, recurrent, and sometimes malignant
  - • Excess catecholamine secretion causes paroxysmal or chronic headache, sweating, tachycardia, hypertension, anxiety, dizziness, tremor, weakness, nausea, emesis diarrhea, dilated pupils
  - • Plasma-free metanephrine is 3X normal limit. Serum and urine catecholamines (VMA, HVA) elevated during symptoms
  - • Biologic imaging with I^{123} MIBG helps localize tumors

10

- ■ Differential Diagnosis
  - • Anxiety, psychosis
  - • Other causes of hypertension
  - • Carcinoid syndrome
  - • Drug abuse—amphetamines

- ■ Treatment
  - • α-Blockers and β-blockers to stabilize prior to surgery
  - • Surgical removal of tumor is treatment of choice but carries high risk of intra- and postoperative catecholamine excess or deficit
  - • Prognosis good after successful complete surgical resection
  - • Prognosis poor with metastatic disease usually associated with large extra-adrenal pheochromocytoma

- ■ Pearl

Pheochromocytoma is associated with 4 autosomal dominant pediatric syndromes-multiple endocrine neoplasia type IIA and IIB, von Hippel-Lindau syndrome, and type 1 neurofibromatosis.

Syndrome of Inappropriate Antidiuretic Hormone (SIADH)

- **Essentials of Diagnosis**
    - Anorexia, vomiting, headache, weakness, irritability, confusion, hallucinations, seizures, lethargy, coma
    - Expanded extracellular volume with inappropriately high vasopressin, low serum osmolality (<270 mOsm/L and low serum sodium
    - Decreased urine output with urine osmolality usually between 250 and 1400 mOsm/L

- **Differential Diagnosis**
    - CNS abnormalities—brain and meningeal infection, brain tumor or abscess, head trauma, hydrocephalus, neurosurgery, perinatal asphyxia, Guillain-Barré syndrome, postictal state
    - Paraneoplastic syndrome—oat cell carcinoma, bronchial carcinoid, lymphoma, Ewing sarcoma, and other tumors of the GI and renal system
    - Drugs-carbamazepine, lamotrigine, chlorpropamide, vinblastine, vincristine, tricyclic antidepressants
    - Acute intermittent porphyria

- **Treatment**
    - Fluid restriction (1 L/m^2/day)
    - When hyponatremia produces seizure or coma, 3% saline may be used

- **Pearl**

Increase sodium level by no more than 0.5 mM/L/h or 12 mM/L/day. Rapid correction of hyponatremia is associated with central pontine myelinolysis.

Type 1 Diabetes Mellitus

- Essentials of Diagnosis
  - Genetically determined disorder of glucose regulation due to immunologic destruction of insulin producing β cells of the pancreas with probable environmental trigger(s)
  - 90% of patients have islet cell, insulin, glutamic acid decarboxylase, and other autoantibodies present before clinical onset of diabetes. Role in β-cell destruction is not clear
  - Antibody screening identifies children at risk, but presentation with polyuria, polydipsia, and weight loss still occurs
  - Fasting plasma glucose >200 mg/dL or random plasma glucose >300 mg/dL suggests this diagnosis

- Differential Diagnosis
  - Low T_{max} for glucose causes glucosuria—glucose/galactose malabsorption, renal tubular disease
  - Reducing substances may cause a false-positive urine Clinitest—galactose, amino and acetyl salicylates, levadopa, ascorbate, large-dose nicotinamide, some antibiotics (sulfonamides, streptomycin, nitrofurantoin, cephalothin)
  - Transient hyperglycemia during stress, eg, infections, drug abuse

- Treatment
  - Cyclosporine A may preserve islet tissue for 1–2 years in new patients by inhibiting immune response but renal toxicity precludes its use
  - 5 modalities to maintain euglycemia—insulin replacement, appropriate diet, exercise, stress management, and monitoring of glucose and ketones
  - Insulin pumps have significantly improved glucose control in brittle type 1 patients
  - Monitor for complications—infection, renal function, retinopathy
  - Angiotensin-converting enzyme inhibitors may reverse or delay renal damage at the stage of microalbuminuria
  - Laser treatment to coagulate proliferating capillaries may prevent retinal detachment and vision loss

- Pearl

Free antibody screening is available for families of patients with type 1 diabetes (1-800-425-8361) and intervention trials are in progress to attempt to delay or prevent disease onset.

Type 2 Diabetes Mellitus

- **Essentials of Diagnosis**
    - Disorder of glucose regulation caused by insulin insensitivity. Strong genetic component. Risk increased by obesity (particularly central) and insufficient exercise
    - Blood sugar high but only 30% have ketonuria
    - Prevalence higher in females. Onset usually in midpuberty but may be as young as 4 years
    - Obese children of African, Asian, Hispanic, and Native American ethnicity at higher risk for type 2 diabetes
    - Findings include hyperglycemia, polycystic ovary syndrome, and acanthosis nigricans

10

- **Differential Diagnosis**
    - Insulin antibodies associated with other autoimmune disorders may cause apparent insulin resistance
    - Metabolic syndrome refers to individuals with hypertension, type 2 diabetes, hyperlipidemia, obesity, and elevated serum insulin

- **Treatment**
    - Prevent or reverse type 2 diabetes with weight loss and exercise.
    - Metformin reduces risk of type 2 diabetes by 31%
    - Other oral hypoglycemics may be used
    - Insulin may eventually be required in those in whom insulin secretion becomes insufficient

- **Pearl**

The incidence of type 2 diabetes is increasing dramatically. It is assumed that the increase is related to the concurrent increase in childhood obesity.

Ketoacidosis

- **Essentials of Diagnosis**
  - Ketonemia defined as blood ketone (β-hydroxy butyrate) >1 mM/L with hyperglycemia
  - Ketoacidosis defined as venous pH <7.30 with hyperglycemia and ketonemia
  - Symptoms of ketoacidosis—dehydration, fever, vasodilation, hyperglycemia, Kussmaul respiration, neurologic signs of cerebral edema (lethargy, headache, dilated pupils), severe abdominal pain (usually a result of hepatic swelling)
  - Cerebral edema may result from ketoacidosis or may be secondary to overhydration with hypotonic fluids

- **Differential Diagnosis**
  - Drug-induced hyperglycemia (ketosis rare)—steroids, thiazides, minoxidil, diazoxide, β-blockers
  - Glucagon-secreting tumors elevate blood sugar (ketosis rare)
  - Hyperthyroidism, fever, stress elevate blood sugar (ketosis rare)
  - Patients with type 2 diabetes may be hyperglycemic enough to have hyperosmotic symptoms without ketosis
  - Alcoholic ketoacidosis occurs with sudden alcohol withdrawal. Rare in children
  - Extremely high fat diet or starvation causes ketosis with normoglycemia
  - The abdominal pain associated with ketoacidosis may suggest a surgical abdomen, especially appendicitis

- **Treatment**
  - Principles of therapy in ketoacidosis—restore fluid volume, inhibit lipolysis, restore normal glucose utilization using insulin, correct total body sodium and potassium depletion, correct acidosis, prevent or treat cerebral edema
  - Ketonemia without acidosis—give 10–20% of total daily insulin dose subcutaneously (H, NL, or regular insulin) every 2–3 hours with oral fluids until ketonuria resolves
  - Caution must be exercised in treating fluid deficits in diabetic ketoacidosis to avoid hyponatremia and cerebral edema

- **Pearl**

Hypocalcemia can occur during treatment of diabetic ketoacidosis if all IV potassium is given as potassium phosphate. Hypophosphatemia results if no potassium phosphate is given. Use 50% potassium chloride or acetate and 50% potassium phosphate.

10

11

Inborn Errors of Metabolism

Glycogen Storage Diseases

- ■ Essentials of Diagnosis
  - Caused by enzyme defects in the synthesis and degradation of glycogen
  - Hepatic forms (I, III, IV, VI, IX) usually produce hepatomegaly, growth failure, fasting hypoglycemia, and acidosis
  - Myopathic forms produce weakness, rhabdomyolysis
  - Screening tests—low serum glucose with fasting. Elevated serum lactate, triglycerides, cholesterol, uric acid, and creatine kinase (in myopathic forms). Generally normal transaminases (except in type IV)
  - Confirmation by specific enzyme assay on leukocytes, liver, or muscle

- ■ Types of Glycogen Storage Disease
  - Type Ia (von Gierke disease) glucose-6-phosphatase deficiency produces typical hepatomegaly, hypoglycemia, acidosis
  - Type Ib glucose-6-phosphatase transporter deficiency also produces neutropenia with recurrent infection
  - Type II acid maltase deficiency (Pompe disease). Infantile form produces hypertrophic cardiomyopathy and macroglossia
  - Type III—debrancher enzyme deficiency, less severe symptoms
  - Type IV—brancher enzyme deficiency causes progressive cirrhosis
  - Type V and VII—muscle phosphorylase deficiency and phosphofructokinase deficiency
  - Type VI—hepatic phosphorylase deficiency—similar to Ia but milder
  - Type IX—phosphorylase kinase deficiency

- ■ Treatment
  - In hepatic forms, prevent fasting hypoglycemia and lactic acidosis. Frequent meals by day; support blood glucose during sleep with cornstarch feeding or enteral/parenteral carbohydrate administration
  - In hepatic forms—monitor for late development of hepatic adenoma, gout, focal segmental glomerulosclerosis
  - Enzyme replacement therapy may be effective in infantile Pompe disease, but cardiomyopathy usually requires cardiac transplant

- ■ Pearl

Hypoglycemia and massive hepatomegaly with normal spleen and normal serum transaminases should prompt evaluation for glycogen storage disease in infants, especially in the presence of acidosis, "unexplained" seizures, or failure to thrive.

Galactosemia

■ Essentials of Diagnosis

- Autosomal recessive defect in galactose-1-phospate uridyltrans-ferase
- Galactose-1-phosphate accumulates in liver and renal tubules after lactose ingestion causing liver damage and renal Fanconi syndrome
- Milk-fed infants develop emesis, acidosis, direct hyperbiliru-binemia, high transaminases, hepatomegaly, and hepatic dys-function
- Cataracts develop secondary to galactitol accumulation in the lens
- In severe enzyme deficiency, there is increased risk of language deficit, ovarian failure, mental retardation, tremor, and ataxia even with adequate dietary therapy
- Lactosuria, proteinuria, aminoaciduria, and hematuria present. Reducing substances present in urine without glucosuria
- Diagnosis by elevated galactose-1-phosphate in red cells or enzyme assay on red blood cells. Newborn screening available

■ Differential Diagnosis

- Sepsis of the newborn
- Milder variants of galactosemia have better prognosis
- Hereditary fructose intolerance, urea cycle abnormalities produce neonatal liver dysfunction and emesis

■ Treatment

- Newborn screening allows for early dietary therapy
- Lifelong avoidance of lactose with calcium supplementation
- Monitor compliance with diet by measuring galactose-1-phosphate concentration in red blood cells

■ Pearl

Newborns with Escherichia coli *septicemia should be evaluated for galactosemia.*

Hereditary Fructose Intolerance

- **Essentials of Diagnosis**
  - Autosomal recessive deficiency of fructose-1-phosphate aldolase
  - Hypoglycemia and tissue accumulation of fructose-1-phosphate after ingestion of fructose
  - Symptoms—failure to thrive, vomiting, direct hyperbilirubinemia, hepatomegaly, fructosuria, proteinuria, aminoaciduria, and liver failure upon ingestion of fructose or sucrose
  - Fructose-1-phosphate aldolase is assayed in liver biopsy
  - IV fructose loading test causes a diagnostic hypoglycemia and hypophosphatemia but is a significant risk to the patient

- **Differential Diagnosis**
  - Galactosemia
  - Glycogen storage disease (especially type IV)
  - Neonatal severe bacterial infections
  - Acute or chronic hepatitis
  - Neonatal iron storage disease

- **Treatment**
  - Strict dietary avoidance of fructose and sucrose
  - Vitamin supplementation
  - Monitor dietary compliance by transferrin glycoform analysis

- **Pearl**

Sucrose (disaccharide of fructose and glucose) is found in so many foods and medications that diet management of fructose intolerance is difficult. Later, children voluntarily avoid fruits and sweets. They develop dental caries so rarely that a dentist sometimes makes this diagnosis.

Disorders of Energy Metabolism

- **Essentials of Diagnosis**
  - Most of the common disorders of mitochondrial metabolism involve pyruvate dehydrogenase (PD) and mitochondrial respiratory chain complexes
  - Disorders of gluconeogenesis are less common—pyruvate carboxylase deficiency, fructose-diphosphatase deficiency, glycogen storage disease type I
  - Elevated lactate in blood or cerebrospinal fluid (CSF) with normal lactate/pyruvate ratio in PD deficiency and increased ratio in respiratory chain abnormalities
  - Symptoms involve many systems—variable dysfunction of brain, muscles, kidney, endocrine, cardiac, gastrointestinal, liver, pancreas
  - Inheritance is both autosomal recessive and maternal via the mitochondrial genome
  - Ragged red fibers and abnormal mitochondria are found in skeletal muscle. Enzyme assay in fibroblasts or muscle available in some cases

- **Differential Diagnosis**
  - Secondary lactic acidosis caused by hypoxia, ischemia, or sampling error
  - Multiple carboxylase deficiency
  - D-Lactic acidosis—bacterial fermentation in the intestine produces D-lactate, which causes encephalopathy when absorbed in large quantities. D-lactic acidosis is often missed because most laboratories measure only L-lactate.
  - Fatty acid oxidation defects

- **Treatment**
  - Treatments for PD deficiency have variable effectiveness—ketogenic diet, lipoic acid, dichloroacetate, and thiamine
  - Treat coenzyme Q deficiency with exogenous coenzyme Q
  - Treatment of respiratory chain defects—coenzyme Q and riboflavin occasionally helpful

- **Pearl**

Suspect disorders of energy metabolism when infants present with acidosis accompanied by chronic dysfunction or deterioration of several organ systems at the same time.

Disorders of the Urea Cycle

- ■ Essentials of Diagnosis
    - Ammonia produced during catabolism of amino acids is excreted as urea through the action of the urea cycle enzymes
    - Defects in ornithine transcarbamoylase, carbamoyl phosphate synthetase, arginosuccinate synthase, and arginosuccinate lyase present in neonates with hyperpnea, emesis, alkalosis, hyperammonemia, and fatal encephalopathy
    - Milder defects in these enzymes have milder encephalopathy and hyperammonemia during intercurrent illness or high protein intake
    - Arginase deficiency presents with spastic tetraplegia and behavioral changes in childhood
    - Elevated serum ammonia is the key to initial diagnosis
    - Newborn screening available in many states

- ■ Differential Diagnosis
    - Glutaric acidemia type II and other fatty acid oxidation defects
    - Acute or chronic liver failure causes hyperammonemia
    - Propionic acidemia and other organic acidopathies
    - Transient hyperammonemia of the newborn
    - Mitochondrial ornithine transporter defect produces high serum ammonia, ornithine and homocitrulline (HHH syndrome)

- ■ Treatment
    - Hemodialysis required in severely affected neonates
    - In hyperammonemic crisis, protein intake should be stopped and glucose given
    - IV arginine increases nitrogen excretion in citrullinemia and arginosuccinic aciduria
    - Sodium benzoate and sodium phenylacetate increase ammonia excretion in all urea cycle defects
    - Long-term therapy—low protein diet, supplemental oral arginine, citrulline, sodium benzoate, or sodium phenylacetate
    - Liver transplantation may be curative but does not reverse brain injury caused by neonatal hyperammonemia

- ■ Pearl

A neonate with tachypnea, alkalosis, and vomiting should be evaluated immediately for a urea cycle defect. Stop oral protein intake and give IV glucose while awaiting initial laboratory evaluation.

Phenylketonuria (PKU)

- ■ Essentials of Diagnosis
  - • Deficiency of phenylalanine hydroxylase occurs in 1:10,000 Caucasian births. Autosomal recessive
  - • Symptoms—mental retardation, hyperactivity, seizures, light complexion, eczematoid skin rash
  - • Severe deficiency associated with serum phenylalanine >20 mg/dL on regular diet. Low or normal serum tyrosine and normal pterins
  - • Newborn screening is highly reliable

- ■ Differential Diagnosis
  - • Normal offspring of mothers with PKU may have transient hyperphenylalaninemia at birth
  - • Dihydropteridine reductase deficiency produces elevated pterin metabolites, seizures, and psychomotor regression secondary to neuronal serotonin and dopamine deficiency in affected infants
  - • Defects in biopterin synthesis produce low serum pterins and variable phenylalanine. Symptoms include myoclonus, tetraplegia, dystonia, oculogyric crises
  - • Benign tyrosinemia with moderate hyperphenylalaninemia occurs in premature infants due to transient 4-hydroxyphenylpyruvic acid oxidase deficiency

- ■ Treatment
  - • Lifelong limitation of dietary phenylalanine to maintain serum level <6 mg/dL
  - • Dietary therapy is most effective when started at birth, but may also improve hyperactivity, irritability, and distractibility if started later in life
  - • Poorly controlled diet during pregnancy causes mental retardation, microcephaly, growth retardation, and congenital heart disease in the fetus

- ■ Pearl

Control of PKU during pregnancy is important as elevated phenylalanine is teratogenic. Female patients should be encouraged to use contraceptives to prevent accidental conception and accidental injury to the fetus.

Hereditary Tyrosinemia

- **Essentials of Diagnosis**
  - Type 1 (infantile) tyrosinemia caused by deficiency of fumaryl-acetoacetase
  - Symptoms of type 1 tyrosinemia—severe hepatic synthetic failure, porphyria, renal tubular dystrophy, aminoaciduria, hypophosphatemic rickets, and neuropathic crises—caused by accumulation of toxic metabolites maleylacetoacetate, fumarylacetoacetate, and succinylacetone
  - Key diagnostic test is elevated urinary succinylacetone
  - Late presenting forms have milder symptoms. Hepatocellular carcinoma is a late complication
  - Newborn screening is possible but not routine in some areas

- **Differential Diagnosis**
  - Galactosemia, hereditary fructose intolerance, mitochondrial disease
  - Tylenol overdose
  - Many chronic liver diseases have elevated serum amino acids including tyrosine
  - Niemann-Pick type C
  - Neonatal hemochromatosis

- **Treatment**
  - 2-(2-nitro-4-trifluoromethylbenzoyl)-1,3-cyclohexanedione (NTBC) decreases production of toxic metabolites and improves liver, renal, and neurologic disease
  - When started early, NTBC reduces the risk of hepatocellular carcinoma
  - Low phenylalanine, low tyrosine diet improves liver disease but does not prevent development of hepatocellular carcinoma
  - Liver transplant is curative

- **Pearl**

This autosomal recessive condition is especially common in Scandinavia and in the Chicoutimi-Lac St. Jean region of Quebec.

Maple Syrup Urine Disease (Branched-Chain Ketoaciduria) (MSUD)

- **Essentials of Diagnosis**
  - Autosomal recessive deficiency of enzyme catalyzing oxidative decarboxylation of keto acid forms of leucine, isoleucine, and valine
  - Only leucine and its keto acid cause central nervous system (CNS) dysfunction
  - Feeding problems, seizures, coma develop at 4–10 days of age. Fatal if not treated
  - Affected patients have increased serum branched chain amino acids. Alloisoleucine in serum is pathognomonic
  - Newborn screening is available

- **Differential Diagnosis**
  - Variants of this condition are milder, intermittent, and thiamin dependent
  - Other neonatal CNS disease—infection, trauma, degenerative disorders may mimic MSUD
  - Other organic acidopathies such as propionic aciduria
  - Urea cycle defects present at a similar age with CNS dysfunction

- **Treatment**
  - Formula deficient in branched-chain amino acids is supplemented with small amounts of normal milk
  - Serum levels of branched-chain amino acids monitored frequently
  - Isoleucine and valine are usually supplemented
  - Normal growth and development are achieved if therapy started within 10 days of birth
  - Thiamine is effective in rare (milder) forms

- **Pearl**

This condition gets its name from the sweet smell of the keto acids of isoleucine.

Homocystinuria

- ■ Essentials of Diagnosis
  - Autosomal recessive deficiency of cystathionine β-synthase
  - Patients have mental retardation, arachnodactyly, osteoporosis, and dislocated ocular lens
  - Thromboembolism is a major cause of morbidity and mortality
  - Diagnosis confirmed by finding homocystinuria, elevated blood homocysteine and methionine in the setting of vitamin B_{12} sufficiency
  - Newborn screening available

- ■ Differential Diagnosis
  - Vitamin B_{12} deficiency
  - Marfan syndrome patients have similar arachnodactyly and lens dislocation
  - Defects in methionine synthase or methylene tetrahydrofolate reductase deficiency (remethylation defects) cause elevated homocysteine with low methionine

- ■ Treatment
  - 50% of patients with cystathionine β-synthase deficiency respond to high-dose pyridoxine
  - Neurologic prognosis better in pyridoxine responders
  - Treat pyridoxine nonresponders with dietary restriction of methionine
  - Surgical correction of dislocated lens is often required
  - Betaine and vitamin B_{12} supplementation

- ■ Pearl

Early dietary restriction of methionine in pyridoxine nonresponders may improve or prevent mental retardation, thromboembolic events, and lens dislocations.

Nonketotic Hyperglycinemia (NKH)

- **Essentials of Diagnosis**
  - Autosomal recessive deficiency of various subunits of the glycine cleavage enzyme system
  - Glycine accumulation in brain disturbs neurotransmission of the glycinergic and N-methyl-D-aspartate receptor
  - In severe disease, newborns display hypotonia, lethargy, myoclonic seizures, apnea requiring ventilatory support, coma, hiccups, burst suppression pattern on electroencephalogram (EEG)
  - Some patients have agenesis of corpus callosum or posterior fossa malformations
  - High CSF glycine with high ratio of CSF to serum glycine is diagnostic

- **Differential Diagnosis**
  - Sulfite oxidase deficiency
  - Molybdenum cofactor deficiency
  - Pyridoxine responsive seizures
  - Folinic acid responsive seizures
  - Hypoxic-ischemic encephalopathy
  - Sepsis

- **Treatment**
  - Prenatal diagnosis by chorionic villus samples or molecular analysis is possible if the genetic mutation is known
  - High-dose sodium benzoate improves serum glycine levels but does not correct CSF levels
  - Dextromethorphan or ketamine blocks seizures
  - Treatment does not improve mental retardation

- **Pearl**

NKH should be suspected in any infant with intractable seizures, especially when accompanied by hiccups. Mothers may report that the infant has hiccups in utero.

Propionic and Methylmalonic Acidemia

- **Essentials of Diagnosis**

  - *Propionic acidemia*—deficiency of propionyl-CoA carboxylase activity
  - *Methylmalonic acidemia*—deficiency of methylmalonyl-CoA mutase
  - Neonates with severe deficiency of either enzyme have life-threatening metabolic acidosis, hyperammonemia, and bone marrow depression
  - Late complications—failure to thrive, emesis, mental retardation, pancreatitis, cardiomyopathy, basal ganglia strokes, and interstitial nephritis (methylmalonic acidemia)
  - Mass spectrometry on urine reveals elevated propionic or methylmalonic acid
  - Newborn screening available

- **Differential Diagnosis**

  - Defects in processing of vitamin B_{12} cause elevated serum methylmalonic acid
  - Genetically normal newborns of mothers with B_{12} deficiency during pregnancy have abnormal newborn screening tests for propionic and methylmalonic acidemia
  - Isovaleric acidemia or MSUD

- **Treatment**

  - Large-dose vitamin B_{12} is effective in some patients with methylmalonylic acidemia
  - Dietary restriction of threonine, valine, methionine, and isoleucine
  - Carnitine supplementation enhances propionyl-carnitine excretion
  - Intermittent metronidazole reduces propionate absorbed from the gut
  - Combined renal and liver transplant has been performed without significant success

- **Pearl**

Methylmalonic and propionic acidemia cannot be distinguished from each other by newborn screening.

Isovaleric Acidemia

- **Essentials of Diagnosis**
    - Autosomal recessive deficiency of isovaleryl-CoA dehydrogenase in the leucine oxidative pathway
    - Presentation in infancy—poor feeding, metabolic acidosis, and seizures. Coma and death if untreated
    - Patients with partial deficiency have bouts of emesis, hair loss, lethargy, and pancreatitis during intercurrent illness or excess protein intake
    - Isovalerylglycine present in urine
    - Intrauterine diagnosis is available
    - Newborn screening available

- **Differential Diagnosis**
    - May resemble other mild organic acidemia or mitochondrial defects

- **Treatment**
    - Low protein diet or diet low in leucine is effective
    - Conjugation of isovaleric acid with glycine or carnitine
    - Outcome is good with adequate dietary therapy

- **Pearl**

Excess isovalerylglycine in the urine and body secretions reminds some clinicians of the smell of sweaty feet.

Multiple Carboxylase Deficiency

- ■ Essentials of Diagnosis
    - • Defect in synthesis of biotin, biotin-containing carboxylases (holo-carboxylase synthetase deficiency), and recycling of enzyme-linked biotin (biotinidase deficiency)
    - • Holocarboxylase deficiency becomes symptomatic at 2–6 weeks, biotinidase deficiency at 2–6 months
    - • Presentation of holocarboxylase deficiency—lethargy, hypotonia, vomiting, seizures, lactic acidosis, and hyperammonemia
    - • Biotinidase deficiency—ataxia, seizures, progressive hearing loss, seborrhea, and alopecia
    - • Newborn screening for biotinidase deficiency available

- ■ Differential Diagnosis
    - • Pyruvate carboxylase deficiency has similar laboratory findings
    - • Organic acidopathies such as propionic acidemia

- ■ Treatment
    - • Treat holocarboxylase synthetase deficiency with high-dose biotin and dietary protein restriction
    - • Biotinidase deficiency is well controlled with exogenous biotin
    - • Early use of biotin prevents hearing loss in biotinidase deficiency
    - • Once established, hearing loss in biotinidase deficiency persists despite therapy

- ■ Pearl

The urine of patients with multiple carboxylase deficiency has been described as smelling like cat urine.

Glutaric Acidemia Type I

- ■ Essentials of Diagnosis
    - • Autosomal deficiency of glutaryl-CoA dehydrogenase
    - • Progressive extrapyramidal movement disorder with episodic acidosis and encephalopathy in first 4 years of life
    - • Diagnosis by assay of glutaryl-CoA dehydrogenase in fibroblasts; increased glutaric and 3-OH-glutaric acid in urine, serum or amniotic fluid, or by mutation analysis
    - • Brain magnetic resonance imaging (MRI) shows frontotemporal atrophy, macrocephaly, and large sylvian fissures
    - • Newborn screening available

- ■ Differential Diagnosis
    - • Glutaric acidemia type II caused by deficiency in electron transfer flavoprotein with glutaric and other organic acids and sarcosine in serum and urine
    - • Type II symptoms—episodic hypoglycemia, acidosis, hyperammonemia, polycystic, dysplastic kidneys
    - • Other organic acidemias, primary lactic acidosis, and urea cycle disorders may mimic symptoms
    - • Nonaccidental head trauma may cause similar MRI findings

- ■ Treatment
    - • Prevention of catabolism during intercurrent illness and supplemental carnitine may prevent basal ganglia degeneration in type I
    - • Restriction of dietary lysine and tryptophan
    - • Symptomatic treatment of severe dystonia is sometimes required

- ■ Pearl

Children with type I glutaric acidemia may present with retinal hemorrhages, intracranial bleeding, and encephalopathy, which may be attributed to child abuse unless metabolic screening is performed.

Long- and Medium-Chain Acyl-CoA Dehydrogenase Deficiency

- **■ Essentials of Diagnosis**
  - Deficiency of very-long- and medium-chain acyl-CoA dehydrogenase (VLCAD, MCAD, and long-chain 3-hydroxyacyl-CoA dehydrogenase [LCHAD]) cause episodic hypoketotic hypoglycemia, hyperammonemia, hepatomegaly, and encephalopathy with elevated liver chemistries
  - LCHAD deficiency may cause progressive hepatic cirrhosis, peripheral neuropathy, and retinitis pigmentosa
  - MCAD deficiency is relatively common (1:9000 live births)
  - MCAD deficient patients excrete hexanoylglycine, suberylglycine, and phenylpropionylglycine in urine during episodes and are measurable by mass spectrometry
  - Screening test of choice is analysis of acylcarnitine esters. **11** Newborn screening available

- **■ Differential Diagnosis**
  - Carnitine palmitoyltransferase I and II and carnitine acylcarnitine translocase deficiency cause similar episodes with hypotonia, myopathy, cardiomyopathy, and ventricular arrhythmia
  - Glutaric acidemia type II
  - Trifunctional protein deficiency is a rare disorder with multiple defects in long-chain fat metabolism

- **■ Treatment**
  - Prevent and/or treat hypoglycemia by avoiding fasting
  - Oral carnitine is sometimes helpful
  - Restrict nonessential long-chain fats in VLCAD, LCHAD, and possibly MCAD
  - Medium-chain triglycerides contraindicated in MCAD but are essential in VLCAD and LCHAD deficiency
  - Outcome in MCAD deficiency is excellent with treatment. Outcome less optimistic in VLCAD and LCHAD deficiency

- **■ Pearl**

Rarely, "sudden infant death syndrome" has been shown to be the result of hypoglycemia secondary to VLCAD, MCAD, or LCHAD deficiency. Mothers carrying fetuses affected by LCHAD may develop HELLP syndrome (hypertension, elevated liver function tests, and low platelets).

Hypoxanthine-Guanine Phosphoribosyl Transferase Deficiency (Lesch-Nyhan Syndrome)

- **Essentials of Diagnosis**
  - Hypoxanthine-guanine phosphoribosyltransferase (HPRT) converts hypoxanthine and guanine to inosine and guanosine monophosphate
  - Complete deficiency causes purine overproduction with hyperuricemia and increased urinary uric acid/creatinine ratio
  - X-linked recessive
  - Affected males have choreoathetosis, spasticity, aggressiveness, cognitive deficits, compulsive lip and finger biting, gouty arthritis, renal and ureteral stones, subcutaneous urate tophi
  - Enzyme assayed in erythrocytes, fibroblasts, and amniotic cells

- **Differential Diagnosis**
  - Cerebral palsy
  - Dystonia
  - Behavioral abnormalities, autism

- **Treatment**
  - Hydration and alkalinization prevent kidney stones and nephropathy
  - Allopurinol and probenecid reduce hyperuricemia and gout but do not treat neurologic disease
  - Benzodiazepines may reduce extrapyramidal symptoms
  - Physical restraint may be needed to prevent self-mutilation

- **Pearl**

Self-injurious behavior is rarely the presenting symptom of Lesch-Nyhan syndrome but eventually emerges in almost all patients and may point to the diagnosis in children with unexplained growth failure and developmental delay.

Lysosomal Disorders

- **Essentials of Diagnosis**
  - Lysosomes contain acid hydrolases needed to degrade numerous complex macromolecules
  - Deficiency in lysosomal enzymes causes accumulation of mucopolysaccharides, complex lipids, or mucolipids
  - Hurler syndrome (α-iduronidase) is a typical mucopolysaccharidosis—mental retardation, hepatosplenomegaly, coarse facies, corneal clouding, vertebral degeneration, cardiac disease
  - Mannosidosis (α-mannosidase) is a typical mucolipidosis—coarse facies, bony deformities, mental retardation
  - Niemann-Pick disease (sphingomyelinase) is a typical lipidosis—hepatosplenomegaly, degenerative neurologic disease, macular cherry red spot

- **Differential Diagnosis**
  - Cystinosis and Salla disease are caused by defects in lysosomal proteins transporting material from lysosome to cytoplasm
  - Urine screening tests can detect mucopolysaccharides and oligosaccharides, which point to specific enzyme deficiency diagnosis

- **Treatment**
  - Stem cell transplantation holds some promise especially in Hurler syndrome, Gaucher disease, Fabry disease, and Pompe disease
  - Enzyme replacement therapy is commercially available for Pompe disease, Fabry disease, Gaucher disease, Hunter disease, Hurler syndrome, and Maroteaux-Lamy syndrome. This therapy is only effective for non-neurologic symptoms

- **Pearl**

Accumulation of abnormal mucopolysaccharides and lipids causes abnormalities of bone, viscera, CNS, and RE system. Growth failure, neurodegeneration, organomegaly, and coarse facies are typical findings in many of these conditions.

Peroxisomal Disorders

- **Essentials of Diagnosis**
  - Peroxisomal enzymes catalyze β-oxidation of very-long-chain (VLC) fatty acids, metabolize phytanic acid, and synthesize ether phospholipids, bile acids, and other products
  - Peroxisomal disorders caused by defects in generation of peroxisomes (Zellweger spectrum) or defects in individual peroxisomal enzymes
  - All peroxisomal enzymes are deficient in Zellweger disease—profound neonatal hypotonia, seizures, tower skull, cholestasis, renal cystic disease, ocular disease, bone disease death in first year of life
  - VLC fatty acids elevated
  - Peroxisomes are absent in liver biopsy in Zellweger disease
  - Isolated peroxisomal enzyme deficiencies include
    - Primary hyperoxaluria—renal stones and nephropathy
    - Adrenoleukodystrophy—VLC fatty acid transporter deficiency
    - Adrenomyeloneuropathy
    - Infantile Refsum disease—phytanic acid oxidative defect
    - Abnormal plasmalogen synthesis causes rhizomelic chondrodysplasia punctata

- **Differential Diagnosis**
  - Mitochondrial defects
  - Lysosomal storage diseases

- **Treatment**
  - Bone marrow transplantation may be effective in early adrenoleukodystrophy
  - Lorenzo's oil, very low fat diet and essential fatty acid supplementation but may help prevent symptoms in presymptomatic adrenoleukodystrophy
  - Zellweger disease is almost always fatal
  - Diet therapy for adult Refsum disease
  - Liver transplantation protects kidneys in primary hyperoxaluria

- **Pearl**

Hypotonia in patients with Zellweger disease may be apparent in utero. It is so profound that these neonates may be unable to suck or swallow.

Carbohydrate-Deficient Glycoprotein (CDG) Syndromes

- **Essentials of Diagnosis**

  - Many enzymes require glycosylation for normal function. If glycosylation enzyme systems are abnormal, many organs and functions are affected
  - *Type Ia* is the most common form—in utero growth retardation (small for gestational age [SGA]), abnormal fat distribution, cerebellar hypoplasia, dysmorphic features, and psychomotor retardation
  - *Type Ia* disease has abnormalities of liver function, peripheral and CNS, endocrine function, and retina
  - *Type Ib* disease has liver fibrosis, protein-losing enteropathy, and hypoglycemia
  - Isoelectric focusing of serum transferrin (an easily measured glycosylated protein) is needed for diagnosis

11

- **Differential Diagnosis**

  - >12 forms of CDG disease recognized
  - Other findings include coloboma, cutis laxa, epilepsy, ichthyosis, Dandy-Walker malformation

- **Treatment**

  - Supportive treatment for functional deficiencies
  - Mannose supplementation may benefit patients with type Ib disease

- **Pearl**

When multiple organ system functions in the neonate are affected, especially in association with hepatic functional abnormalities, consider type Ia CDG syndrome.

Smith-Lemli-Opitz (SLO) Syndrome

- **Essentials of Diagnosis**
    - Autosomal recessive deficiency of 7-dehydrocholesterol δ^7-reductase
    - Neonatal onset microcephaly, poor growth, mental retardation, dysmorphic facies, 2–3 toe syndactyly, heart and renal abnormalities
    - Intrauterine demise or neonatal death occurs in severe cases
    - Routine serum cholesterol may be low but a normal level does not exclude SLO syndrome. Fractionation of cholesterol reveals diagnostic elevation of 7- and 8-dehydrocholesterol in serum, amniotic fluid, or other tissues

- **Differential Diagnosis**
    - Conradi-Hünermann syndrome—low cholesterol with chondrodysplasia punctata and atrophic skin
    - Mevalonic aciduria—low cholesterol and developmental delay
    - Trisomy 13 or trisomy 18 sometimes resembles severe SLO syndrome

- **Treatment**
    - Postnatal therapy does not resolve the prenatal injury
    - Cholesterol supplementation improves growth and behavior in SLO syndrome. Most effective in mildly affected patients

- **Pearl**

Cholesterol is covalently bound to the embryonic signaling protein "sonic hedgehog" and is necessary for its normal function. Abnormal function of SHH in early gestation probably causes the multiple congenital abnormalities in SLO syndrome.

12

Genetics and Dysmorphology

Trisomy 21 (Down Syndrome)

- ■ Epidemiology and Clinical Diagnosis
  - 1:600 live births. Incidence greater with maternal age >35 years
  - Microcephaly, upslanting palpebral fissures, epicanthal folds, midface hypoplasia, small pinnae, minor limb anomalies
  - 30% have congenital heart disease (endocardial cushion, other septal defects). 15% have gastrointestinal (GI) anomalies (esophageal atresia, duodenal atresia, Hirschsprung disease, and others)
  - Mental retardation, hypotonia, short stature, delayed puberty, male sterility, neonatal jaundice, polycythemia, transient leukemoid reactions, leukemia

- ■ Diagnostic Testing
  - Postnatal diagnosis is made by chromosome analysis of infant
  - Second trimester maternal serum showing ↓unconjugated estriol, ↓serum α-fetoprotein, and ↑human chorionic gonadotropin compared to mothers of same age and week of pregnancy suggests Down syndrome
  - Most characteristic intrauterine ultrasound finding in fetuses with Down syndrome is increased nuchal fold thickness (edema). Other cardiac, skeletal, and GI anomalies can be detected
  - Cytogenetic analysis of chorionic villus sample or amniocentesis is the only certain prenatal test

- ■ Genetic Mechanisms
  - Risk increases with maternal age >35 years
  - Aneuploidy causing trisomy of chromosome 21 is most common mechanism
  - Mosaic Down syndrome—nondisjunction of chromosome 21 early in embryogenesis produces 1 normal cell line and 1 with trisomy 21
  - Translocation Down syndrome (familial)—translocation of long arm 21 to chromosome 14 (or rarely chromosome 21)
  - Duplication of long arm of 21—rare disorder with Down syndrome phenotype

- ■ Pearl

Paternal age is not a risk factor for Down syndrome, but translocation Down syndrome may be transmitted by the father.

Trisomy 18

- **Essentials of Diagnosis**
  - Incidence 1:4000 live births. Male/female ratio is 1:3
  - Second most common aneuploid disorder after Down syndrome caused by nondisjunction during meiosis. Mosaic forms also occur
  - Prenatal and postnatal growth retardation, hypertonicity, facial dysmorphism, small jaw, low-set ears, microcephaly, overlapping fingers, rocker bottom feet, renal and genital anomalies, brain malformations, severe developmental retardation
  - Cardiac anomalies—ventricular septal defect, atrial septal defect, patent ductus arteriosus, coarctation of the aorta
  - 50–90% of fetuses with trisomy 18 die in utero. 5–10% of live born infants survive more than 1 year
  - Death usually caused by inanition, apnea, heart failure, renal failure, or infection in infancy
  - Confirmation of diagnosis by simple chromosome analysis

12

- **Differential Diagnosis**
  - Little doubt about this diagnosis based on typical features

- **Treatment**
  - There is no treatment
  - Supportive care with attention to nutrition
  - Medical therapy of cardiac disease may prolong life. Surgical intervention is decided upon after careful consideration of ultimate long- and short-term survival
  - Recurrence risk in subsequent pregnancies very low for full trisomy 18

- **Pearl**

Increased maternal age is a risk factor for trisomy 18. The additional chromosome is almost always maternal in origin.

Fragile X Syndrome

- ■ Epidemiology and Clinical Diagnosis
  - Affects 1:1000 males
  - Affected males have developmental delay, hyperactivity, autistic traits, oblong facies, large ears, large testicles, hyperextensible joints, mitral valve prolapse
  - 50% of affected females have normal IQ. 50% have mild/moderate learning disabilities and behavioral problems
  - Male and female patients with premutation may have mild physical traits, developmental and behavioral problems
  - Females with premutation may have premature ovarian failure. Older males with premutation may develop tremor and ataxia

- ■ Diagnosis
  - DNA analysis can identify the amplified area in affected individuals and carriers
  - Prenatal diagnosis by chorionic villus sampling or amniocentesis is possible
  - Consider this diagnosis in male children with behavioral problems, learning disabilities or autism, and mild facial dysmorphism

- ■ Genetic Mechanism
  - Triplet instability—excess number of cytosine-guanine-guanine (CGG) repeats (51–200) at the 5' end of *FMR-1* gene causes a premutation that may become a full mutation (>200 repeats) in successive generations
  - "Anticipation"—symptoms become manifest at earlier ages and with increasing severity in successive generations
  - Premutation can become a full mutation only when passed through a female

- ■ Pearl

Aggressive behavior stimulated by anxiety, impulsivity, hyperarousal, and mood instability affects 40% of males with fragile X. It may worsen during puberty.

Myotonic Dystrophy (DM1)

- ■ Essentials of Diagnosis
  - • Autosomal dominant disorder associated with anticipation. Unstable CTG triplet in the *DMPK* gene on chromosome 19 expands with each generation
  - • Adults with 50–100 repeats have cataracts without myotonia. Adults with >100 repeats have myotonia. Myotonia develops in childhood with >400 repeats
  - • Intrauterine (800–2000 repeats) myotonus causes polyhydramnios and arthrogryposis which may be fatal
  - • Symptoms in children—progressive distal weakness and muscle stiffness, facial weakness with dysphagia and ptosis, muscle wasting, fatigue, constipation, cognitive problems
  - • DNA analysis can identify genetic defect and number of repeats

- ■ Differential Diagnosis
  - • Other forms of myotonic dystrophy have been associated with mutations on chromosomes 16 and 21
  - • DM2 myotonic dystrophy is a milder phenotype. Number of repeats very high. No anticipation phenomenon. No correlation between number of repeats and symptom severity
  - • Other muscular dystrophies
  - • Early symptoms are sometimes very nonspecific—weakness, constipation, fatigue. Emotional problems may be suspected

- ■ Treatment
  - • No specific therapy
  - • Genetic counseling
  - • Nutrition support in very affected children may require tube feedings

- ■ Pearl

The diagnosis of myotonic dystrophy can sometimes be made on a handshake. The patient grips your hand but has difficulty releasing the grip.

Friedreich Ataxia

- **Essentials of Diagnosis**
  - Autosomal recessive disorder with anticipation. Unstable triplet (GAA) in the *FDRA* gene on chromosome 9 expands with successive generations
  - Normal individuals carry 7–33 GAA repeats. 96% of affected patients are homozygous for >66 repeats
  - Mutation in *FDRA* suppresses synthesis of frataxin, a protein needed in nerve and muscle mitochondria for iron removal
  - In adolescence—onset of ataxia, nystagmus, abnormal gait, scoliosis, ↓reflexes, ↓light touch and position sense, dysarthria, cardiomyopathy, diabetes mellitus, high arched feet (pes cavus)
  - Death occurs 30–40 years from heart failure or dysrhythmia

- **Differential Diagnosis**
  - Other forms with point mutations of the *FDRA* gene occur
  - Dominant hereditary ataxia—CAG trinucleotide repeats
  - Ataxia telangiectasia
  - Wilson disease
  - Refsum disease
  - Rett syndrome
  - Vitamin E deficiency—celiac disease, a-β-lipoproteinemia

- **Treatment**
  - No effective therapy
  - Antiarrhythmic medications for late cardiac disease
  - Some reports that idebenone (coenzyme Q-like drug that improves antioxidant function) improves heart disease

- **Pearl**

Cardiac disease associated with Friedreich ataxia is a hypertrophic cardiomyopathy.

12

Turner Syndrome

- ■ Essentials of Diagnosis
  - 1:10,000 live female births
  - Monosomy of the X chromosome is the most common mechanism. 45X mosaicism also occurs with similar phenotype
  - Only 5% of fetuses with Turner syndrome are live born. Most are spontaneously aborted
  - Newborn findings—webbed neck, generalized edema, coarctation of aorta, triangular facies
  - Older patient findings—short stature, shield chest, wide set nipples, streak ovaries, amenorrhea, absent puberty, infertility, renal anomalies, late gonadoblastoma
  - Learning disabilities are common. Caused by defects in perceptual motor integration
  - Postnatal diagnosis by standard chromosome analysis

- ■ Differential Diagnosis
  - Pseudohypoparathyroidism—similar skeletal findings
  - Noonan syndrome—similar phenotype with normal chromosomes

- ■ Treatment
  - Monitor and treat perceptual problems early
  - Short stature treated with human growth hormone (GH)
  - At puberty estrogen replacement therapy prevents osteoporosis, permits normal secondary sex characteristics and normal menses

- ■ Pearl

Women with Turner syndrome have low fertility and high rate of spontaneous abortion or stillbirth. Live infants of mothers with Turner syndrome have increased chromosomal and congenital anomalies.

Klinefelter Syndrome (XXY)

- **Essentials of Diagnosis**
  - Incidence 1:1000 male births. Accounts for 1% of retarded males and 3% of infertile males
  - Klinefelter syndrome is not a cause of spontaneous abortions
  - Normal phenotype in preadolescence delays diagnosis
  - Findings after puberty—micro-orchidism, normal penis, azoospermia, gynecomastia, ↓facial hair, ↓libido, tall eunuchoid body habitus
  - Chromosomal variants with 3–4 X chromosomes have more severe mental retardation, radioulnar stenosis, abnormalities of external genitalia
  - Multiple X chromosomes may allow expression of normally recessive X-linked genes
  - Increased risk of germ cell tumors
  - Karyotyping is the only secure diagnostic test

- **Differential Diagnosis**
  - Fragile X syndrome
  - Hypogonadism
  - Marfan syndrome

- **Treatment**
  - Testosterone replacement therapy during puberty
  - Monitor for germ cell tumors
  - Psychosocial counseling

- **Pearl**

Increased maternal age is a risk factor for Klinefelter syndrome.

Wolf-Hirschhorn Syndrome (4p-)

- **Epidemiology and Clinical Diagnosis**
  - Females more often affected. Incidence 1:50,000 live births
  - No family history in 85%
  - Typical facial features—microcephaly, high frontal hairline, frontal bossing, wide-set eyes, hooked nose, cleft lip and palate, coloboma
  - Other features—hypotonia; hearing loss; seizures; ataxia; mental retardation; renal and cardiac anomalies; short stature; malformations of hands, feet, spine, and chest
  - Risk of Wolf-Hirschhorn syndrome in subsequent pregnancies very low

- **Diagnosis**
  - Diagnosis can be suspected in utero from bony abnormalities
  - 4p- abnormality can be seen by routine karyotype analysis and high-resolution chromosome analysis
  - Confirmation of diagnosis by fluorescence in situ hybridization (FISH) assay using a Wolf-Hirschhorn critical region probe

- **Genetic Mechanism**
  - Structural abnormality of chromosome 4
  - Deletion of 4p16 (also called 4p-)

- **Pearl**

The developmental abnormalities of nose, orbits, and forehead are said to resemble the ancient Greek warrior helmet.

12

Cri Du Chat Syndrome (5p-)

- **Epidemiology and Clinical Diagnosis**
  - 1:20,000–50,000 live births
  - Neonates have high-pitched cat-like cry, which disappears by age 2 years
  - Facial features—microcephaly, hypertelorism, synophrys, downward slanting palpebral fissures, small jaw, small mouth, low-set ears, preauricular tags
  - Other features—low birth weight, hypotonia, feeding problems due to poor suck and swallow, webbing of fingers or toes, single palmar crease, mental and motor retardation, hyperactivity
  - Cardiac defects include ventricular septal defect, atrial septal defect, tetralogy of Fallot, and patent ductus arteriosus
  - Gastroesophageal (GE) reflux disease often develops with esophageal strictures

- **Diagnosis**
  - Diagnosis is usually clinical based upon typical appearance
  - Diagnosis can be made by high-resolution chromosome analysis
  - Patients with very small deletions diagnosed by fluorescent in situ hybridization (FISH) using specific genetic markers associated with cri du chat

12

- **Genetic Mechanisms**
  - Deletion in the short arm of chromosome 5 (5p-) probably eliminates several genes—semaphorine F, δ-catenine telomerase, and reverse transcriptase needed in cerebral development
  - 30–60% of the genetic material deleted from 5p in most patients
  - 80% of mutations are sporadic
  - 10–15% of cases due to translocation, mosaicism, ring formation

- **Pearl**

The 5p deletion is of paternal origin in about 80% of de novo cases.

Williams Syndrome (7q-)

- **Essentials of Clinical Diagnosis**
  - At birth—small for gestational age, elfin facies with prominent lips, feeding problems, failure to thrive, hypercalcemia, hypercalciuria, developmental delay
  - Cardiac disease includes supravalvular aortic stenosis, supravalvular pulmonic stenosis, hypertension
  - Irritability in infancy gives way to outgoing, impulsive, garrulous, mildly obsessive behavior in childhood
  - Older children and adults develop diabetes, sensorineural hearing loss, abnormality in spatial relations and abstract thinking, attention-deficit hyperactivity disorder, phobias

- **Diagnosis**
  - Typical facies and hypercalcemia at birth are often the first clue
  - FISH technology reveals the chromosomal deletion
  - Hypercalcemia and hypercalciuria may be absent or of very short duration and always resolve by age 2 years. Perform genetic evaluation in infants with phenotypic features even if the calcium is normal

- **Genetic Mechanisms**
  - Most cases are new mutations
  - Autosomal structural disorder—deletion of genetic material from chromosome 7q11.2
  - As many as 25 contiguous genes may be deleted including elastin, CLIP2

- **Pearl**

Williams syndrome children may have excellent vocabularies and unusual musical skills such as perfect pitch.

Spectrum of 22q Deletion (DiGeorge Syndrome, Velocardiofacial Syndrome, Shprintzen Syndrome)

- **Essentials of Diagnosis**
  - Autosomal dominant condition with microdeletion of the long arm of chromosome 22 (22q11) with variable phenotype. ~1:1000 live births
  - This is not a contiguous gene deletion syndrome. Length of deletion does not correlate with extent of abnormalities
  - *DiGeorge syndrome*—tetralogy of Fallot, transposition of the great arteries, other cyanotic congenital heart disease, thymic hypoplasia, immunodeficiency, absent parathyroids, and hypocalcemia
  - *Velocardiofacial syndrome/Shprintzen syndrome;*—microcephaly; small mandible; flat cheekbones; long face; narrow palpebral fissures; hypoplastic alae nasae; cleft palate (85%); dysplastic ears and hearing problems; ventricular septal defect; learning disability; hypospadias; umbilical hernia; and many other organ anomalies
  - As many as 25% of patients with 22q deletion develop schizophrenia in adolescence
  - High-resolution chromosome examination and FISH analysis with specific probes

12

- **Differential Diagnosis**
  - Pierre Robin sequence—micrognathia, cleft soft palate, glossoptosis, cardiac defects has multifactorial inheritance
  - Cleft palate can occur in isolation, but a surprising percentage may have 22q deletion
  - Isolated tetralogy of Fallot and transposition of the great arteries occur, but all patients should be screened for DiGeorge syndrome

- **Treatment**
  - Surgery indicated for cleft palate, congenital heart disease, micrognathia, ear anomalies, GI anomalies, and other organ malformations
  - In DiGeorge syndrome—monitor and treat hypoparathyroidism, monitor and treat infections associated with T-cell dysfunction

Pearl

22q deletion complex is one of the most common genetic disorders of humans. In some studies it is reported to be second only to trisomy 21.

Neurofibromatosis (NF) Type 1

- **Essentials of Diagnosis**
    - Autosomal dominant mutation of gene on chromosome 17 coding for tumor suppressor-like factor. Occurs in 1:3000 live births
    - Diagnosis requires at least 2 of the following:
        - >6 café au lait spots ≥15 mm postpuberty or ≥5 mm prepuberty
        - >2 neurofibromas of any type or 1 plexiform type
        - Axillary or inguinal freckling
        - ≥2 Lisch nodules (hamartoma of the iris)
        - Optic glioma—15% of patients
        - Bone lesions—sphenoid dysplasia, pseudarthroses
        - Affected first-degree relative
    - Most affected children have only skin lesions and few other problems
    - Common features—large head, bony abnormalities on x-ray, scoliosis, developmental problems, and learning disabilities
    - Less common features—seizures, short stature, precocious puberty, hypertension, slight increased risk (5%) of malignancies

- **Differential Diagnosis**
    - Type 2 NF is caused by a different gene mutation. Patients have bilateral acoustic neuromas and no skin changes
    - Hyperpigmented skin macules can occur in Albright syndrome, Noonan syndrome, LEOPARD syndrome but usually easily differentiated
    - Familial café au lait spots
    - Isolated nonsyndromatic neurofibromas

- **Treatment**
    - Neurofibromas causing cosmetic or functional problems can be removed
    - Regular monitoring for orthopedic, neurologic, ocular, and developmental problems is required

- **Pearl**

Plexiform neurofibromas are invasive. They grow rapidly during growth spurts and, when present on face or limbs, may cause significant hypertrophy of the underlying bony and soft tissues.

Craniosynostosis Syndromes

- ### Essentials of Diagnosis
  - Dominant mutations of the fibroblast growth factor receptor (*FGFR*) genes cause premature fusion of cranial sutures and other bony abnormalities
  - *Crouzon syndrome* (*FGFR2* mutation)—multiple suture fusions, normal limbs, exophthalmos, hypertelorism, beak nose, maxillary hypoplasia with relative prognathism
  - *Pfeiffer syndrome* (*FGFR* 1, 2 mutation)—craniosynostosis with broad thumbs and great toes, cutaneous syndactyly
  - *Apert syndrome* (*FGFR* 2 mutation) coronal synostosis, bony and cutaneous syndactyly of 2, 3, 4 digits, midfacial, spine, and limb abnormalities, obstructive sleep apnea, visual and auditory problems
  - Prenatal ultrasound of the head can detect some of these disorders

- ### Differential Diagnosis
  - Hyperthyroidism, hypophosphatasia can cause premature fusion of cranial sutures
  - Underlying failure of brain growth causes apparent premature fusion of sutures but usually with a symmetric skull
  - Some severe variants exist with infantile tracheal stenosis and life-threatening skeletal abnormalities

- ### Treatment
  - Surgery for craniosynostosis in the first 6 months of life gives the best cosmetic results
  - Coronal suture synostosis causes brachycephaly which poses the most severe risk to eyesight
  - Saggital synostosis produces scaphocephaly which is corrected mainly for cosmesis

- ### Pearl

Multiple cranial synostoses severely restrict brain growth and may cause a so-called clover leaf skull with intracranial hypertension and mental retardation if untreated.

Treacher Collins Syndrome

- **Essentials of Diagnosis**
  - Autosomal dominant mutation of *TCPF1* gene on chromosome 5. Gene product assists in protein sorting during embryogenesis. More than 50% are new mutations
  - Variable severity of facial dysmorphism with normal intelligence
  - Facial features—downward slanting eyes, lower lid notching (coloboma), small mandible, cleft palate, malformed, small or absent ears with conductive hearing loss, prominent nose, cleft palate
  - Major facial bones involved are zygomatic arch and mandible
  - Other features—apnea, airway obstruction, feeding problems due to small mouth, and hypopharynx and nasal passages

- **Differential Diagnosis**
  - Variable penetrance of facial features makes visual diagnosis difficult in some cases with very mild features

- **Treatment**
  - Plastic surgery can improve facial abnormalities
  - Monitoring for hearing loss
  - Maintain nutrition and monitor for airway obstruction especially during sleep and intercurrent infection
  - Evaluation of parents to detect mutations is important for genetic counseling

- **Pearl**

Very good cosmetic improvement may be obtained through orthopedic, plastic, and ear, nose, throat (ENT) surgery. A series of operations may be required over several years to obtain the best results.

Spinal Muscular Atrophy (SMA)

■ Essentials of Diagnosis

- 1:6000–12000 live births
- Autosomal recessive deletion of *SMN1* gene on chromosome 5q
- Degeneration of the anterior horn cells of the spinal cord
- Three clinical types
  - (SMA I)—progressive fatal motor weakness of infants
  - (SMA II)—milder weakness with onset age 2 years
  - (SMA III)—weakness onset in adolescence
- Decreased fetal movements may be an early sign of SMA
- Death in SMA I occurs by age 2 from inanition, aspiration, pneumonia, respiratory failure
- Diagnose by detection of *SMN1* gene mutation or by electromyographic findings (fibrillations)

■ Differential Diagnosis

- Birth injury with hypotonia
- Neonatal drug toxicity or systemic illness
- Neonatal myasthenia gravis or myotonic dystrophy
- Muscular glycogen storage diseases
- Duchenne muscular dystrophy or Charcot-Marie-Tooth disease may resemble SMA II or III
- SMA with respiratory distress—mutation of the *SMARD* gene on chromosome 11
- Distal SMA with upper limb predominance—mutation of glycyl tRNA synthase gene on chromosome 7

■ Treatment

- No specific therapy
- Physical therapy, attention to respiratory hygiene and nutrition are important
- Some experimental experience in treating SMA with butyrates, valproate, hydroxyurea
- Careful genetic counseling required before attempt at prenatal diagnosis because of compound heterozygosity, de novo mutations, and duplications of *SMN I* gene

■ Pearl

Intellect is preserved in all forms of SMA.

Duchenne Type Muscular Dystrophy

- **Essentials of Diagnosis**
  - Sex-linked disorder occurs in 1:4000 male births
  - Gene on X chromosome controls synthesis of cytoskeletal protein dystrophin. New mutations account for ~30% of cases
  - The absence of dystrophin in skeletal and cardiac muscle allows unregulated calcium ingress, overproduction of reactive oxygen species, and muscle destruction by oxidant injury
  - Muscle destruction causes swelling and weakness of calf muscles by age 5–6 years, inability to walk in midteens, and death from cardiac failure or respiratory infection/insufficiency in midtwenties
  - Diagnosis can be made on muscle biopsy but genetic testing for deletions in dystrophin gene now commonly used

- **Differential Diagnosis**
  - Becker muscular dystrophy is a less severe form with partial expression of the dystrophin gene
  - Myotonic dystrophy
  - Limb girdle muscular dystrophy—affects sexes equally 8–15 years old
  - Fascioscapulohumoral muscular dystrophy affects sexes equally

- **Treatment**
  - No specific therapy
  - Nutritional monitoring—older patients become obese from inactivity
  - Treat respiratory illness aggressively
  - Involve cardiologist to manage progressive cardiac failure and arrhythmias

- **Pearl**

The incidental finding of a high serum glutamic-oxaloacetic transaminase (SGOT) or serum glutamic-pyruvic transaminase (SGPT) in a healthy boy suggests the possibility of liver disease. Always measure the creatine phosphokinase (CPK) in such a patient. It will be high in muscular dystrophy and normal in liver disease.

12

Beckwith-Wiedemann Syndrome

- **Essentials of Diagnosis**
  - Non-Mendelian disorder of imprinting—preferential expression of paternal genes on chromosome 11p15 due to paternal duplication of 11p15 region or paternal uniparental disomy (UPD)
  - Infant findings—macrosomia, macroglossia, omphalocele
  - Other findings—hypertelorism, abnormal ear creases, hypoglycemia, transient hyperinsulinemia, cleft palate, urinary tract anomalies, hepatomegaly
  - ↑risk of Wilms tumor (7–10% of cases) hepatoblastoma, adrenocortical tumors, and other embryonal tumors
  - Large tongue may cause feeding and respiratory problems

- **Differential Diagnosis**
  - Glycogen storage disease—hypoglycemia and large liver but no other dysmorphisms
  - Infants of diabetic mothers—macrosomic and hypoglycemic

12

- **Treatment**
  - Monitor and support blood glucose in neonates
  - Large tongue may necessitate tube feedings, ventilatory support, and sometime surgical debulking
  - Regular tumor surveillance for Wilms' and other tumors (abdominal ultrasound) until age 7 years

- **Pearl**

Increased secretion of insulin-like growth factor 2 seems to be the final common pathway of the abnormalities of Beckwith-Wiedemann syndrome.

Prader-Willi Syndrome

- **Essentials of Diagnosis**
  - Lack of expression of several imprinted genes on 15q11 caused by chromosomal rearrangements and mutations
  - Deletion of the paternal allele for SNRPn is the most common cause with maternal uniparental disomy (UDP) second
  - Infants—profound hypotonia necessitating tube feedings, undescended testicles, and micropenis in males
  - Older children—characteristic facies (almond-shaped eyes, strabismus) short stature, obesity, hyperphagia, hypogenitalism, small hands and feet
  - Problems secondary to obesity—diabetes mellitus, orthopedic problems, sleep apnea, and cor pulmonale

- **Differential Diagnosis**
  - Exogenous obesity from overfeeding
  - Congenital hypothyroidism causes hypotonia, macroglossia, obesity, and growth failure
  - Down syndrome
  - Other causes of the "floppy infant" must be ruled out in the neonatal period

- **Treatment**
  - Prevention of obesity is the major goal of therapy
  - GH increases muscle mass and promotes linear growth but adverse effects must be considered
  - Micropenis in males—testosterone is effective
  - Serum ghrelin is increased in Prader-Willi syndrome and may cause the increased appetite. Ghrelin can be suppressed with octreotide. Not much clinical experience with this therapy
  - Hormone replacement at adolescence to promote secondary sexual characteristics

- **Pearl**

These children are good examples of the Pickwickian syndrome of obesity, apnea, and right-sided heart failure.

CHARGE Syndrome

- Essentials of Diagnosis

  - Autosomal dominant mutation or deletion of the *CHD7* gene on chromosome 8q (chromodomain helicase DNA-binding protein 7)
  - Midline structures derived from rostral neural crest cells affected with early arrest of embryologic differentiation
  - Major features—coloboma, cyanotic congenital heart disease, choanal atresia, growth retardation, hypogenitalism, ear abnormalities
  - Minor features—facial asymmetry, hand dysmorphology, hypotonia, urinary tract anomalies, orofacial cleft, deafness, tracheoesophageal (TE) fistula, mild-to-moderate developmental delay
  - Clinical diagnosis requires 3 major features or 2 major and 3 minor features
  - Neonatal tip-off to diagnosis is inability to pass nasogastric tube in a dysmorphic baby because of choanal atresia
  - High-resolution karyotype and FISH can detect mutation

- Differential Diagnosis

  - Some common features of VACTERL syndrome are minor features of CHARGE—renal anomalies, TE fistula, hemivertebrae
  - 22q11 deletion syndrome also has some similar features of cyanotic heart disease (DiGeorge) and facial anomalies (Shprintzen)
  - Smith-Lemli-Opitz—hypotonia and facial dysmorphism

- Treatment

  - Assessment for associated skeletal, head, chest, and abdominal anomalies
  - Cyanotic heart disease may require immediate evaluation/treatment
  - Bilateral choanal atresia is a neonatal emergency because of obligate nose breathing. Relieve respiratory obstruction surgically or by choanal stenting
  - TE fistula and tracheomalacia may cause feeding and respiratory problems in neonates

- Pearl

It took a twisted mind to fit the acronym CHARGE to the common features of this disorder. Now that the gene defect is known a better name is needed.

Cornelia de Lange Syndrome

■ Essentials of Diagnosis

- Some patients have mutations of *NIPBL* gene. >99% of cases are sporadic
- Distinct facial appearance—synophrys, microcephaly, low anterior and posterior hairline, long eyelashes, anteverted nares, thin lips, high arched palate, micrognathia
- Other features—pre- and postnatal growth deficiency, feeding difficulties, mental retardation, hyperactivity, hypoplastic forearms, oligodactyly, hirsutism, severe GE reflux, renal anomalies, hearing loss, endocrine abnormalities
- Usually a clinical diagnosis based on facial features. Sometimes the facial dysmorphism is subtle

■ Differential Diagnosis

- Duplication of 3q—rare syndrome with similar facial features and retardation
- Coffin-Siris syndrome—rare syndrome of unknown cause with dysmorphic facies, digital abnormalities, and retardation

■ Treatment

- Anatomic abnormalities of head and neck may cause hypoxia or asphyxia at delivery
- High index of suspicion for GE reflux and aggressive therapy may prevent esophageal peptic stricture
- Full radiologic and biochemical evaluation to detect skeletal, renal, cardiac, GI, endocrine, and central nervous system (CNS) abnormalities
- Food refusal behavior and/or micrognathia may require tube feedings or gastrostomy
- Major speech and communication problems require therapy
- Hyperactive and destructive behavior may require medication and therapy

■ Pearl

Life expectancy can be normal in children with no major anomalies.

Goldenhar Syndrome
(Vertebro-Auriculo-Facial Syndrome)

- **Essentials of Diagnosis**
  - Multiple head and neck anomalies:
    - Hemifacial microsomia—often severe oral, malar, and mandibular asymmetry, cleft palate, facial and oral motor dysfunction
    - Ears—unilateral abnormalities of pinna and ear (absence of ear common) with deafness, preauricular tags
    - Eyes—benign epibulbar dermoid, eye on affected side may be small or absent
    - Cervical spine—fused vertebrae, Arnold Chiari type I
    - Cardiac anomalies—in severe cases
    - Hydrocephalus—in severe cases
  - Cause unknown—possibly toxin exposure, recurrence risk very low
  - Mildly affected cases are common occurrences. Mental development is normal

12

- **Differential Diagnosis**
  - Other syndromes with multiple facial anomalies—Treacher Collins syndrome, Pierre Robin syndrome
  - Hemifacial microsomia is probably a mild form of Goldenhar syndrome

- **Treatment**
  - Can be diagnosed on intrauterine ultrasound
  - Surgery may be required in neonates to correct oral and mandibular abnormalities that interfere with nutrition and respiration
  - Arnold-Chiari type I may require surgery
  - Plastic surgical repair of the hemifacial asymmetry and ear anomalies
  - Speech therapy may be required in those with extreme asymmetry of tongue

- **Pearl**

Both sides of the face are affected in 10–33% of patients with Goldenhar syndrome.

Noonan Syndrome

- **Essentials of Diagnosis**
  - Autosomal dominant mutations in *PTPN11* (50%), *SOS1* (10%), or *KRAS* (<5%). Mutations of these regulator genes for organ development cause overgrowth phenomena
  - New mutations common. Incidence 1:2500 births. Sex distribution equal. Variable penetrance of abnormalities
  - Symptoms—short stature, delayed puberty, hypertelorism and other eye problems, low-set ears, mild mental retardation (25%), micropenis and cryptorchidism in males, delayed puberty pectus excavatum with low-set wide-spaced nipples, webbed neck, coagulation defects
  - 50–80% have pulmonary valve stenosis or hypertrophic cardiomyopathy
  - Increased risk of myeloproliferative disorders and juvenile myelomonocytic leukemia (JMML)
  - Usually a clinical diagnosis in newborns. Molecular genetic testing by sequence analysis is available. Intrauterine ultrasound often detects edema

- **Differential Diagnosis**
  - Turner syndrome—very similar phenotype
  - LEOPARD syndrome—mutations in other exons of the *PTPN11* gene causes lentigines, cardiac arrhythmia, pulmonary stenosis, hypertelorism, growth failure, genital abnormalities, and deafness
  - Costello syndrome—similar features but gene defect not identified
  - Cardio-facial-cutaneous syndrome—heart, skin, and growth problems

- **Treatment**
  - GH therapy is helpful, but some patients have GH resistance
  - Monitoring for bleeding disorders, myeloproliferative disorders
  - Hormone therapy may be required at puberty
  - Cardiac defects may require specialty care. Hypertrophic cardiomyopathy can develop at any time

- **Pearl**

Noonan syndrome used to be called "male Turner syndrome" because of the similarities in phenotype. Now that the autosomal dominant gene defects have been identified, this misnomer should be discontinued.

VACTERL Association

- ### Essentials of Diagnosis
  - **V**ertebral defects—butterfly vertebrae, hemi and fused vertebrae
  - Imperforate **A**nus
  - **C**ardiac malformations—mainly ventricular septal defect
  - **T**racheo-**E**sophageal fistula—often with severe tracheomalacia
  - **R**enal—agenesis, fused kidneys, other upper tract anatomic defects
  - **L**imb anomalies—mainly radial defects, polydactyly, club hand
  - Cause unknown. Monozygotic twin concordance and multiple organ anomalies suggest defect during blastogenesis or defect in the sonic hedgehog pathway (SHH)-regulating organogenesis
  - Defects often life threatening. Hydrocephalus is often associated
  - Intra-uterine ultrasound detects vertebral anomalies, TE fistula, and limb anomalies in first trimester pointing to diagnosis

- ### Differential diagnosis
  - Syndromes with multiple anomalies—trisomy 13, trisomy 18,
  - Syndromes with radial anomalies—thrombocytopenia-absent-radius syndrome, Fanconi syndrome, Holt-Oram syndrome

- ### Treatment
  - After prenatal diagnosis, delivery should be at a tertiary center
  - Surgical treatment of TE fistula required at birth
  - Respiratory problems due to TE fistula, vertebral anomalies, and tracheo-bronchomalacia often require mechanical ventilation
  - Other anomalies require surgical correction electively
  - Monitor for urinary tract infection and renal function

- ### Pearl

50% of infants with tracheo-esophageal fistula have other features of VACTERL syndrome.

12

Alport Syndrome

- **Essentials of Diagnosis**
    - X-linked defect—progressive glomerulonephritis (hypertension, hematuria, proteinuria), renal failure by age 30–40 years, sensory-neural hearing loss and anterior lenticonus develop in childhood
    - Autosomal dominant forms occur. Affected females have less severe disease
    - Several mutations of type IV collagen gene cause abnormalities of the glomerular basement membrane
    - Diagnosis may be clear because of family history
    - Electron microscopy reveals glomerular basement membrane thickening. Absence of type IV collagen by immunostain
    - Hearing tests may reveal subclinical sensorineural deficits

- **Differential Diagnosis**
    - Acute poststreptococcal glomerulonephritis becomes chronic in rare cases
    - Immunoglobulin (IgA) nephropathy—very rarely progresses to renal failure
    - Nongenetic chronic glomerulonephritides—systemic lupus, Henoch-Schönlein (HS) purpura, membranoproliferative glomerulonephritis
    - Mutations of connexin 26, a gap junction protein, causes sensorineural hearing loss
    - Other causes of sensorineural hearing loss—ototoxic medication, meningitis, congenital cytomegalovirus (CMV) and other viral infections, autoimmune or neoplastic disease, noise exposure, trauma

- **Treatment**
    - Angiotensin-converting enzyme (ACE) inhibitors may improve hypertension and proteinuria
    - Some reports of cyclosporine A use to decrease proteinuria
    - Most male patients will require kidney transplant

- **Pearl**

Avoid the use of ototoxic medications in patients with Alport syndrome.

12

13

Dermatology

Acne

- ■ Essentials of Diagnosis
  - Obstruction of the sebaceous follicle neck produces closed comedone (white head). Obstruction of follicular mouth produces open comedone (black head)
  - Pathogenic factors—individual immune responses, androgen-promoted proliferation of keratinocytes, and sebum production leading to plugging of sebaceous follicles, proliferation of *Propionibacterium acnes* causing follicular inflammation
  - Severe and deep chronic inflammatory lesions may interconnect causing cystic acne and scarring
  - Generally a visual diagnosis. Lesions of different ages in an adolescent starting on face but also involving upper chest and back

- ■ Differential Diagnosis
  - Drug-induced acne (corticotrophin, glucocorticoids, androgens, hydantoins, isoniazid)
  - Rosacea
  - Seborrheic dermatitis
  - Consider endocrinopathy in older girls with sudden-onset resistant acne especially if associated with hirsutism, striae, and other signs of adrenal disease
  - Staphylococcal folliculitis

- ■ Treatment
  - Therapy targeting all pathogenic factors is most effective
  - Topical keratolytics (tretinoin, adapalene, benzoyl peroxide) and topical antibiotics (1% clindamycin) are sufficient for most patients
  - Most organisms are resistant to topical erythromycin and cillins
  - Treat more severe acne with systemic antibiotics (tetracycline, minocycline, doxycycline) and oral retinoids
  - Oral contraceptive therapy is effective for perimenstrual acne flares and for girls with polycystic ovaries

- ■ Pearl

Ask about doxycycline and minocycline use in any teenager with sudden severe midesophageal dysphagia. When taken before bed without sufficient water, these pills get caught in the esophagus and cause painful "pill ulcers."

Warts

- **Essentials of Diagnosis**
    - Skin-colored papules with irregular surface. Intraepidermal tumors caused by 1 of the many types of human papillomavirus (HPV)
    - Warts on the face (flat warts), dorsa of extremities, plantar surfaces or genitals (condylomata acuminata) are caused by specific HPV species
    - Risk of warts increased by immunosuppression and chronic debilitation
    - Visual diagnosis is usually adequate. However, HPV type can be determined if important (child sexual abuse cases)

- **Differential Diagnosis**
    - Molluscum contagiosum—papular lesion produced by a poxvirus. Umbilication of lesion is a helpful differential finding
    - Scabies lesions of the hand may be mistaken for warts. Pruritus is a helpful differential finding

- **Treatment**
    - No therapy is ideal. 30% of warts clear in 6 months regardless of therapy
    - Common warts—liquid nitrogen
    - Plantar warts—local application of 40% salicylic acid plaster with careful removal of macerated tissue. Repeat procedure weekly
    - Flat warts—topical 0.05% tretinoin cream or imiquimod
    - Venereal warts—imiquimod. Podophyllin should be used very carefully to protect adjacent skin
    - Periungual—cantharidin often useful but satellite (ring warts) may develop

- **Pearl**

Infants with condylomata acuminata may be victims of sexual abuse. However, maternal-infant transmission occurs. Serotyping the HPV is helpful in this situation.

Scabies

■ Essentials of Diagnosis

- Linear burrows about the wrists, ankles, finger webs, areolas, anterior axillary folds, genitalia, or face created by skin mites
- Intense generalize or localized pruritus
- Skin scraping over a burrow may show diagnostic female mites, eggs, or feces
- Generalized allergic reaction to mite protein may exacerbate itching and produce a confusing generalized rash

■ Differential Diagnosis

- Allergic reaction to food, drug, or inhalants
- Neurotic scratching
- Mastocytosis
- Biliary obstruction, bile acid synthetic defects, and hepatitis produce severe pruritus
- Lymphoma, leukemia, polycythemia vera may be associated with pruritus more often in adults
- Uremia

13

■ Treatment

- 5% topical permethrin single overnight application usually sufficient
- Antihistamines, topical menthol rarely effective and delay the diagnosis
- Check siblings—person-to-person spread and single-source infection are common

■ Pearl

In a child with constant scratching, check the material under the fingernails for mites. You may avoid having to scrape the skin.

Atopic Dermatitis/Eczema

- **Essentials of Diagnosis**
  - General term for chronic superficial pruritic scaly skin inflammation. Cause unknown. Role of allergy not always clear
  - Infantile eczema—onset 2–3 months involves cheeks, scalp, and extensor surfaces of extremities
  - Childhood eczema (2 years to adolescence) involves flexural creases, neck, wrists, and sometimes hands and feet. 30% continue as adolescents with flexural and hand eczema
  - Faulty epidermal barrier with dry skin, allergic family history, deficient antimicrobial skin proteins, hyperimmunoglobulin E, defective neutrophil and monocyte chemotaxis, and abnormal T-cell function all predispose to eczematoid rashes
  - Eczema >age 30 years is fairly rare

- **Differential Diagnosis**
  - Nummular eczema
  - Primary irritant contact dermatitis
  - Allergic contact dermatitis—poison ivy
  - Seborrheic dermatitis
  - Xerosis
  - Pityriasis alba—scaly macules over cheeks and extensor surfaces. Depigmentation should discriminate this from infantile eczema
  - β-Hemolytic streptococcus infection (impetigo) may be primary or occur in the setting of underlying eczema

- **Treatment**
  - Skin hydration is key—wet dressings, avoid soaps and detergents, lubrication
  - Reduce skin injury—prevent scratching and avoid harsh clothing
  - Topical corticosteroids
  - Topical tacrolimus and pimecrolimus should be reserved for children >2 years with eczema unresponsive to standard therapy

- **Pearl**

Topical tacrolimus and pimecrolimus may increase the risk of malignancy in immunologically compromised children. Since immunocompromise may not be obvious, and since transdermal absorption of theses potent compounds may be increased in immunologically immature infants, caution in using these preparations is a good idea.

Seborrheic Dermatitis

- **■ Essentials of Diagnosis**
  - Erythematous, greasy, scaly dermatitis in the sebum-producing areas of face, scalp, intertriginous folds, and perineum
  - Affects mainly newborns (scalp and intertriginous areas) and adolescents (face, intertriginous areas, perineum)
  - *Pityrosporum ovale* (yeast organism) often found in affected areas. Possibly pathogenic
  - Leiner disease—severe, widespread, infantile seborrheic dermatitis associated with functional defect in C5 complement. Wasting, diarrhea, failure to thrive, superimposed infections
  - Visual diagnosis is key. Skin biopsy findings are nonspecific

- **■ Differential Diagnosis**
  - May resemble atopic dermatitis of the scalp in infants
  - Psoriasis occurs in seborrheic areas in older children
  - Pityriasis rosea—herald patch and distribution should distinguish
  - Tinea (dermatophytoses) infections

13

- **■ Treatment**
  - Low-potency topical corticosteroids usually suffice
  - Leiner disease may require therapy with fresh frozen plasma (FFP)
  - Disease severity is usually worse in adults than children

- **■ Pearl**

Seborrhea (cradle cap) is not *treated the same as dandruff in adults. Vigorous scrubbing of the scalp, adult dandruff shampoos, and picking the scales may damage the infant's delicate skin and increase the risk of infection. A little warm olive oil to loosen scales followed by gentle shampoo is a time-honored, harmless therapy.*

Pityriasis Rosea

- **Essentials of Diagnosis**
  - Papulosquamous eruption of school-aged children with small, red oval plaques with fine scales often aligned parallel to skin tension lines
  - In 20–80% , the generalized rash is preceded for up to 30 days by a single larger scaly plaque with central clearing (herald patch) often on the trunk (in whites) or extremities (in blacks)
  - Human herpes virus 7 may be a pathogen
  - Lasts about 6 weeks with mild-moderate pruritus
  - History and visual diagnosis are key. Biopsy may be required in confusing cases

- **Differential Diagnosis**
  - Herald patch looks like ringworm
  - Secondary syphilis should be ruled out in high-risk situations, especially if palms and soles are affected. Obtain VDRL
  - Psoriasis
  - Lichen planus
  - Dermatomyositis, systemic lupus erythematous (SLE)

- **Treatment**
  - Exposure to sunlight may hasten resolution
  - Oral antihistamines for pruritus
  - Spontaneous resolution is expected

- **Pearl**

If pityriasis rosea lasts >12 weeks, refer to dermatologist for more in-depth evaluation of alternative diagnoses.

Psoriasis

- ■ Essentials of diagnosis
  - Erythematous papules covered by thick white scales
  - *Guttate psoriasis* (3–8 mm, drop-like papules with pearly white covering) is the common form of childhood often occurring 3–4 weeks after streptococcal pharyngitis
  - *Chronic psoriasis*—larger plaques over elbows, knees, scalp, and sites of trauma. Pinpoint pits in nails and yellow discoloration from onycholysis
  - *Other forms*—pustular, acral, follicular are rarer in children
  - Family history often positive. Underlying cause unclear. May be T-cell–mediated release of cytokines which stimulates keratinocyte proliferation
  - Visual diagnosis is usually accurate. Biopsy shows hyperkeratosis, parakeratosis, acanthosis, epidermal hyperplasia, and pericapillary inflammatory infiltrate

- ■ Differential Diagnosis
  - Other papulosquamous eruptions—pityriasis rosea, tinea corporis, lichen planus, dermatomyositis, lupus, secondary syphilis
  - Lesions in infants may look like diaper dermatitis
  - Drug dermatitis especially β-blocker (practolol)

- ■ Treatment
  - Topical steroids initial treatment of choice. High-potency preparations required to penetrate skin. Guttate psoriasis usually responsive
  - Topical calcipotriene (vitamin D derivative) with steroids used in severe cases but hypercalcemia may complicate therapy
  - Topical skin and scalp preparations contain retinoids, anthralin, coal tar, tar gels for exfoliation
  - Topical anticytokine therapy has been used in some patients—etanercept, infliximab

- ■ Pearl

Scraping the scales of a psoriatic lesion with the edge of a glass slide leaves minute bleeding points. This may help differentiate from seborrhea.

13

Erythema Multiforme

- **Essentials of Diagnosis**
  - Hypersensitivity reaction involving dermal vascular endothelium following medication, infection, or other illnesses
  - Sudden-onset, wide distribution (legs, arms, palms, hands, feet, face, and mucous membranes often with truncal sparing). Initial red macules, papules, or blisters gradually enlarge developing concentric rings of pallor and erythema (target lesions)
  - Skin usually heals spontaneously over 2–8 weeks. Common precipitants are sulfonamides, penicillins, barbiturates, phenytoin, *Herpes simplex*, *Mycoplasma,* and many other infections

- **Differential Diagnosis**
  - Stevens-Johnson syndrome—very extensive erythema multiforme rash with mucous membrane and conjunctival involvement, fever, malaise, and arthralgia
  - Toxic epidermal necrolysis—erythema multiforme with large bullae and epidermal sloughing
  - Fixed drug eruption—anticonvulsants, nonsteroidal anti-inflammatory drugs (NSAIDs), sulfonamides cause a variety of skin responses that may resemble erythema multiforme
  - DRESS syndrome—fixed drug eruption with fever, eosinophilia, and systemic symptoms usually after anticonvulsants

- **Treatment**
  - Conservative measures—cool, moist compresses, antihistamines, antipyretics, mild analgesics
  - Topical anesthetics to reduce dysphagia and dysuria
  - Prophylactic acyclovir prevents recurrence of rash during herpes reactivation
  - In severe Stevens-Johnson, dehydration, shock, electrolyte imbalance, superinfection, and hypoproteinemia from skin slough may require intensive care unit admission
  - Intravenous immunoglobulin (IVIG) has been used to prevent progression of rash in Stevens-Johnson syndrome

- **Pearl**

Corticosteroids are not effective in treating or preventing erythema multiforme.

Erythema Nodosum

- **Essentials of Diagnosis**
  - Reactive inflammation of subcutaneous fatty tissue causing single or multiple tender red/violaceous lumps usually over the shins. Resolving nodules look bruised
  - Occurs in isolation but often after medications (oral contraceptive pills, estrogens, sulfa), infections (strep throat, Yersinia, tuberculosis, mycoplasma, cat scratch, fungal infections, Epstein-Barr virus, inflammatory bowel disease, autoimmune hepatitis
  - Resolution usually occurs in 6 weeks but chronic/recurrent disease occurs
  - Visual diagnosis usually sufficient. Biopsy showing septal inflammation in fatty layers is diagnostic

- **Differential Diagnosis**
  - Nodular vasculitis
  - Fat necrosis—with corticosteroid therapy and severe pancreatitis
  - Panniculitis—with SLE, cold injury
  - Henoch-Schönlein purpura
  - Scleroderma or dermatomyositis may cause firm dermal patches that resemble erythema nodosum
  - Factitious lesion or child abuse

13

- **Treatment**
  - Most lesions resolve spontaneously or with treatment of underlying condition
  - Anti-inflammatory medications and corticosteroids (oral or local injection) if lesions are very painful or extensive
  - Corticosteroids may be contraindicated with underlying infection

- **Pearl**

A rare form of erythema nodosa in childhood affects only the palms or soles.

Epidermolysis Bullosa (EB)

- **Essentials of Diagnosis**
  - Inherited bullous disorder with intraepidermal blister formation in response to mechanical trauma. 4 major histologic types—EB simplex (92%), junctional EB (1%), dystrophic EB (5%), and hemidesmosomal (<1%) with many variants
  - Mutations in genes for keratins 5 and 14 (simplex), laminin (junctional), type VII collagen (dystrophica) produce fragility at various sites in the epidermal basal layer with separation and blistering
  - EB simplex—usually mild presentation in infancy with hemorrhagic blisters on legs especially with walking
  - Junctional and dystrophic forms present at birth with variable, often widespread blistering and slough. Complications include infection, fluid and electrolyte abnormalities, malnutrition, dysphagia, esophageal strictures (mostly dystrophic EB), limb contractures, syndactyly (recessive dystrophic EB), oral contractures, and facial scarring
  - Biopsy needed to clearly define the epidermal structures affected in each subtype

- **Differential Diagnosis**
  - Some mild patients with EB simplex only have palmar and plantar dyshydrosis
  - Epidermolytic hyperkeratosis may look like EB at birth

- **Treatment**
  - Most EB simplex patients are not severely affected. Protect skin from injury, especially hands, feet, knees, and elbows. Reduce skin friction points with 5% glutaraldehyde every 3 days. Skin cooling can prevent blisters
  - Treatment of junctional and dystrophic types is supportive— protect skin from injury, daily wound care with nonstick dressings, treat infections, physical therapy, nutritional support, emotional support
  - Monitor for complications—highly malignant squamous cell carcinoma is a late complication of recessive dystrophic EB
  - Gene therapy directed at the collagen VII, laminin, and keratin genes has been attempted in experimental models

- **Pearl**

Autosomal recessive junctional EB (Herlitz or EB letalis) is the most severe EB subtype with blistering and slough of epithelia of skin, gastrointestinal (GI), respiratory, eye, and urinary tract causing inanition, infection, and early death.

Ichthyosis

- ## Essentials of Diagnosis
  - Inherited disorder with excessive scaliness of skin
  - *Ichthyosis vulgaris*—most common form with variable severity. Scaly dry skin on trunk, abdomen, legs, and buttocks; deep palmar and plantar creases. Autosomal dominant defect in filaggrin
  - *X-linked ichthyosis*—thick scales sparing palms and soles, corneal opacities in patient and carrier mother. X-lined defect in cholesterol sulfatase
  - *Epidermolytic hyperkeratosis*—rapid epidermal turnover. Skin red, moist, and blistered at birth with subsequent warty scaling especially in flexural areas, palms and soles. Autosomal dominant defect in keratins 1 and 10
  - *Lamellar ichthyosis*—autosomal recessive defect in transglutaminase 1 with erythroderma, ectropion, rapid epidermal turnover, large skin scales, thick palms and soles. Sepsis, dehydration, dyshydrosis, heat intolerance, corneal damage are complications
  - Visual diagnosis confirmed by skin biopsy, genetic testing, and enzyme analysis

- ## Differential Diagnosis
  - Atopic dermatitis—occurs in isolation but often complicates ichthyosis vulgaris
  - Psoriasis
  - KID syndrome—keratitis, ichthyosis, deafness, and sometimes notched teeth
  - Sjögren-Larsson syndrome—ichthyosiform dermatitis, spastic diplegia, retinitis pigmentosa, and mental retardation
  - Human immunodeficiency virus (HIV) patients may develop acquired ichthyosis

- ## Treatment
  - Medications to control scaling (lactic acid with ammonium hydroxide, salicylic acid, topical retinoic acid lubricants), avoidance of injury
  - Topical products must be used with caution because of skin absorption
  - Treat associated atopic dermatitis
  - Protect eyes in lamellar ichthyosis—artificial tears, protective covering during sleep, surgery for ectropion may be required
  - Antibiotics in infants with epidermolytic hyperkeratosis
  - KID syndrome may respond to topical cyclosporine

- ## Pearl

Newborns with lamellar ichthyosis may be completely encased in a collodion membrane, which sheds at 10–14 days of age revealing the erythematous skin condition.

Milia

- **Essentials of Diagnosis**
  - 1–2 mm benign, keratin-filled epidermal cysts on the face of 40% of normal newborns
  - Cysts arise in immature or obstructed sebaceous glands around and on the nose (neonates) and around the eye (children and adults). Small vesicles may be present
  - Intraoral counterpart seen in 60–85% of neonates (Epstein pearls, Bohn nodules)
  - Secondary milia occurs in areas of skin trauma—dermabrasion, burns, EB, lichen planus, porphyria cutanea tarda, strong topical steroids
  - Visual diagnosis is sufficient in neonates. Secondary milia requires diagnostic evaluation. Biopsy rarely needed

- **Differential Diagnosis**
  - Neonatal acne
  - Sebaceous gland hyperplasia of neonates due to maternal androgens
  - Miliaria—obstruction of eccrine sweat ducts in neonates cause tiny grouped vesicles or red papules in intertriginous areas and contiguous skin
  - Pustular melanosis—neutrophil containing pustules leave pigmented macules upon spontaneous rupture

- **Treatment**
  - No treatment required in neonates. Cysts usually rupture and disappear in the first month
  - Identify and treat causes of secondary milia

- **Pearl**

Vigorous washing of these "whiteheads" in neonates is not helpful and may worsen the condition.

Erythema Toxicum

■ Essentials of Diagnosis

- Benign rash in 50% of term newborns onset 24–48 hours
- 2–3 cm blotchy red macules on chest; also back, face, and extremities
- May be up to 100 lesions
- Macular erythema may fade or may progress to urticarial wheals or pustules filled with eosinophils. Blood eosinophilia up to 20%

■ Differential Diagnosis

- Intrauterine infection (rubella, cytomegalovirus [CMV], toxo)—rash usually present at birth with purpuric component
- Postnatally acquired herpes simplex usually associated with severe illness and vesicular lesions. Neonatal varicella
- Pustular melanosis—may appear on palms and soles
- Insect bites
- Bacterial pyoderma

■ Treatment

- Spontaneous resolution usually in 5–7 days but may last for 6 weeks

■ Pearl

The cause of this condition is unknown. The presence of eosinophilic pus suggests an allergic reaction to something. Oddly, the longer the length of labor in vaginal deliveries, the higher the incidence and duration of erythema toxicum. Go figure.

13

Pigment Cell Skin Lesions

- **Essentials of Diagnosis**
    - *Mongolian spot*—blue-black macule over lumbosacral area (occasionally over shoulders and back) in infants of Native American, African American, and Asian descent. Migratory defect in neural crest melanocytes. Benign and fades with time
    - *Café au lait macule*—light brown oval macule found anywhere on body in 10% of white and 22% of black children. >6 macules >1.5 cm may indicate NF-1. Patients with McCune-Albright syndrome have large single irregular macules
    - *Spitz nevus*—red brown solitary benign nodule consists of bizarre pigment producing cells with many mitoses
    - *Acquired melanocytic nevus*—common mole. Increases with age. Clones of melanocytes at dermo-epidermal junction. Benign
    - *Melanoma*—rare before puberty. Malignant collections of melanocytes. Local excision and pathologic examination of suspicious lesions especially with ulceration and bleeding is essential
    - *Congenital melanocytic nevus*—larger and darker than acquired nevi and may contain hairs. A nevus covering >5% of body surface is called a giant nevus. 1–5% may become malignant

- **Differential Diagnosis**
    - A Mongolian spot may be mistaken for bruising and raise the suspicion of child abuse
    - Epidermal nevi may be brown, resembling common moles

- **Treatment**
    - No therapy required for Mongolian spots, café au lait macules, Spitz nevus, or common moles
    - Congenital melanotic nevi should be monitored for change in size or coloration, which may indicate malignant transformation
    - Melanoma in children with congenital melanotic nevus may develop in areas other than skin
    - Surgical removal of large acquired or congenital moles for cosmetic reasons may be considered but scarring and keloid may result

- **Pearl**

The presence of hair in a mole does not carry any greater risk of malignancy. Hairs are found in common moles as well as congenital melanocytic nevi.

Vascular Birthmarks

- **Essentials of Diagnosis**

  - *Capillary malformations*—localized red/pink area of capillary hypertrophy in neonates found over glabellum, eyelid, forehead, or nape of neck (stork bites)
  - *Port wine stain*—dark red capillary malformation usually an isolated lesion. Unilateral facial lesion suggests Sturge-Weber syndrome. Extremity lesions produce underlying limb hypertrophy (Klippel-Trénaunay syndrome)
  - *Hemangioma*—red rubbery benign tumor of capillary endothelium. May not be present at birth, appearing as a blanched area that becomes a red nodule by 2–3 weeks. Lesions may be superficial, deep, or mixed. 90% resolve by age 9 years
  - *Lymphatic malformation*—loose fluid-filled superficial multiloculated masses or deep, irregular masses in neck, parotids, mouth, axilla, retroperitoneum, mediastinum (cystic hygroma). May be very large and disfiguring. May cause oral or airway obstruction
  - Careful magnetic resonance imaging (MRI) evaluation to determine extent of lesion before any treatment

13

- **Differential Diagnosis**

  - Branchial cleft cyst, thyroglossal duct cyst, ranula, goiter, mediastinal tumor, cervical lymphadenitis may mimic deep cystic hygroma and hemangioma in the neck.
  - Secondary lymphangiomas may develop after trauma or surgery

- **Treatment**

  - Small capillary malformations usually disappear. Larger lesions become less apparent as the skin thickens and rarely need treatment
  - Hemangiomas causing airway obstruction, visual obstruction amblyopia, cardiac decompensation ($\uparrow$output), or bleeding may be treated with prednisolone, interferon-α-2a, pulsed dye laser
  - Life-threatening cystic hygromas treated with injection of picibanil or surgery
  - Port wine stains treated with dye laser

- **Pearl**

Kasabach-Merritt syndrome (platelet trapping with consumptive coagulopathy) does not occur in solitary cutaneous hemangiomas. It occurs only with internal hemangiomas, hemangioendotheliomas, and tufted angiomas.

Acanthosis Nigricans (AN)

- **Essentials of Diagnosis**
  - Acquired symmetric velvety hyperpigmented patches in skin creases of axilla, groin, neck and sometimes face, umbilicus, thighs, genitalia. May be slightly pruritic. Small skin tags may develop in affected areas
  - Associated with obesity and insulin-resistant diabetes. Severity of AN may relate to severity of insulin resistance
  - Insulin or insulin-like growth factors are the probable stimulus for keratinocyte proliferation
  - More common in highly pigmented skin
  - Also occurs in polycystic ovary syndrome, hyperandrogen states, autoimmune conditions in which anti-insulin antibodies are present, nicotinic acid, and OCPs

- **Differential Diagnosis**
  - Addison disease
  - Hemochromatosis
  - Pellagra

- **Treatment**
  - Treatment is not required
  - Weight loss with associated drop in insulin resistance may be associated with improvement
  - Identify and evaluate associated conditions
  - Identify and discontinue suspect medications

- **Pearl**

In rare children, black or white, obese or slim, growth factors (possibly transforming growth factor-α [TGF-α]) released from malignant cancers may provoke AN. In a nonobese child with sudden-onset AN, consider this rare possibility.

Impetigo

- ■ Essentials of Diagnosis
  - Initial pruritic papule that vesiculates and then ruptures leaving denuded area covered by honey-colored crust. Often perioral or in nasolabial folds
  - Lesions spread readily. Systemic symptoms rare
  - *Staphylococcus aureus* and group A β-hemolytic streptococcus (GAS) can be isolated but cultures sometimes negative
  - Glomerulonephritis may follow impetigo caused by nephritogenic strains of GAS

- ■ Differential Diagnosis
  - Perianal cellulitis—red circumanal rash with scant rectal bleeding. Pain on defecation. Anal swab culture yields GAS
  - Streptococcal vaginitis—Prepubertal girls, dysuria, pain, erythema, and tenderness of the introitus with blood-tinged discharge. Culture yields GAS
  - Bullous impetigo—flaccid bullae on trunk and extremities caused by epidermolytic exotoxin-producing strains of *S aureus*. Children <2 years most commonly affected. Often with fever and toxicity
  - Herpes simplex may cause perioral painful, pruritic vesicles
  - Consider also—burns, candida, scabies, contact or atopic eczema, insect bites, erythema multiforme

13

- ■ Treatment
  - Cleanse skin gently
  - Mild, limited impetigo responds to topical antibiotics—mupirocin, fusidic acid
  - Widespread infection, recurrent infections, systemic toxicity, deep infection may require systemic antibiotics—penicillin, erythromycin, clarithromycin, azithromycin depending upon patient and organism sensitivities
  - Methicillin resistant strains of *S aureus* are prevalent. Clindamycin may be required

- ■ Pearl

The relative roles of staphylococcus and streptococcus in this common infection are still not clearly delineated. The old theory that streptococcus is the primary pathogen and staphylococcus a superinfection doesn't seem uniformly true, but a unifying explanation that covers all impetigo hasn't appeared yet.

14

Ophthalmology

14

Conjunctivitis

- **Essentials of Diagnosis**
  - *Viral*—general hyperemia. Profuse tearing. Upper respiratory infection (URI) symptoms and preauricular adenopathy. Mild, mucoid eye discharge with lymphocytes, plasma cells, multinucleated giant cells, eosinophilic intranuclear inclusions
  - *Bacterial*—general hyperemia. Purulent exudate with bacteria and neutrophils. Occasional fever and sore throat
  - *Allergic*—hyperemia and itching. Minimal thin exudate with eosinophils. URI symptoms rare
  - *Chlamydial*—hyperemia. Profuse mucoid discharge with neutrophils, plasma cells, basophilic intracytoplasmic inclusions. Neonates may have preauricular adenopathy, pneumonia, and eosinophilia

- **Differential Diagnosis**
  - Conjunctivitis in neonates also caused by silver nitrate, gonococcus, staphylococcus, pneumococcus, and viruses (herpes simplex)
  - Erythema multiforme
  - Stevens-Johnson syndrome
  - Reiter syndrome
  - Kawasaki disease
  - Conjunctival or corneal trauma
  - Periorbital and orbital cellulitis
  - Oculoglandular syndrome with *Staphylococcus aureus*, group A β-hemolytic streptococcus, *Mycobacterium tuberculosis*, atypical mycobacteria, *Bartonella* (cat scratch), and *Francisella* infections (tularemia)

14

- **Treatment**
  - Accurate diagnosis needed before therapy
  - Viral—supportive treatment for adenovirus. Treat *Herpes simplex* with topical trifluridine or vidarabine. Oral acyclovir reduces recurrence
  - Bacterial—topical antibiotics for common infections (nontypeable *Haemophilus*, *Streptococcus pneumoniae*, *Moraxella catarrhalis,* and *S aureus*). Systemic therapy for *Neisseria gonorrhoeae* and *Neisseria meningitidis*
  - Allergic—topical antihistamine and mast cell stabilizers. Topical vasoconstrictors, nonsteroidal anti-inflammatory drugs (NSAIDs), and corticosteroids occasionally indicated
  - Chlamydia—in neonates, systemic and topical erythromycin

- **Pearl**

Vernal conjunctivitis is a seasonal allergic conjunctivitis. Dramatic cobblestone changes on the superior palpebral conjunctiva help confirm the diagnosis.

Hyphema

- **Essentials of Diagnosis**
  - Blunt trauma to the globe causes bleeding in the anterior chamber
  - Juvenile xanthogranuloma and bleeding disorders increase the risk of hyphema
  - Ophthalmologic examination in any case where extensive eye injury is suspected
  - Prognosis worsens with extensive ocular injury and with rebleeding

- **Differential Diagnosis**
  - Consider the possibility of additional ocular injury—iritis, lens subluxation, retinal detachment, glaucoma
  - Child abuse

- **Treatment**
  - Prevention is key. Protective eyewear during sports, in the laboratory, industrial arts classes, and when operating power tools
  - If patient is otherwise uninjured, test visual acuity, assess integrity of globe and orbit, keep head elevated and eye covered
  - Resolution of hyphema covering <50% of the anterior chamber is likely
  - In large hyphemas, cycloplegics may prevent pupillary synechiae

- **Pearl**

Patients with sickle cell anemia or trait are at higher risk for optic atrophy and loss of vision from the elevated intraocular pressure due to hyphema. Any African American with hyphema should have his/her sickle cell status checked if it is not known so that treatment can be adjusted for the increased risk.

Dacryocystitis

■ Essentials of Diagnosis

- Infection of nasolacrimal duct or sac by upper respiratory bacteria in association with acute or chronic duct obstruction
- Presents with erythema, swelling, tenderness, pain over the lacrimal sac, fever, purulent discharge, and tearing
- In chronic dacryocystitis, there may be mucopurulent debris on lids and lashes, tearing, palpebral and conjunctival injection, reflux of pus at the puncta
- Culture often shows *S aureus*, *S pneumoniae*, *Streptococcus pyogenes*, *Streptococcus viridans*, *M catarrhalis,* and *Haemophilus* species

■ Differential Diagnosis

- Congenital dacryocystocele—often has bluish hue
- Incomplete canalization of the duct in infants
- Hordeolum
- Congenital glaucoma
- Allergies

■ Treatment

- Treat severe acute dacryocystitis with specific intravenous antibiotics after culture of discharge
- Oral antibiotics for mild cases
- Warm compresses improve drainage
- Probing the duct or surgery is sometimes needed to relieve duct obstruction

■ Pearl

Daily gentle massage over the nasolacrimal sac in the newborn with "goopy" eyes may help remove inspissated secretions and promote complete canalization of the duct.

14

Uveitis

- ### Essentials of Diagnosis
  - *Anterior* (iritis)—syphilis, tuberculosis, sarcoidosis, relapsing fever, Lyme disease, juvenile spondyloarthropathy, Reiter syndrome, psoriatic arthritis, Crohn's disease, pauciarticular rheumatoid arthritis
  - *Posterior* (choroiditis and retinitis)—toxoplasma, rubella, cytomegalovirus, herpes simplex, varicella-zoster, syphilis, lymphocytic choriomeningitis virus, candida, *Toxocara canis* and *Toxocara cati*
  - *Intermediate*—(pars planitis)—*Toxocara*, inflammatory bowel disease, multiple sclerosis, sarcoid
  - Anterior symptoms—photophobia, pain, and blurred vision
  - Slit lamp examination shows inflammatory cells and protein flare in anterior uveitis and retinal and vitreous exudates in posterior uveitis

- ### Differential Diagnosis
  - Retinoblastoma and other ocular neoplasms
  - Traumatic iridocyclitis
  - Human immunodeficiency virus (HIV)-associated acute retinal necrosis

- ### Treatment
  - Patients with immunodeficiency, rheumatoid arthritis, inflammatory bowel disease require routine ophthalmologic examination
  - Some inflammatory eye conditions associated with Crohn disease (uveitis, episcleritis) are treated with topical steroid. Others (cataracts, herpetic infections) are the consequence of long-term steroid use
  - Serologic testing may reveal the cause of neonatal posterior uveitis
  - Toxocara infections may be treated with periocular corticosteroid and vitrectomy

- ### Pearl
  Children acquire T canis *or* T cati *ocular infection (ocular larva migrans) by ingesting dirt contaminated with parasite eggs. They usually have unilateral disease with a red eye, leukocoria, and decreased vision.*

Papilledema

- ■ Essentials of Diagnosis
  - Bilateral optic disc edema associated with increased intracranial pressure
  - Central nervous system (CNS) causes include tumor, infection, inflammation, bleed, hydrocephalus, venous sinus thrombosis
  - Pseudotumor cerebri associated with obesity, steroid use or withdrawal, viral infection, tetracycline, growth hormone, idiopathic intracranial hypertension
  - Disc margins appear elevated and indistinct, increased vessel diameter, hyperemia, retinal hemorrhages or exudates. Optic atrophy in long-standing cases
  - Symptoms—visual disturbances, brief periods of blindness, enlarged blind spot, headache, vomiting, and other symptoms of intracranial hypertension

- ■ Differential Diagnosis
  - Papillitis—optic neuritis secondary to cat scratch disease, multiple sclerosis, acute disseminated encephalomyelitis, Devic disease
  - Pseudopapilledema is a normal optic disc variant
  - Optic atrophy may be secondary to brain injury, intraventricular hemorrhage, glioma, craniosynostosis, methyl alcohol, metabolic diseases

14

- ■ Treatment
  - Identify specific causes by radiologic examination and sometimes spinal fluid analysis
  - Shunting may be needed to prevent permanent optic nerve injury
  - Symptoms of idiopathic intracranial hypertension may respond immediately to lumbar puncture or to acetazolamide or corticosteroid

- ■ Pearl

Although the optic discs in papillitis and papilledema may look the same, papillitis is usually unilateral and papilledema is almost always bilateral.

Orbital and Periorbital Cellulitis

- **Essentials of Diagnosis**
  - Periorbital infections cause eyelid edema, swelling, erythema, pain, fever. Usually caused by exogenous infections—skin, hordeolum, dacryocystitis, chalazion—with *S aureus, S pyogenes*
  - Orbital infections cause additional symptoms of proptosis, pain with and restriction of eye movement, high fever. Infection arises via perforating veins from contiguous sinuses. *S aureus* and respiratory pathogens
  - Young children may be bacteremic with orbital and periorbital infection
  - Computed tomography (CT) scan differentiates periorbital cellulitis from orbital cellulitis/abscess
  - Sinus imaging should be done at the time of diagnosis

- **Differential Diagnosis**
  - Severe conjunctivitis—viral, bacterial, or allergic
  - Trauma or foreign body

- **Treatment**
  - Systemic antibiotics required
  - Orbital infection/abscess may require surgical drainage
  - Drainage of infected sinuses

- **Pearl**

Careful examination of the entire eye is essential when there is significant cellulitis of the eyelids. Sedation or anesthesia may be required to accomplish the necessary radiologic and ophthalmologic examinations.

Amblyopia

- ■ Essentials of Diagnosis
  - Unilateral or bilateral reduction in central visual acuity due to deprivation of well-formed retinal images during early visual development
  - In testable children, visual acuity is different in the 2 eyes
  - In preverbal child, suggestive findings are strabismus, media opacities, unequal papillary red reflexes, positive family history
  - Causes include muscle imbalance (strabismic), refractive errors (ametropic, anisometropic), stimulus deprivation (dense cataract, severe ptosis)

- ■ Differential Diagnosis
  - Convergence insufficiency

- ■ Treatment
  - The earlier treatment is initiated the better the outcome
  - Address refractive errors
  - Remove congenital cataracts
  - Strengthen extraocular musculature or operate if strabismus is severe
  - Patching or producing temporary cycloplegia in the sound eye causes the visual cortex to process input from the amblyopic eye and promotes development

14

- ■ Pearl

The worst prognosis for vision occurs when there is total deprivation of visual input as with dense cataracts or severe ptosis.

Hordeolum (Stye)

- ■ Essentials of Diagnosis
  - • Staphylococcal infection of the sebaceous glands of Zeis or Moll in the upper or lower eyelid
  - • Infection of the meibomian glands on the internal aspect of tarsa are also called styes
  - • Warmth, tenderness, erythema, and local swelling at edge of lid
  - • Recurrent infections common

- ■ Differential Diagnosis
  - • Eyelid warts secondary to papillomavirus
  - • Pediculosis of the lid
  - • Rosacea involves the lid, conjunctivae, and cornea
  - • Blepharitis—(staphylococcus infection of lid margin) may cause corneal erosion and ulcers if severe and may arise as an extension of a single stye
  - • Chalazion—(meibomian gland inflammation) produces tender nodule on the upper or lower lid tarsus. Palpebral conjunctiva underneath the nodule displays yellow lipogranuloma

14

- ■ Treatment
  - • Warm compresses
  - • Topical antibiotics of questionable value
  - • Hordeolum may require incision and drainage
  - • Blepharitis treated with local cleansing and topical antistaphylococcal ointment
  - • Most chalazions respond to warm compresses. Incision and curettage occasionally needed

- ■ Pearl

Most styes drain spontaneously. The complications of styes almost all arise as a result of poor technique in drainage—loss of tarsal tissue, loss of eyelashes, fistula through the tarsal plate from improper puncture of the stye.

15

Dental and Oral Medicine

15

Dental Caries

■ **Essentials of Diagnosis**

- The most common dental disease of childhood which exists even in absence of "cavities" in the teeth
- Infection usually after oral colonization with *Streptococcus mutans* transmitted from mother to child
- Caries is promoted by bacterial acid production stimulated by carbohydrate intake
- The "cavity-prone child" is usually a normal child with a cariogenic diet and poor oral hygiene

■ **Differential Diagnosis**

- The teeth of children with hyperbilirubinemia may be stained brown
- Ectodermal dysplasia syndromes are associated with abnormal enamel and increase in caries
- Gastroesophageal (GE) reflux does not cause caries
- Bulimia may produce erosions of the inner aspect of the teeth

■ **Treatment**

- Filling cavities does not remove the cause of caries. Prevention and early diagnosis are key
- Reduce acidogenesis of oral flora by reducing frequent carbohydrate ingestion
- If drinking water contains <0.3 ppm fluoride, oral fluoride supplement is 0.25 mg/day (<3 years), 0.5 mg/day (3–6 years), 1 mg/day (6–16 years)
- If drinking water contains >0.6 ppm fluoride, no supplement needed
- Start tooth brushing as soon as teeth appear
- Avoid sticky carbohydrate-rich foods—caramel, raisins, gum drops
- Topical fluoride in toothpaste can retard the development of caries

15

■ **Pearl**

A baby with extensive caries of the maxillary incisors probably has "nursing bottle teeth." This can be prevented by appropriate education!

Periodontal Disease

- ■ Essentials of Diagnosis
    - Inflammation or infection of dental-supporting tissues—bone, gums, ligaments
    - Plaque deposits in the sulcus between tooth and gum support bacterial growth causing gingivitis
    - Gingivitis causes soft tissue destruction, bone loss, and inflammation extending to the tooth apex
    - Often no symptoms. May present with fever, foul breath, tooth loss, mouth pain, easy bleeding

- ■ Differential Diagnosis
    - Herpes, candida, varicella, and other oral infections
    - Aphthous mouth ulcers associated with inflammatory bowel disease
    - Drug effects—dilantin, cyclosporine A cause gingival hypertrophy
    - Erythema multiforme drug reactions
    - Immune deficiency, human immunodeficiency virus (HIV), graft-versus-host disease, cancer chemotherapy all predispose to gingivitis. Leukemia causes gingival infiltrates
    - One symptom of trench mouth (Vincent's angina) is severe gingivitis

- ■ Treatment
    - Good oral hygiene—brushing and flossing—can prevent most gingivitis. Professional cleaning, medication, or surgery may be required
    - Topical or systemic antiviral agents for herpes gingivostomatitis
    - Babies with mild oral thrush require no therapy
    - Prevent gingivitis in children with congenital valvular heart disease or intravascular foreign bodies

- ■ Pearl

There is an association between maternal periodontal disease and premature delivery. No mechanism yet determined but possibly both are phenomena associated with malnutrition.

Vincent's Angina (Trench Mouth)

- ■ Essentials of Diagnosis
  - Necrotizing oral/pharyngeal infection due to combined infection with *Fusiformis* (gram-negative bacteria) and *Borrelia vincentii* (spirochete)
  - Often associated with poor oral hygiene, malnutrition, and immunodeficiency
  - Fever, pain, dysphagia, regional adenopathy, deep ulcers of mouth and pharynx, tissue necrosis with slough and bleeding
  - Diagnosed by gentian violet stain of ulcer exudates

- ■ Differential Diagnosis
  - Immunodeficiency with opportunistic infection
  - Allergic reaction
  - Inflammatory bowel disease
  - Herpes simplex
  - Candida
  - Oral gonococcal infection
  - Diphtheria

- ■ Treatment
  - Penicillin, clindamycin, topical antibiotics, careful mouth hygiene
  - Repair nutritional defects and support ongoing nutritional needs
  - Protect the airway if tissue slough is severe
  - Treat pain locally or systemically

15

- ■ Pearl

The "trench" in trench mouth refers to the frequent infections suffered in World War I by the soldiers who spent long days in the trenches with inadequate food and hygiene.

Orodental Trauma

- **Essentials of Diagnosis**
  - Blow to the chin is the most common orofacial trauma of childhood
  - Lip, gingival, tongue, or mucosal trauma is sometimes associated with embedded tooth fragments or foreign bodies
  - Tooth trauma includes luxation (tooth displacement), fracture, or avulsion (complete loss)
  - Pain on opening the jaw or deviation of the jaw suggests condylar fracture

- **Differential Diagnosis**
  - Facial cellulitis

- **Treatment**
  - Simple subluxation (mobility without displacement) requires no intervention
  - Intrusive (displacement into the socket) or extrusive luxation of primary teeth usually resolves in several months. Removal required for periodontal infection or major displacement
  - Intrusive and extrusive luxation of permanent teeth usually require orthodontic or surgical repositioning and splinting
  - Avulsed primary teeth are not reimplanted. Reimplantation of avulsed tooth into alveolar bone within 1 hour is often successful
  - Tooth fractures should be covered and protected by a dentist to prevent pain and infection

- **Pearl**

If there is injury to a tooth, be sure to check the soft tissues for foreign bodies and the jaw for fractures, especially condylar fracture.

16

Ear, Nose, and Throat

16

Acute Rhinosinusitis

- **Essentials of Diagnosis**
  - Viral upper respiratory infections (URI) worse after 7 days or unimproved after 10 days suggests this diagnosis
  - Mucociliary clearance depressed by viral URI allows bacterial sinus infection (*Streptococcus pneumoniae*, nontypeable *Haemophilus influenzae, Moraxella catarrhalis,* β-hemolytic streptococci, and rarely anaerobes)
  - Maxillary and ethmoid sinuses affected in children <5 years. Frontal and sphenoid sinuses also affected in children >5 years
  - Symptoms—nasal congestion, nasal and postnasal drainage, facial pressure/pain, fever, cough, malaise, ear and maxillary tooth pain
  - Sinus aspiration can identify responsible agent. Sinus aspiration, x-rays or computed tomography (CT) scan not indicated in first episode of acute rhinosinusitis

- **Differential Diagnosis**
  - Allergy may cause rhinitis
  - Tension headache, cluster headache
  - Caries/abscesses of maxillary teeth, cheek cellulitis, popsicle paniculitis may resemble maxillary sinusitis
  - Orbital/periorbital cellulitis, dacryocystitis may resemble ethmoid sinusitis
  - Recurrent rhinosinusitis—episodes of acute bacteria rhinosinusitis clear with antibiotics but recur with each or most URIs
  - Chronic rhinosinusitis—acute sinusitis that does not clear with treatment. CT scan may be useful adjunct to diagnosis
  - Conditions that may present with rhinosinusitis—immotile cilia syndrome (Kartagener syndrome), cystic fibrosis, nasal polyp, septal deviation, nasal foreign body

- **Treatment**
  - Topical decongestants and oral vasoconstrictor/decongestants often used in acute rhinosinusitis but efficacy has not been proven
  - Allergic rhinitis—intranasal cromolyn or corticosteroids may be helpful
  - First-line antibiotics—amoxicillin-clavulanate, cefpodoxime proxetil, cefuroxime axetil, cefdinir, trimethoprim-sulfamethoxazole, clindamycin (in proven strep infection)
  - Second-line antibiotic therapy for resistant symptoms—increase dose of first-line drugs or ceftriaxone for 5 days

- **Pearl**

Limited extraocular movement, proptosis, chemosis, and ↓visual acuity are warning signs of severe ethmoid sinusitis with penetration into the orbit.

16

Acute Otitis Media (AOM)

- **Essentials of Diagnosis**
  - Middle ear inflammation with effusion, otalgia, fever, irritability, anorexia, or vomiting
  - Physical signs—erythema, bulging, and ↓mobility of tympanic membrane (TM), air-fluid level behind the TM, otorrhea
  - Viral URI causes adenoid swelling, ↑nasopharyngeal colonization by bacterial pathogens, and ↓Eustation tube drainage
  - Viral antigens found in 40% of effusions (mainly respiratory syncytial virus [RSV] and influenza)
  - Nasal organisms *S pneumoniae, H influenzae,* and *M catarrhalis* found in 50% of effusions
  - Clinical diagnosis of AOM requires cerumen removal, pneumatic otoscopy, and occasionally tympanocentesis and culture
  - Tympanometry useful in diagnosis of effusion, not infection

- **Differential Diagnosis**
  - Simple otitis media with effusion. This condition does not require antibiotic therapy
  - External otitis with purulent otorrhea
  - Relapse of chronic or recurrent otitis media

- **Treatment**
  - Pain management—Tylenol or ibuprofen usually suffices
  - Overuse of antibiotics for simple otitis media has promoted nasal colonization with antibiotic resistant bacteria
  - Infants <6 months with clinical diagnosis of AOM should receive antibiotics
  - Other situations requiring antibiotics—AOM with proven bacterial effusion, children <2 years with AOM, children >2 years with AOM causing severe pain, fever, or purulent discharge
  - Children >2 years with uncomplicated AOM can be observed for 48–72 hours before using antibiotics
  - First-line antibiotics—amoxicillin or cefuroxime. After 48–72 hours observation, treat clinical failures with amoxicillin-clavulanate
  - Pneumococcal vaccine and intranasal influenza vaccine reduce frequency of AOM

- **Pearl**

Risk factors for AOM include household cigarette smoke, propping of nursing bottles for infant feeding, pacifier sucking, daycare, low cord-blood pneumococcal antibody titer, immunoglobulin (IgA) deficiency, and other immune deficiencies.

Chronic Otitis Media

- **Essentials of Diagnosis**
  - *Otitis media with persistent effusion (OME)*—occurs in 30% of AOM regardless of antibiotic therapy. May be serous, mucoid, or purulent. Diagnosable by tympanometry. May cause mild conductive hearing loss
  - *Unresponsive AOM*—persistent signs of acute infection despite antibiotic use. Tympanocentesis for culture should be performed
  - *Otitis media with TM perforation*—a result of AOM usually heals in 2 weeks. Persistent perforation may require surgical repair
  - *Chronic suppurative otitis media*—persistent middle ear discharge in a child with tympanostomy tubes or TM perforation. Often associated with middle ear colonization by *Pseudomonas* or anaerobes.

- **Differential Diagnosis**
  - Tympanosclerosis—chronic inflammation or trauma of the TM produces granulations sometimes mistaken for infection
  - Cholesteatoma—white malignant TM mass at the site of retraction or perforation is a late complication of chronic perforation and effusion. CT examination to assess extent of tumor invasion is indicated
  - Chronic otorrhea secondary to otitis externa
  - Chronic otorrhea secondary to foreign body or trauma

16

- **Treatment**
  - Persistent OME (>2–4 months) with conductive hearing loss—treat with corticosteroids for 7 days or culture the middle ear and treat pathogenic bacteria
  - Ventilating tubes are indicated for bilateral hearing loss ≥20 dB
  - Reculture unresponsive AOM and treat with antibiotics
  - Acute perforation of TM usually heals spontaneously as AOM resolves. Avoid swimming while perforation is present
  - Surgical repair may be indicated in children >7 years with perforations lasting >3 months
  - Treat chronic suppurative OM with antibiotics after culturing the middle ear drainage. Quinolones used in older children

- **Pearl**

Repeated broad spectrum antibiotic treatment of persistent middle ear effusions is a major cause of increased antibiotic resistance among respiratory pathogens.

Stomatitis

- **Essentials of Diagnosis**
  - Aphthous stomatitis—painful, small ulcers on inner aspect of lips or tongue. Possibly allergic, infectious, or autoimmune. Seen in Crohn disease, Behçet disease, familial Mediterranean fever, FAPA syndrome, leukemia, cyclic neutropenia
  - Herpes simplex gingivostomatitis—small ulcers on buccal mucosa, anterior tonsillar pillars, inner lips, tongue, and gingiva. Fever, tender cervical adenopathy, pain, dysphagia. Ulcer base contains microscopic viral inclusions
  - Oral candidiasis—common in healthy infants and immunosupressed patients. Adherent white plaques on buccal mucosa sometimes painful. ↑infection risk with immunodeficiency, antibiotic use, inhaled or systemic corticosteroids. Organisms can be seen in plaques
  - Herpangina—infectious stomatitis caused by Coxsackie A virus. Patients have small ulcers with an erythematous halo on the tonsillar pillars, soft palate and uvula, but not the anterior mouth or the tonsils themselves. Polymerase chain reaction (PCR) diagnosis available
  - Drugs and trauma—accidental bites, hot food or drink, irritants, chemotherapeutic agents, especially cytoxan cause mouth ulcers

- **Differential Diagnosis**
  - Parotitis, oral hairy leukoplakia (seen in HIV)
  - Geographic tongue may look like tongue ulcers
  - Periodontal disease, trench mouth (mixed bacterial gingivitis)
  - Hand-foot-and-mouth disease (enterovirus)—oral ulcers may predominate but usually also involves palms and soles
  - Kawasaki disease, erythema multiforme may cause desquamation in the mouth

- **Treatment**
  - Aphthous stomatitis usually resolves spontaneously without scarring. Bland diet and local analgesics for pain. Treat underlying diseases. Betamethasone valerate ointment sometimes hastens healing
  - Herpes stomatitis—monitor for dehydration, laryngotracheitis. Corticosteroids contraindicated. Antihistamine mouthwash helps pain
  - Oral candidiasis—no therapy for healthy infants. Use oral nystatin suspension in sick infants or immunosupressed patients

- **Pearl**

Recurrent blisters of lips, tongue, or buccal mucosa may be thermal burns caused by child abuse.

Cervical Adenitis

■ **Essentials of Diagnosis**

- Ear, nose, and throat (ENT) infections can spread to cervical lymph node causing inflammation or abscess. Typically single anterior cervical node involved
- 70% of adenitis is due to β-hemolytic streptococcus, 20% to staphylococci, and 10% to viruses, atypical mycobacteria, and *Bartonella henslae* (cat scratch disease)
- Atypical mycobacteria—node usually violaceous, matted, often associated with infected teeth. Purified protein derivative (PPD) mildly positive; second strength PPD positive
- Testing—throat culture, complete blood culture (CBC) and differential (look for atypical lymphocytes), Epstein-Barr serology, cat scratch serology, PPD, chest x-ray
- Aspirate fluctuant nodes to obtain diagnostic bacterial culture

■ **Differential Diagnosis**

- Systemic bacterial, viral, parasitic, fungal infections associated with adenopathy
- Malignancy—leukemia, thyroid carcinoma, rhabdomyosarcoma, Hodgkin's and non-Hodgkin's lymphoma
- Structural anomalies—thyroglossal duct cyst, branchial cleft cyst, cystic hygroma
- Parotitis—swelling is at the angle of the jaw, but may look like a neck mass
- Ranula—cyst in the floor of the mouth may extend below the mylohyoid and appear as a neck mass
- Sternocleidomastoid muscle hematoma
- Kawasaki disease—multiple, nonfluctuant nodes in a febrile child

16

■ **Treatment**

- Drain fluctuant nodes. It speeds resolution
- Treat streptococcal and staphylococcal infection according to sensitivity with cillins or cephalosporins. Methicillin-resistant *Staphylococcus aureus* is a growing problem
- Cat scratch disease may respond to azithromycin, rifampin, and other drugs
- Treat atypical mycobacteria by surgical excision of node. Treat recurrent infection with macrolide in combination with either rifampin or ethambutol (children >5 years) for 3–6 months

■ **Pearl**

Malignant nodes are usually firm, cool, nontender, fixed to underlying tissues, often multiple and extracervical. Don't give antibiotics, think biopsy.

Pharyngitis and Tonsillitis

- **Essentials of Diagnosis**
  - 90% of sore throat and fever in childhood is viral. Most viruses cannot be identified but some have typical features:
    - *Epstein-Barr virus* (EBV)—exudative tonsillitis, generalized cervical adenitis, fever, child >5 years, positive mono spot or EBV titers, atypical lymphocytes on peripheral smear
    - *Herpangina (Coxsackie A viruses)*—small ulcers on anterior pillars, soft palate, and uvula, sparing mouth and tonsils
    - *Hand-foot-and-mouth disease (enteroviruses)*—small mouth ulcers with vesicles, papules, and pustules on palms and soles
    - *Pharyngoconjunctival fever (adenovirus)*—epidemic exudative tonsillitis and conjunctivitis with lymphadenopathy and fever
  - Bacterial pharyngitis usually due to group A β-streptococcus (GAS) but also *Mycoplasma pneumoniae, Chlamydia pneumoniae,* group C and G streptococcus, *Arcanobacterium hemolyticum. Neisseria gonorrhoeae* may cause sexually transmitted oral infection

- **Differential Diagnosis**
  - Peritonsillar cellulitis or abscess—fever, pain, unilateral tonsillar bulge with displacement of uvula and soft palate away from the affected side
  - Retropharyngeal abscess—usually due to β-hemolytic streptococcus or *S aureus.* Fever, systemic toxicity, drooling, neck hyperextension, dyspnea. Neck CT shows anterior displacement of posterior pharyngeal wall
  - Oral burns from hot liquid or caustics
  - Varicella may involve the oropharynx but skin lesions are usually obvious
  - Erythema multiforme or other allergic stomatitis

- **Treatment**
  - Treat tonsillitis with antibiotics only if pathogenic bacteria are identified
  - Treat group A streptococcal tonsillitis with 10 days of oral penicillin V potassium, cephalosporin, or intramuscular penicillin G benzathine LA
  - Retropharyngeal abscess is a surgical emergency requiring hospitalization because of potential for airway obstruction
  - Tonsillectomy for massive hypertrophy or recurrent infection

- **Pearl**

Recently, sleep apnea has become a major indication for tonsillectomy and adenoidectomy.

Epiglottitis

- **Essentials of Diagnosis**
  - Infection of the epiglottis with *H influenzae* type B, nontypeable *H influenzae, S pneumoniae*, group A streptococcus, *Streptococcus pyogenes*, *Neisseria meningitides,* and *S aureus*
  - Swelling of epiglottis and arytenoids progresses rapidly and can produce fatal upper airway obstruction
  - Blood culture is often positive, especially in *H influenzae*
  - Symptoms—fever, drooling, dysphagia, muffled voice, inspiratory retractions, and stridor; patient leans forward to ease breathing
  - Fatal respiratory obstruction can occur during attempts to culture or visualize the pharynx or if the child becomes anxious. First be sure that the airway is protected

- **Differential Diagnosis**
  - Viral croup—slower development of stridor, URI prodrome with cough. Less stridor at rest. Infants are at highest risk for respiratory compromise
  - Bacterial tracheitis—exudative laryngotracheobronchitis due to *S aureus, H influenzae*, GAS, *S pyogenes*, *Neisseria* species. *M catarrhalis,* and others. Sometime follows viral croup
  - Aspirated laryngeal foreign body—lateral neck and chest films are indicated
  - Rapidly growing neck or mediastinal mass may produce acute respiratory obstruction

- **Treatment**
  - Emergent endotracheal intubation as soon as diagnosis is confirmed in the operating room with general anesthesia
  - Culture blood and epiglottis after airway is secured
  - Initially intravenous (IV) antibiotics to cover *H influenzae* and change according to culture results
  - Extubation after epiglottis decreases in size
  - After 2–3 days, oral antibiotics may be used

- **Pearl**

H influenzae type B (HIB) vaccine has made this dreaded condition rare. However, other organisms can still produce life-threatening swelling of the epiglottis.

16

17

Rheumatic Disorders

17

Juvenile Rheumatoid Arthritis (JRA)

■ Essentials of Diagnosis

- *Acute febrile form*—episodic, evanescent pink macular rash, arthritis, hepatosplenomegaly, elevated white blood cell count (WBC), polyserositis
- *Polyarticular form*—chronic pain and swelling of many joints, symmetrical distribution, low-grade fever, fatigue, rheumatoid nodules anemia, occasional iridocyclitis
- *Pauciarticular form*—asymmetric chronic arthritis of a few joints, few systemic symptoms, painless synovitis, iridocyclitis in 30% of patients
- Rheumatoid factor positive in 15% of patients, usually older children with polyarticular disease
- Antinuclear antibody (ANA) often positive in pauciarticular disease with iridocyclitis
- Joint fluid with normal glucose and 5000–60000 neutrophils/μL

■ Differential Diagnosis

- Traumatic joint injury
- Reactive arthritides—Henoch-Schönlein purpura, reactive arthritis, toxic synovitis of the hip, viral-associated synovitis, rheumatic fever
- Acute joint infections
- Collagen-vascular disease—systemic lupus erythematous (SLE), dermatomyositis
- Neoplastic disease—leukemia, lymphoma, neuroblastoma, bone and joint tumors

■ Treatment

- Restore function and maintain joint mobility with physical therapy
- Nonsteroidal anti-inflammatory (NSAIDs) medications
- May use methotrexate, leflunomide, etanercept, infliximab in patients unresponsive to NSAIDs
- Iridocyclitis must be treated to prevent blindness. Local corticosteroid drops or ointment may be used. Unresponsive inflammation treated with methotrexate
- In selected patients, use local corticosteroid in affected joints, synovectomy, joint replacement

■ Pearl

Iridocyclitis may develop insidiously in pauciarticular disease. Activity of eye disease does not correlate with arthritis. Routine ophthalmologic screening by slit lamp every 3 months is recommended.

17

Spondyloarthropathy

- **Essentials of Diagnosis**
  - Lower extremity arthritis, sacroiliitis, and low back pain
  - Affects males over 10 years
  - Inflammation of tendinous insertions characteristic
  - Human leukocyte antigen (HLA)-B27 positive in 80% of patients, elevated erythrocyte sedimentation rate (ESR) and C-reactive protein (CRP)
  - Episodic symptoms
  - Acute uveitis may occur but not chronic iridocyclitis

- **Differential Diagnosis**
  - Other collagen-vascular disorders—JRA, SLE, dermatomyositis
  - In boys, ulcerative colitis may be associated with HLA-B27 positive ankylosing spondylitis
  - Traumatic or overuse injury
  - Acute infection or postinfectious arthropathy
  - Leukemia, lymphoma, bone, or joint tumor
  - Spine or disc disease

- **Treatment**
  - Indomethacin and naproxen are more effective than salicylates
  - Refractory cases may respond to methotrexate, etanercept, or infliximab
  - Local corticosteroid injections contraindicated in Achilles tendonitis

17

- **Pearl**

Pure spondyloarthropathy in childhood (in contrast to adults with the disorder) rarely progresses to joint destruction or ankylosis.

Enteropathic Arthritis

- ■ Essentials of Diagnosis
  - Reactive arthritis usually of lower extremities several weeks after gastrointestinal (GI) infection with *Salmonella, Shigella, Yersinia,* and *Campylobacter*
  - HLA-B27 individuals at greatest risk
  - May be associated with active inflammatory bowel disease (Crohn disease, ulcerative colitis, collagenous colitis) and celiac disease
  - Intestinal bypass surgery and intestinal bacterial overgrowth are risk factors
  - Other inflammatory symptoms—uveitis, stomatitis, hepatitis, erythema nodosum (Crohn disease), pyoderma gangrenosa (ulcerative colitis), urethritis

- ■ Differential Diagnosis
  - Behçet disease
  - Gonococcus and other bacterial joint infections
  - Lyme disease
  - JRA
  - Sarcoid

- ■ Treatment
  - Sulfasalazine and/or corticosteroids in patients with inflammatory bowel disease controls both GI disease and arthritis
  - Gluten-free diet for patients with celiac disease
  - NSAIDs helpful in postinfection arthritis. Infliximab, methotrexate have been used
  - Bacterial or parasitic pathogens in the stool should be treated

17

- ■ Pearl

Intestinal parasitic infestations also cause enteropathic arthritis. Check stools for Strongyloides stercoralis, Taenia saginata, Giardia lamblia, Ascaris lumbricoides, *and* Cryptosporidium *species when no obvious source is present.*

Systemic Lupus Erythematosus

- **Essentials of Diagnosis**
  - Soluble immune complexes deposited in tissues attract lymphocytes and neutrophils. Complement fixation then produces inflammation in multiple systems—joints, serous linings, skin, kidneys, central nervous system, heart, lungs, liver
  - Fatigue, weight loss, fever, amenorrhea, joint pains, malar "butterfly" rash. Hypertension, encephalitis, renal disease, carditis also occur
  - ANA always positive in active, untreated disease. Leucopenia, anemia, thrombocytopenia, elevated ESR, elevated γ-globulin, antigen-antibody complexes found in most cases
  - SLE most common in girls 9–15 years
  - Early diagnosis, diagnosis of milder cases, more aggressive therapy has increased survival to 90% at 5 years

- **Differential Diagnosis**
  - Rheumatic fever
  - Rheumatoid arthritis
  - Viral infections
  - Collagen-vascular diseases and mixed connective tissue disease

- **Treatment**
  - Corticosteroids reduce morbidity and mortality from renal, cardiac, and central nervous system (CNS) disease
  - Dermatitis, arthritis, and fatigue may respond to hydroxychloroquine
  - Pleuritic pain or arthritis treated with NSAIDs
  - Resistant cases may require azathioprine, cyclophosphamide, mycophenolate mofetil
  - Anticogulants may be required in patients with anticardiolopin or lupus anticoagulant antibodies to prevent or treat thrombotic events
  - Side effects of all therapies may be severe

- **Pearl**

Elevated titers of anti-DNA antibody and depressed serum C3 accurately reflect activity of disease, especially renal, CNS, and skin disease.

Dermatomyositis

- ■ Essentials of Diagnosis
  - Vasculitis of small arteries and veins leads to intimal proliferation and thrombus formation in skin, muscle, kidney, retina, and GI tract with postinflammatory calcinosis
  - Pelvic and shoulder girdle weakness predominate. Dysphagia and dysphonia also occur due to esophageal and laryngeal motor weakness
  - 50% have muscular pain
  - Purplish (heliotrope) rash on upper eyelids and extensor surfaces of knuckles, elbows, and knees progresses to scaling, atrophy, and calcinosis
  - Muscle enzyme levels elevated. ANA often positive. Electromyogram (EMG) shows myopathic change. Muscle biopsy indicated if characteristic skin rash is absent
  - Anti-Jo-1 antibodies associated with interstitial lung disease. Anti-Mi-2 antibodies specific for dermatomyositis but present in only 25% of cases

- ■ Differential Diagnosis
  - Postviral myopathy
  - Endocrine myopathies (Addison disease, hyperthyroid)
  - Other dermatologic conditions share some features—lichen planus, polymorphous light eruptions, seborrhea, SLE, psoriasis, contact and atopic dermatitis, drug eruption
  - Other connective tissue disease and autoimmune diseases with myopathic component
  - Muscular dystrophy, myasthenia gravis, mitochondrial myopathy, glycogen storage disease V and VII
  - Rhabdomyolysis

17

- ■ Treatment
  - Childhood dermatomyositis usually responds to corticosteroids
  - Methotrexate, intravenous immune globulin, cyclosporine in refractory cases
  - Physical therapy critical to prevent and treat muscle contractures
  - Nutritional supplementation with calories and protein may be helpful in maintaining quality of life
  - Calcium channel blockers of unproven efficacy in preventing calcinosis

- ■ Pearl

In adults, there is a sixfold increase in malignancy associated with dermatomyositis, mainly ovarian, gastric, and lymphoma. This is not the case in affected children.

Polyarteritis Nodosa

- **Essentials of Diagnosis**
  - Vasculitis of medium-sized arteries with fibrinoid degeneration in media, intima, and adventitia
  - Aneurysms may develop in affected vessels. Thrombosis and infarcts occur
  - Symptoms involve many organ systems—fever, hypertension, conjunctivitis, cardiomyopathy, CNS, GI, and renal disease
  - Biopsy needed to demonstrate vasculitis. Magnetic resonance imaging (MRI) or angiography may demonstrate aneurysms

- **Differential Diagnosis**
  - Wegener granulomatosis
  - Hypersensitivity vasculitis
  - When symptoms of 1 organ system predominate, the overarching diagnosis may be missed as a single (more common) organ disease is sought—eg, endocarditis, inflammatory bowel disease

- **Treatment**
  - Treat with corticosteroids, immunosuppressants, and immune globulin
  - Cyclophosphamide may be used in systemic vasculitis
  - Azathioprine used for maintenance
  - Treat complications of infarct and thrombosis
  - Surgery may be needed for aneurysms

17

- **Pearl**

Carditis greatly increases the morbidity and mortality of this condition.

Scleroderma

- ■ Essentials of Diagnosis
  - Localized disease (linear scleroderma and morphea) most common in childhood. Progressive systemic sclerosis rare
  - *Linear scleroderma*—streaks of indurated skin on extremities with slow progression to subcutaneous atrophy and joint contractures
  - *Morphea*—patchy induration and depigmentation
  - *Systemic sclerosis*—patients may have Raynaud phenomenon, fatigue, joint pain, contractures, dysphagia, abdominal pain, diarrhea, pulmonary fibrosis, hypertension, cardiac and renal failure
  - ANA usually positive. Anticollagen antibodies I–V usually negative. Skin biopsy sometimes needed to confirm diagnosis

- ■ Differential Diagnosis
  - Other skin disorders—vitiligo, acrocyanosis, atopic dermatitis, pityriasis
  - Dermatomyositis and other connective tissue disorders
  - Graft-versus-host disease
  - Amyloidosis

- ■ Treatment
  - Physical therapy to retain motor function and prevent contracture
  - Methotrexate and vitamin D analogues may limit extension of skin lesions especially in linear form
  - Systemic corticosteroids of questionable value in progressive systemic sclerosis. Penicillamine helpful in some cases
  - Specific therapy for hypertension. Calcium channel blockers for Raynaud phenomenon. Acid suppression for gastroesophageal reflux disease
  - Avoid skin trauma and sun exposure, protect extremities from cold, no smoking, avoid vasoconstrictors (pseudoephedrine), and avoid harsh skin cleansers and lotions

17

- ■ Pearl

A recent study found that 25% of children with localized scleroderma had some extracutaneous symptoms including joint contractures (47%), seizures and other neurologic symptoms (17%), vascular insufficiency (9.3%), and eye disease, especially uveitis (8.3%).

Reflex Sympathetic Dystrophy
(Complex Regional Pain Syndrome)

- Essentials of Diagnosis
  - Nonrheumatic pain syndrome involving an extremity with associated autonomic dysfunction—color change, temperature difference, dyshydrosis, swelling, cutaneous hyperesthesia, changes in hair and nail growth
  - Symptoms may worsen with psychic stress
  - Diagnosis is clinical. Laboratory tests and x-rays negative. Bone scan may show increased or decreased blood supply in the affected extremity
  - Disuse of limb may cause osteopenia and muscle wasting

- Differential Diagnosis
  - Nerve entrapment, neuritis, spinal disc disease
  - Fibromyalgia
  - Chronic fatigue syndrome
  - Psychosomatic illness

- Treatment
  - In mild cases, use physical therapy and desensitization techniques
  - Corticosteroids or sympathetic ganglionic blockade with local anesthetic occasionally used
  - Most medications have no scientific proof of efficacy—topical anesthetics, opioids, antiseizure medications, α-blockers, antidepressants
  - Counseling of patient and family often helpful to improve coping and quality of life

17

- Pearl

Unlike adults, children with this syndrome rarely have a history of trauma to the affected limb.

Fibromyalgia

- **Essentials of Diagnosis**
  - Diffuse pain syndrome with absence of physical findings
  - Insomnia or prolonged night-time waking periods very common
  - Trigger points at muscular insertions especially along spine, neck, and pelvis
  - Laboratory tests negative, cause unknown

- **Differential Diagnosis**
  - Chronic fatigue syndrome, reflex sympathetic dystrophy
  - Clinical depression
  - Ehlers-Danlos syndrome or other hypermobility disorder
  - Viral infection—Lyme disease, Epstein-Barr virus, influenza
  - Thyroid disease
  - Rheumatoid arthritis
  - Whiplash injury

- **Treatment**
  - Physical therapy
  - Medication or other therapy to improve sleep
  - Low-dose antidepressants helpful
  - Analgesics provide poor pain relief and may become addictive
  - Counseling to improve coping and quality of life

- **Pearl**

17

Many patients indicate that weather changes and fatigue provoke symptoms.

Ehlers-Danlos Syndrome (EDS)

- **Essentials of Diagnosis**
  - Large group of genetic disorders of collagen synthesis
  - Major symptoms—lax joints, chronic joint pains, hyperelastic skin, fragile blood vessels with easy bruising, poor wound healing with "cigarette paper" scars, corneal deformity
  - Serious complications of some genotypes include—mitral valve prolapse, periodontal disease, platelet aggregation disorder with bleeding tendency and, in vascular-type EDS, spontaneous rupture of uterus, intestines, eyeball, or major blood vessel
  - Diagnostic tests—collagen typing of skin biopsy. Lysyl hydroxylase or lysyl oxidase activity may be reduced. Collagen gene mutation testing

- **Differential Diagnosis**
  - Fibromyalgia, chronic fatigue

- **Treatment**
  - No specific therapy
  - Protect skin, joints, and eyes from injury
  - Avoid unnecessary surgery, instrumentation such as GI endoscopy, rectal enemas, cystoscopy
  - Careful monitoring during pregnancy
  - Physical therapy

17

- **Pearl**

Premature rupture of membranes at birth is characteristic of infants with EDS.

18

Orthopedics

18

Club Foot (Talipes Equinovarus)

- ## Essentials of Diagnosis
  - Plantar flexion of the foot at the ankle joint (equinus), inversion deformity of the heel (varus), and medial deviation of the forefoot (varus)
  - Incidence 1:100 live births
  - In idiopathic cases, 1 affected child increases subsequent sibling risk to 2:100. Probably hereditary component
  - Spina bifida and other spinal and muscle defects may cause in club foot

- ## Differential Diagnosis
  - Larsen syndrome has associated club feet—flat facies, congenital dislocations, accessory carpal bones, short distal phalanges, syndactyly, pseudoclubbing, short stature
  - Arthrogryposis congenita—many joint abnormalities including club feet

- ## Treatment
  - Manipulate the foot to stretch contracted medial and posterior tissues
  - Treatment instituted directly after birth improves correction
  - After full correction, night bracing maintains normal positioning
  - If the foot cannot be manipulated sufficiently to attain normal positioning, surgery is required

- ## Pearl

The normal foot becomes rigid within several days of birth. Manipulation of the club foot should be performed early to improve the effectiveness of nonsurgical correction.

18

Infantile Dysplasia of the Hip Joint

- Essentials of Diagnosis
  - Abnormal relationship of femoral head and acetabulum in utero. Severe cases have complete dislocation
  - 1:1000 live births. Female/Male ratio 9:1
  - Femoral head and acetabulum both usually dysplastic. Dysplasia progresses during skeletal growth if dislocation is not corrected
  - Flexion and abduction of the femur while lifting the greater trochanter forward reveals unstable femoral head (Ortolani sign) in infants <6 weeks
  - Medial pressure on the thigh during adduction reveals posterior slip of the femoral head (Barlow sign) in infants >6 weeks
  - Ambulatory older children with unilateral dislocation develop painless lurching gait on the affected side, unequal leg length, positive Trendelenburg sign, lumbar lordosis
  - Hip x-rays are most accurate after 16 weeks of age. Ultrasound is accurate in infancy

- Differential Diagnosis
  - Spinal abnormalities
  - Arthrogryposis, congenital joint laxity
  - Functional joint laxity—maternal hormones loosen the joint ligaments in neonates and cause a "hip click" on examination that can be mistaken for congenital dislocation

- Treatment
  - In infants, splint the hip in flexion and abduction. Double diapering is not sufficient for splinting of the hips
  - Avoid any forced abduction. It may produce avascular necrosis of the femoral head
  - Surgical correction is possible if splinting or casting is ineffective or if anatomic abnormalities are severe

- Pearl

Asymmetrical thigh skin folds are present in 40% of normal newborns and not uniformly present in neonates with hip dysplasia. It is not a reliable diagnostic sign. Examine the hips and repeat the examination several times during the first 4 months.

Torticollis

- ■ Essentials of Diagnosis
  - Unilateral contracture of the sternocleidomastoid muscle causes the chin to rotate away from the contracture and the head to tilt toward the contracture
  - Causes—diseases of the cervical spine, injury to the sternocleidomastoid during delivery, or intrauterine pressure
  - Sternocleidomastoid mass is often palpable. It is a fibrous transformation within the muscle, not tumor
  - Hip dysplasia associated in 20% of cases
  - Diagnosis is by physical examination, but magnetic resonance imaging (MRI) may be needed to completely evaluate

- ■ Differential Diagnosis
  - Arthrogryposis
  - Klippel-Feil syndrome
  - Cervical spine tumor or syrinx
  - Brain tumor
  - Rheumatoid arthritis—older children
  - Trauma and mild respiratory illness may precede onset
  - Unilateral flattened occiput from intrauterine pressure or back sleeping causes apparent torticollis when infant is supine
  - Motor weakness, cerebral palsy, dystonia, spasticity produce torticollis

- ■ Treatment
  - Passive stretching is usually effective <1 year
  - Surgical release after 1 year is effective in uncomplicated cases
  - Excision of the fibrous "tumor" is unnecessary

18

- ■ Pearl

Infants with gastroesophageal reflux may assume a position of comfort known as Sandifer syndrome with neck extended and head tilted. Give an acid blocker to healthy children with torticollis to see if Sandifer syndrome is the cause.

Arthrogryposis Multiplex Congenita

- **Essentials of Diagnosis**
  - Congenital fibrous ankylosis of many joints—shoulders adducted, elbows extended, wrists flexed, fingers stiff, dislocated hips, knees extended, club feet, scoliosis
  - Usually bilateral involvement
  - Infants usually have normal mental and sensory development but severe physical disability
  - Variable inheritance—may be associated with other somatic abnormalities
  - Diagnosable by intrauterine ultrasound

- **Differential Diagnosis**
  - Intrauterine pressure with unilateral decrease in fetal limb movement causes joint contractures
  - In utero abnormalities of muscle tone, muscle development (amyoplasia), lower motor neuron or spinal cord function may cause multiple joint contractures
  - Intrauterine bands may cause contractures

- **Treatment**
  - Passive mobilization early
  - Prolonged casting is contraindicated because of further stiffness
  - Surgical joint release, tendon transplant, capsulotomies, osteotomies sometimes needed

- **Pearl**

Fetal akinesia (lack of muscle movement) can also produce polyhydramnios, pulmonary hypoplasia, micrognathia, hypertelorism, shortened umbilical cord depending on severity of the akinesia.

Marfan Syndrome

- Essentials of Diagnosis
  - Connective tissue disorder—tall stature, long fingers and toes, hypermobile joints, scoliosis, high arched palate, pectus carinatum, thoracic aortic aneurysm, mitral valve prolapse
  - Ocular abnormalities include subluxation of the lens, cataract, coloboma, megalocornea, strabismus, myopia, and nystagmus
  - Defect is in genes coding for fibrillin. One-third of cases are sporadic mutations, two-thirds are familial. Sex distribution equal
  - Diagnosis is usually clinical but testing shows ↓serum mucoproteins, ↑urinary hydroxyproline excretion. Genetic testing available
  - Diagnosis is much more obvious as children grow. Tall stature is the most common reason for investigation

- Differential Diagnosis
  - Homocystinuria—patients look marfanoid but urinary homocystine is elevated in homocystinuria
  - Familial tall stature
  - Ehlers-Danlos syndrome shares some findings

- Treatment
  - Regular ophthalmologic evaluation and care
  - Regular orthopedic evaluation and care, especially to prevent scoliosis
  - Regular cardiac evaluation with serial echocardiograms. β-blockers may reduce the progression of aortic root dilation

18

- Pearl

The rate of mutation of the fibrillin gene appears to be related to paternal age. The older the father, the higher the mutation rate.

Klippel-Feil Syndrome

- ■ Essentials of Diagnosis
    - Early in utero failure of segmentation of some or all cervical vertebrae causes multiple bony defects—hemivertebrae, fused vertebrae, scoliosis, cervical rib, spina bifida
    - Short stiff neck, low hairline, low-set ears, deafness, web neck, high scapula
    - Structural and functional renal abnormalities
    - Gene inversion on long arm of chromosome 8. Increased risk in infants with fetal alcohol syndrome

- ■ Differential Diagnosis
    - VACTERL syndrome has many of the same characteristics
    - Sprengel deformity of the scapula causes similar short neck

- ■ Treatment
    - Many patients have no symptoms
    - Fusion of the cervical vertebrae causes neurologic symptoms with growth—tingling, numbness, paralysis of upper extremities
    - All patients require hearing evaluation
    - Renal, orthopedic, neurology, and sometimes cardiology specialists should follow these children

- ■ Pearl

Minor trauma may cause serious injury to the spinal cord in patients with Klippel-Feil syndrome. Spinal fusion can reduce this risk.

18

Osteogenesis Imperfecta

- ■ Essentials of Diagnosis
  - Genetic connective tissue disease with recurrent bone fractures caused by mutations in *COL IA1* and *2* genes encoding for type I procollagen
  - Fetal type has intrauterine and perinatal fractures, blue sclerae, thin skin, joint hypermobility, otosclerosis, hearing loss, hypoplastic teeth, wormian bones, normal intelligence
  - Later presentation (tarda type) is less severe
  - Other forms fatal due to severe skeletal deformities and respiratory insufficiency due to thoracic constriction
  - Intrauterine ultrasound or chorionic villus sampling allow prenatal diagnosis and evaluation of severity

- ■ Differential Diagnosis
  - Child abuse
  - Osteopenia secondary to rickets, metabolic renal disease, renal insufficiency, and nutritional deficiencies all promote easy fractures

- ■ Treatment
  - Avoidance of injury, regular physical therapy
  - Biphosphonates may be helpful
  - Bone marrow transplant, growth hormone, gene therapy are experimental

- ■ Pearl

Osteogenesis imperfecta is a rare disorder. Multiple bone fractures in different stages of healing are a red flag for child abuse first and osteogenesis imperfecta second.

18

Achondroplasia

- ■ Essentials of Diagnosis
    - • The most common form of short-limbed dwarfism. Autosomal dominant. 80% are new mutations on chromosome 4
    - • Caused by delayed ossification of cartilage
    - • Short upper arms and thighs, waddling gait, bowed legs, joint limitation, short fingers of equal length, frontal bossing, hydrocephalus, depressed nasal bridge, lumbar lordosis
    - • Thoracic and skull deformities cause respiratory insufficiency and recurrent otitis
    - • Intelligence normal
    - • Narrowed spinal canal and foramen magnum may lead to progressive spinal cord compression with sudden death in infancy or paraplegia in older individuals
    - • Phenotypic features are nearly diagnostic, even at birth. Prenatal diagnosis is available

- ■ Differential Diagnosis
    - • Other forms of dwarfism and nonsyndromatic short stature

- ■ Treatment
    - • No specific therapy
    - • Patients should be monitored for foramen magnum compression
    - • Growth hormone therapy and limb lengthening surgery have been used with some success to increase final height
    - • Recurrent otitis should be treated aggressively to prevent otosclerosis and hearing loss

- ■ Pearl

Mutations in fibroblast growth factor receptor gene are involved in a number of syndromes with skeletal abnormalities. The mechanism by which the abnormal growth factor receptor protein produces achondroplasia is not yet known.

Scoliosis

■ Essentials of Diagnosis

- Lateral curvature of the spine with rotation of the involved vertebrae.
- Idiopathic scoliosis four to five times more common in girls than boys. Onset 8–10 years
- Convexity of the thoracic curve to the right is the most common deformity in idiopathic scoliosis
- Screen by noting asymmetry of rib height or paravertebral muscles while patient bent at 90º
- Spine x-rays in the standing position useful for diagnosis, staging, and planning therapy

■ Differential Diagnosis

- Scoliosis associated with neurofibromatosis, Marfan syndrome, cerebral palsy, muscular dystrophies, polio, myelodysplasia, chronic vertebral osteomyelitis
- Congenital vertebral anomalies are the cause of scoliosis in 5–7% of patients
- Transient scoliosis may result from splinting of the chest during acute pneumonia or other lung disease

■ Treatment

- Treatment determined by magnitude of curve, skeletal maturity, and risk of progression
- Curvature <20° usually requires no treatment
- Curvature 20°–40° treated by bracing
- Curvature >40° usually resistant to bracing and may require spinal fusion
- Curvature >60° causes poor adult pulmonary function

18

■ Pearl

Idiopathic scoliosis of girls is usually convex to the right and rarely causes pain. The presence of pain or a left convex curvature should dictate careful investigation for other disorders such as bone or spinal cord tumor.

Slipped Capital Femoral Epiphysis

- **Essentials of Diagnosis**
    - Posterior, inferior displacement of the proximal femoral epiphysis with disruption of the proximal femoral growth plate
    - May occur through weakness of the perichondrial ring stabilizing the epiphysis during adolescent growth spurt
    - 30% bilateral disease
    - Most common in obese adolescent males. Other risk factors are hypothyroidism, panhypopituitarism, growth hormone therapy
    - Often becomes symptomatic after a fall, hip trauma, or bending over
    - Symptoms of vague pain in hip, knee, groin, or thigh with or without limp
    - Limitation of internal rotation on physical examination
    - Lateral hip radiographs show posterior and inferior slippage of the proximal epiphysis

- **Differential Diagnosis**
    - Renal osteodystrophy or other metabolic bone disease
    - Lower spine or disc disease causing sciatic pain
    - Bone tumor of the proximal femur may cause hip pain

- **Treatment**
    - Surgical fixation similar to that used in fractures of the femoral neck
    - Forceful reduction should be avoided. It increases the risk of avascular necrosis of the femoral head (AVN)
    - Long-term problems with hip arthritis occur with or without AVN

- **Pearl**

An obese adolescent male with knee pain may actually have slipped capital femoral epiphysis with referred pain to the knee.

Genu Varum/Genu Valgum

- ■ Essentials of Diagnosis
  - Genu varum (bowleg) is normal up to 2 years
  - Genu valgum (knock knee) is normal in children from 2 to 8 years
  - Persistent bowleg, increasing bowleg, unilateral bowing beyond age 2 should be evaluated
  - Knock knee associated with short stature should be evaluated
  - Monitor bowleg by measuring the inter-knee distance at every well-child visit

- ■ Differential Diagnosis
  - Bowleg may be associated with internal tibial torsion, Blount disease (proximal tibial epiphysial dysplasia), metaphysical chondrodysplasia, achondroplasia, nutritional or hypophosphatemic rickets, lead or fluoride intoxication
  - Knock knee >age 8 associated with obesity
  - Asymmetric bone growth following trauma to the growth plate may resemble either knock knees or bowleg depending on site of injury

- ■ Treatment
  - Most bowleg <3 years or knock knee <8 years will resolve spontaneously
  - Night splints, internal or external augmentation of the heel may be useful
  - Severe bowleg or knock knee may respond to bracing or even osteotomy, especially when tibial torsion is the primary cause

18

- ■ Pearl

There is such confusion about the closely related terms genu valgum and genu varum (or is it genu varus and genu valgus?) that many prefer the clarity of good old "bowleg" and "knock knee." The terms may sound insensitive but at least you don't have to know Latin to understand what the problem is!

Tibial Torsion

- **Essentials of Diagnosis**
  - In-toeing is common in infants and is caused by tibial torsion of about 20° which decreases gradually by the age of walking
  - Measure the degree of tibial torsion by measuring the angle between a line from second toe to midheel and a line along the length of the thigh with knee and ankle both flexed 90°

- **Differential Diagnosis**
  - Associated with excess intrauterine pressure, eg, macrosomic infants of diabetic mothers
  - Metatarsus adductus causes curvature of the foot which looks like tibial torsion
  - Femoral anteversion produces toeing in beyond age 2–3 years
  - This condition shouldn't be mistaken for club foot but sometimes is

- **Treatment**
  - Most tibial torsion requires no therapy
  - Discourage belly sleeping with feet turned in
  - Tibial torsion >15° after age 7–10 years may require tibial osteotomy
  - Braces or splints to promote external rotation are sometimes used

- **Pearl**

Neither putting a toddler's shoes on backwards nor using the old Denis-Browne splint to keep the feet at a 45° angle outward are proven to be better than waiting for natural resolution in most infants.

18

Osteomyelitis

- ■ Essentials of Diagnosis
    - Infection of the medullary bone with extension to cortical bone. Lower extremities most commonly affected, often after trauma
    - Most common agents are *Staphylococcus aureus* and *Streptococcus*. ↑risk for *Salmonella* osteomyelitis in sickle cell. ↑risk of *Pseudomonas* after nail punctures through the shoe
    - Infection penetrates across the growth plate in children <1 year causing septic arthritis and long-term growth problems
    - Infection spreads via the periosteum in older children with fused growth plates. Joints are less often involved
    - Symptoms—fever, irritability, pseudoparalysis, local redness, pain, tenderness
    - High erythrocyte sedimentation rate (ESR) and white blood cell count (WBC); positive blood or bone culture
    - X-ray cannot detect early osteomyelitis or small infections. Bone scan and MRI are more sensitive

- ■ Differential Diagnosis
    - Clinical findings may suggest fracture, bone cyst, bone tumor
    - Other serious infections, inflammatory and autoimmune conditions may initially have the same nonspecific fever and systemic symptoms of osteomyelitis

- ■ Treatment
    - Antibiotic therapy depending on culture and sensitivity for at least 3 weeks
    - Splinting the limb minimizes pain and decreases lymphatic spread
    - Aspiration of the affected bone is the best way to culture and to provide surgical drainage if needed

- ■ Pearl

If acute symptoms and signs of osteomyelitis are not resolving within 3 days of initiation of therapy, consider surgical exploration for drainage and debridement.

Pyogenic Arthritis

- ■ Essentials of Diagnosis
  - Arises from adjacent osteomyelitis in infants (*S aureus*)
  - In older children arises during systemic infections with organisms having a predilection for joints (*S aureus*, *Streptococcus* species, *Neisseria gonorrhea*, *Kingella kingae*, tuberculosis, *Salmonella* species)
  - Risk increased in immunodeficiency, intravenous (IV) drug use, and sickle cell disease
  - Symptoms—fever, malaise, emesis, restricted movement
  - Joint aspiration for drainage and culture is key to diagnosis and therapy.
  - Joint fluid WBC >100,000/μL, ESR >50
  - Joint x-rays are insensitive. WBC or gallium scan localizes infection

- ■ Differential Diagnosis
  - Fever of unknown origin
  - Noninfectious arthritis—inflammatory bowel disease, rheumatoid arthritis, Reiter syndrome, Lyme disease, rheumatic fever, systemic lupus, leukemia, drug reactions, autoimmune hepatitis
  - Hemarthrosis with bleeding disorders

- ■ Treatment
  - Antibiotic therapy depends on culture and sensitivity testing of joint fluid
  - Drainage of joint often needed for irrigation and debridement, especially the hip
  - Tuberculous arthritis is usually spinal and requires drainage, immobilization, and sometimes casting for spine stabilization

18

- ■ Pearl

Infants are at higher risk of having multiple joint involvement with pyogenic arthritis than older children.

Transient Synovitis of the Hip

- ■ Essentials of Diagnosis
  - Most common cause of limp and hip pain in children 3–10 years
  - Male predominance
  - Associated with viral infection, mild trauma, or possibly allergy
  - Limitation of motion of hip, especially internal rotation
  - ESR, WBC normal. Fever usually absent
  - Hip joint aspirate yields sterile serous fluid with few WBC

- ■ Differential Diagnosis
  - Pyogenic arthritis
  - Other noninfectious arthritis—inflammatory bowel disease, rheumatoid arthritis, Reiter syndrome, Lyme disease, rheumatic fever, systemic lupus, leukemia, drug reactions, autoimmune hepatitis
  - Slipped capital femoral epiphysis
  - Fracture

- ■ Treatment
  - Rest and gentle traction
  - Pain control with nonsteroidal anti-inflammatory agents
  - Usually self-limited but may recur
  - Monitor by x-ray for slipped capital femoral epiphysis

- ■ Pearl

Aseptic necrosis of the femoral head occurs in 1–2% of patients with **18** *transient tenosynovitis of the hip. Coxa magna (asymptomatic enlargement of the femoral head and broadening of the femoral neck) occurs in 32.1% and may be a precursor of aseptic necrosis or long-term arthritis in the hip.*

Avascular Necrosis (AVN) of the Proximal Femur (Legg-Calvé-Perthes Disease)

■ **Essentials of Diagnosis**

- Highest incidence in 4–8-year-old males
- Persistent pain, limp, limitation of movement
- Joint aspirate normal. Laboratory studies normal. Systemic symptoms absent
- X-ray shows joint effusion early. Later findings are patchy decreased bone density around the joint
- Very late complications—necrotic ossification, collapse of femoral head, fragmentation of the epiphysis, variegated bone density, involvement of metaphysis

■ **Differential Diagnosis**

- Pyogenic arthritis
- Noninfectious arthritis
- Transient synovitis of the hip
- Osteochondritis desiccans

■ **Treatment**

- Protection of the joint is key—decrease weight bearing, trauma, and other factors augmenting disease below
- Prognosis poor with metaphysial involvement, complete involvement of the femoral head, later childhood presentation
- Replacement of the femoral head may be needed in advanced cases. 10% of total hip replacement surgery in the United States is for AVN

18

■ **Pearl**

Vascular occlusion of the macro- and microcirculation of the femoral head is the final common pathway for the many causes of AVN—steroids, trauma, alcoholism, coagulopathy, pancreatitis, storage disease, autoimmune and inflammatory disease, parenchymal bone disease, decompression sickness, microfractures, sickle cell, malignancy, pregnancy, hyperlipidemia, kidney transplant, hemodialysis, systemic lupus erythematous (SLE), rheumatoid arthritis, slipped capital femoral epiphysis.

Osteochondritis Dissecans

- ### Essentials of Diagnosis
    - Wedge-shaped necrotic area next to the articular surface results from vascular occlusion
    - Most common sites are knee (medial femoral condyle), elbow (capitellum), and ankle (talus)
    - Bone or cartilage fragments may separate and enter the joint space (joint mice)
    - Necrotic fragments that remain in place may be resorbed
    - Local swelling and pain, sensation of joint "locking" or "giving way"
    - X-ray of affected joint may show area of necrosis. MRI helpful in finding joint fragments

- ### Differential Diagnosis
    - Other arthritides
    - AVN of the femoral head
    - Sprains, strains, and fractures

- ### Treatment
    - Rest for 6–8 weeks
    - Joint mice may be removed arthroscopically
    - Attached necrotic fragments may be surgically drilled to promote more rapid neovascularization and resorption

- ### Pearl

Arthritis often develops in a joint with mice. Protect the joint from further trauma to reduce the risk of late arthritis.

18

Fibrous Dysplasia

- **Essentials of Diagnosis**
    - Idiopathic disorder. Proliferation of fibrous tissue arising from the medullary canal causes uneven bone growth, pain, fractures, bony deformity (shepherd's crook deformity of the femur is classic)
    - Asymmetric distribution of bony involvement
    - May be monostotic or polyostotic
    - Polyostotic disease with endocrine disturbance (McCune-Albright syndrome) occurs in girls with precocious puberty, café au lait spots, hyperpituitarism, hyperthyroidism, hyperadrenalism
    - Pain is rare, usually associated with fractures

- **Differential Diagnosis**
    - Other fibrous bone lesions—nonossifying fibroma, enchondroma, chondromyxoid fibroma
    - Bone cysts—benign bone cyst, unicameral bone cyst, aneurysmal bone cyst
    - Eosinophilic granuloma
    - Malignancy—primary bone tumor or bone metastases

- **Treatment**
    - No treatment needed for small lesions
    - Large lesions may provoke fractures and may require curettage and bone grafting

18

- **Pearl**

If a young girl with bone pain or fractures has café au lait spots, she probably has McCune-Albright syndrome. Ask about symptoms of precocious puberty.

Infantile Cortical Hyperostosis (Caffey Syndrome)

- **Essentials of Diagnosis**
  - Benign idiopathic inflammation of the periosteum. Usual onset <6 months
  - Familial cases are reported
  - Major symptoms—fussiness, fever, tender swellings of multiple bone shafts (clavicle and mandible most common) without soft tissue involvement
  - Increased WBC, ESR, and alkaline phosphatase with mild anemia
  - Cortical hyperostosis seen on x-ray

- **Differential Diagnosis**
  - Other febrile illnesses
  - Child abuse
  - Osteomyelitis, osteoarthritis
  - Hypervitaminosis A or vitamin C deficiency (scurvy)
  - Congenital syphilis
  - Ewing sarcoma, metastatic neuroblastoma
  - Prostaglandin E_1 or E_2 administration causes hyperostotic swelling

- **Treatment**
  - Resolves spontaneously in weeks or months
  - Steroidal and nonsteroidal medications for symptom relief
  - Occasionally there are long-term abnormalities of bone growth and deformity requiring surgical correction

18

- **Pearl**

For unknown reasons, the frequency of sporadic cases is decreasing. Familial cases are now relatively more likely.

Spondylolysis

- **Essentials of Diagnosis**
  - Injury to the pars interarticularis of the spine. 85% occur at L5
  - Cause is repetitive stress. Common problem of gymnasts, dancers, and football players
  - Most common symptom is back pain worse on extension. Pain radiates to buttock or thigh
  - Oblique x-rays of the spine reveal the posterior "Scottie dog sign"

- **Differential Diagnosis**
  - Spondylolisthesis occurs with bilateral injury. Slippage of the entire vertebra over the adjacent vertebra
  - Tumor—osteoid osteoma, sarcoma, infiltrative bone marrow tumors
  - Infection
  - Intervertebral disc disease or herniation
  - Stress fracture

- **Treatment**
  - Rest
  - Stretching of the hamstrings
  - Spine stabilization exercises
  - Lumbosacral bracing or in severe cases surgical stabilization

- **Pearl**

18

Sports with the highest incidence of back pain and injury are golf, gymnastics, football, dance, wrestling, and weight lifting. Spondylolysis occurs more frequently in patients with spina bifida occulta.

19

Sports Medicine and Rehabilitation

19

Concussion

- **Essentials of Diagnosis**
  - Temporary and immediate impairment of neurologic function with/without loss of consciousness (LOC) after head trauma
    - **Grade 1**—no LOC. Post-traumatic amnesia (PTA) or confusion lasts <15 minutes
    - **Grade 2**—no LOC. PTA or confusion lasts >15 minutes
    - **Grade 3**—any LOC
  - Greater health risks after second concussion due to "second impact syndrome" with loss of vascular auto regulation and cerebral edema

- **Differential Diagnosis**
  - Symptoms appearing after minor head trauma may be a response to underlying brain tumor
  - Consider cardiac arrhythmia, seizure, stroke, or migraine for any LOC occurring during sports
  - Drug abuse

- **Treatment**
  - Return-to-competition guidelines following concussion
    - **Grade 1**—return to play in 15 minutes if examination normal
    - **Grade 2**—return to play in 1 week if symptom free. Hospital evaluation if symptomatic >60 minutes. Computed tomography (CT) or magnetic resonance imaging (MRI) if symptoms persist for >1 week
    - **Grade 3**—return to play in 1 week if LOC <60 seconds and if symptom free. Return to play in 2 weeks if LOC >60 seconds and if symptom free. Hospital evaluation as in Grade 2 for persistent symptoms
  - For a second injury restrictions are greater—Grade 1: no play for 1 week, Grade 2: no play for 2 weeks, and Grade 3: no play for at least 1 month

19

- **Pearl**

The "Standardized Assessment of Concussion (SAC)" is a 5-minute clinical screening instrument that can be used by trained nonmedical sports supervisors to assess the level of injury of a participant. An SAC kit includes a training manual and can be obtained online.

Radiculopathy (Burners and Stingers)

- **Essentials of Diagnosis**
    - Cervical and brachial plexopathy occurs when the head is laterally bent and the shoulder depressed. Common in contact sports
    - Sudden stretch of the upper trunk of the brachial plexus and the roots of cervical nerves V and VI.
    - Immediate burning pain and paresthesias down the arm lasting minutes
    - Weakness of upper trunk muscles—supraspinatus, deltoid, and biceps—can last weeks
    - Recurrent injury is common

- **Differential Diagnosis**
    - Cervical spine injury should be considered and careful evaluation performed if there are persisting symptoms in the arm, shoulder, or neck
    - Cervical nerve compression is suggested if the Spurling maneuver produces arm or hand pain (extension of neck with head rotated to the affected shoulder while weight is applied axially)

- **Treatment**
    - Return to activity when symptoms have resolved, neck and shoulder motion is full and pain free, and Spurling test is negative
    - Prevent these injuries by wearing protective gear, proper blocking and tackling technique, neck and shoulder conditioning

- **Pearl**

19

Athletes of all levels get these common burners or stingers especially in football. Shoulder and neck conditioning to increase strength helps prevent injury. Shoulder pads that ride high with air floatation devices or extra padding also prevent injury.

Rotator Cuff Injury

- **Essentials of Diagnosis**
  - Common injury after activities that require repetitive overhead motions—throwing, reaching, lifting
  - Humeral head forced out of normal position so it impinges on the supraspinatus tendon
  - Most common symptom—pain in anterior and lateral shoulder increases with overhead activity
  - Workup includes plain x-rays and outlet views

- **Differential Diagnosis**
  - Shoulder bursitis, capsulitis, frozen shoulder
  - Arthritis
  - Septic joint
  - Unrecognized fracture

- **Treatment**
  - Reduce inflammation—anti-inflammatory medication, ice, rest
  - Gradually improve flexibility with stretching exercise
  - Increase strength of scapular stabilizers and rotator cuff muscles by isotonic or isokinetic exercise
  - Biomechanic evaluation can assist in recovery by building sport-specific skills and eliminating substitution patterns

- **Pearl**

The shoulder has the greatest range of motion of any joint in the body. The muscles of the rotator cuff hold the humoral head in the socket. They include the subscapularis, supraspinatus, infraspinatus, and teres minor.

19

Anterior Knee Pain

- **Essentials of Diagnosis**
  - Most common cause is "patellofemoral overuse" syndrome in runners causing pain under patella and over medial surface. Swelling and crepitus of knee
  - Plicae alares thickening or fibrosis occurs with repetitive micro-trauma or macro trauma. Pain on flexion and "popping" of the knee
  - Tendonitis of the patellar tendon
  - Osgood-Schlatter disease—inflammation at the tibial tubercle in adolescent boys and girls causes joint pain
  - Patellar chondromalacia—diagnosed by arthroscopy

- **Differential Diagnosis**
  - Hip pathology may refer to the knee
  - Arthritis
  - Neoplasm
  - Tibial stress fracture
  - Meniscus and ligament injuries
  - Tight iliotibial band produces pain over the lateral femoral condyle
  - Gastrocnemius-soleus injury produces posterior knee pain

- **Treatment**
  - Control inflammation with medication, ice, and rest
  - Alignment problems should be treated with stretching and strengthening
  - Orthotics if there are foot deformities producing stress on the joint

19

- **Pearl**

There is no consensus on treatment of patellofemoral overuse syndrome. Quadriceps strengthening and control of inflammation are the most common modalities suggested.

Anterior Cruciate Ligament (ACL) Injury

- Essentials of Diagnosis
  - 3 bands of this ligamentous complex prevent anterior subluxation of the tibia
  - Injury force is encountered during knee hyperextension, excess valgus stress, and external rotation of the femur on a fixed tibia (cutting injury)
  - Lachman test—gentle traction on the tibia with knee bent 30° reveals increased movement (>4 mm)
  - Anterior drawer test similar but with knee bent 90°
  - X-ray and/or MRI needed in knee injuries

- Differential Diagnosis
  - Associated bone fracture at the site of ACL insertion or elsewhere
  - Meniscus injury

- Treatment
  - Conservative measure—bracing, strengthening, restriction of physical activity
  - Surgical repair with patellar tendon graft is possible

- Pearl

Muscular rehabilitation should start immediately after injury with passive range of motion exercises.

Posterior Cruciate Ligament (PCL) Injury

- **Essentials of Diagnosis**
  - 2-part ligament between medial femoral condyle and posterior tibial plateau prevents posterior tibial subluxation
  - Injury caused by forced hyperextension or by fall on flexed knee with ankle in plantar flexion (pointed toe)
  - Pain, swelling, and decreased (ROM)—are milder than with ACL injury
  - Posterior drawer test performed supine with knee flexed 90° reveals excessive posterior mobility of the tibia
  - Sag test—with patient supine, lift both heels. The tibia on the injured side "sags" below the opposite side
  - X-ray and/or MRI needed to fully define injury. Associated injuries are common

- **Differential Diagnosis**
  - Avulsion of the PCL is as common as a tear
  - Bony fracture at the site of avulsion or elsewhere
  - Meniscal injury

- **Treatment**
  - Bracing and progressive rehabilitation are recommended in mild to moderate injuries
  - High-grade injury generally requires surgery

- **Pearl**

Hitting the knee on the dashboard of the car during an accident or sudden stop can cause PCL injury.

19

Medial and Lateral Collateral Ligament Injuries

- ■ Essentials of Diagnosis
    - • Ligaments along either side of the knee act to stabilize and control varus and valgus stress
    - • Excess varus or valgus stress causes injury. Most medial ligament injuries caused by blow to lateral knee
    - • Patient senses a pop or loses sensation over the medial knee. Effusion and local tenderness
    - • Pain reproduced by valgus stress in 20°–30° flexion
    - • Knee x-rays required to rule out other injury

- ■ Differential Diagnosis
    - • ACL or PCL injury
    - • Meniscus tear
    - • Fracture

- ■ Treatment
    - • Initial therapy includes ice and elevation
    - • Bracing with full knee motion in brace after 7 days
    - • Strengthening exercises and weight bearing should begin in first week
    - • Brace should be used until there is pain-free full range of motion

- ■ Pearl

Functional bracing may be required even after the athlete returns to competition in order to permit complete ligament healing.

19

Elbow Pain

- ■ Essentials of diagnosis
  - • *Medial*—medial epicondylitis secondary to overuse and valgus stress, tendonitis, ulnar collateral ligament injury, ulnar neuritis, apophysitis, and fracture
  - • *Lateral*—chronic valgus stress causes focal injury of the capitellum (5–12 year olds), osteochondritis dissecans of the capitellum (13–15 year olds), lateral epicondylitis (racquet sports)
  - • *Posterior*—dislocation, fracture, triceps avulsion, olecranon bursitis
  - • X-rays needed especially to detect avascular necrosis of the capitellum and Panner disease (fragmentation and sclerosis of the capitellum)

- ■ Differential Diagnosis
  - • Infection
  - • Tumor or bone cyst
  - • Fracture
  - • Sprain
  - • Inflammatory disease
  - • Bursitis

- ■ Treatment
  - • Prevention is the key to most of these athletic-related injuries
  - • Acute therapy includes ice, rest, and anti-inflammatory medications
  - • Evaluation of mechanics and physical therapy to strengthen arm musculature
  - • Orthopedic referral and possible surgery for osteochondritis dissecans

19

- ■ Pearl

Little league pitchers are particularly prone to medial epicondylitis. The 85 pitch rule was instituted in response to this problem.

Hip Pain

- ■ Essentials of Diagnosis
  - *Groin pull* (adductor strain) caused by forced abduction causes pain with hip adduction or flexion with tenderness over the adductor tubercle
  - *Quadriceps contusion*—direct injury to the muscle causes local tenderness
  - *Hamstring strain*—forced extension of the knee causes pain in the muscle and on knee flexion against resistance
  - *Trochanteric bursitis*—caused by reduced flexibility of the iliotibial band and gluteus medius tendons. Causes pain on flexion
  - *Hip dislocation*—usually posterior dislocation identified by hip flexion, adduction, and internal rotation. May be associated with acetabular and femoral neck fracture
  - *Stress fracture of the femoral neck*—caused by repetitive microtrauma especially in runners
  - X-rays and bone scans needed to fully evaluate persistent or severe pain

- ■ Differential Diagnosis
  - Infection
  - Slipped capital femoral epiphysis
  - Inflammatory disease
  - Bone cyst or tumor

- ■ Treatment
  - Hip dislocation is an emergency requiring orthopedic evaluation. Bleeding, nerve damage, and avascular necrosis can result
  - Most pulls, strains, contusions are treated with rest, ice, and anti-inflammatory medication
  - Muscle contusions should be fully resolved before stretching exercises to prevent development of myositis ossificans

19

- ■ Pearl

A transverse fracture of the femoral neck almost always requires surgical fixation to prevent avascular necrosis of the femoral head.

Foot Pain

- ■ Essentials of Diagnosis
  - The ankle has 3 lateral ligaments (anterior and posterior talofibular, and calcaneofibular) and a medial deltoid ligament
  - Foot inversion causes anterior talofibular injury. Eversion causes deltoid ligament injury
  - Ankle sprain (ligament overload) is rated (1) stretch without instability, (2) partial tear with some instability, (3) total disruption with unstable joint
  - Sprain causes pain, swelling, and bruising. Anterior drawer test evaluates the anterior talofibular ligament
  - Indications for x-ray evaluation—tenderness over malleoli, tenderness beyond the ligament attachments, excessive swelling
  - Plantar fasciitis from repetitive injury causes heel pain, especially in runners with tight Achilles tendons, pes cavus, poorly fitted shoes. Pain severe upon first standing after period of recumbency

- ■ Differential Diagnosis
  - Infection
  - Fracture
  - Bone tumor or cyst
  - Arthritis or inflammatory disease
  - Gout, calluses, bunions
  - Neuroma

- ■ Treatment
  - Treatment of sprains
    - For sprains, Phase 1—immediate compression and icing. Protected weight bearing
    - Phase 2—after patient can walk without pain, ankle range of motion exercises followed by active isotonic and isokinetic exercises
    - Phase 3—increase strength, improve proprioception, and add ballistic activity
    - Wear protective brace for up to 4 months to prevent further injury
  - Plantar fasciitis—massage, stretching of gastrocsoleus, anti-inflammatory drugs, arch supports, local steroid injection of the plantar fascia

- ■ Pearl

High-heeled shoes or tight shoes may cause a Morton neuroma—perineural thickening involving a digital nerve between the third and fourth toes. These benign swellings cause pain in the ball of the foot and toes, numbness, and the sensation of a small mass on the ball of the foot.

20

Neonatal Disorders

20

Apnea of Prematurity

- Essentials of Diagnosis
  - Respiratory pause >20 seconds, or any pause causing cyanosis, decrease in arterial pulse oxygen saturation or bradycardia
  - Most common in infants <34 weeks' gestation. Usual onset <2 weeks
  - *Central apnea*—brain stem-mediated immature respiratory regulation
  - *Obstructive apnea*—physical obstruction of airway by mucous, airway collapse, extrinsic pressure, aspiration
  - ↑apnea spells may be the first symptom of bacterial infection, necrotizing enterocolitis, intracranial bleeding, other illnesses
  - Apnea spells are worsened by temperature instability, vagal stimulation, gastroesophageal (GE) reflux, hypoxemia, infection, hypoglycemia, hyponatremia, intracranial hemorrhage, drugs

- Differential Diagnosis
  - Periodic breathing is a normal pattern in neonates which has cyclic variation of respiratory rate
  - Primary disease causing central and obstructive apnea such as brain tumor, foreign body
  - Ondine's curse—congenital neurologic disorder characterized by apnea during sleep

- Treatment
  - Evaluate and treat organic causes of apnea
  - Methylxanthines are effective for most apnea of prematurity—caffeine citrate 20 mg/kg loading dose then 5–10 mg/kg/day
  - Nasal continuous positive airway pressure (CPAP) or high-flow nasal cannula is effective in severe cases
  - Intubation and mechanical ventilation is a last resort in resistant cases

20

- Pearl

Prematurity is a risk factor for sudden infant death syndrome (SIDS). However, apnea and bradycardia in the preterm infant are not additional risk factors.

Birth Trauma

- **Essentials of Diagnosis**
  - Most commonly occurs with difficult delivery, increased fetal weight, abnormal fetal position, fetal distress requiring rapid extraction with forceps or vacuum
  - *Head injuries*—scalp bruising, scalp edema, cephalohematoma (usually beneath the parietal periosteum), subgaleal hematoma (severe injury can cause massive blood loss, shock, brain injury and death)
  - *Brain injury*—subdural or subarachnoid bleeding causes alternating somnolence and irritability, poor eating, unexplained fevers
  - *Bone injury*—fractures of clavicle, humerus, femur, and zygomatic arch are most common
  - *Cervical-brachial plexus injury*—usually unilateral paresis due to damage to cervical roots C5–6 or C8–T1
  - *Facial nerve injury*—intrauterine pressure of fetal head against maternal sacrum or forceps application causes asymmetrical mouth during crying and poor eye closure on affected side
  - *Cervical spinal cord injury*—flaccid paresis or paralysis with normal facial tone

- **Differential Diagnosis**
  - Presenting symptoms could possibly be a reflection of another disorder—respiratory, cardiac, muscle disease, metabolic disease, neurologic disease, brain malformation, sepsis, hypoglycemia

- **Treatment**
  - Caput succedaneum, cephalohematoma, bruises—observe for possible elevations of bilirubin and for anemia
  - Nerve injury—physical therapy
  - Fractures—splinting and analgesia
  - Subdural hemorrhage—drain only if there are signs of increased intracranial pressure
  - Subgaleal hemorrhage—intensive care, blood, and clotting factor replacement

- **Pearl**

Birth-related nerve injuries often improve rapidly, but long-term resolution is seldom complete.

20

Respiratory Distress in the Term and Preterm Infant

- ■ Essentials of Diagnosis
  - • This is a clinical description, not a diagnosis
  - • Respiratory rate >60/min, inspiratory chest retractions, expiratory grunting, cyanosis in room air

- ■ Differential Diagnosis
  - • Transient tachypnea of the newborn due to retained lung fluid
  - • Hyaline membrane disease, respiratory distress syndrome
  - • Meconium aspiration
  - • Congenital pneumonia (group B streptococci, *Escherichia coli, Klebsiella*
  - • Spontaneous or traumatic pneumothorax, pneumomediastinum
  - • Space-occupying respiratory lesions—cyst, pleural effusion, upper airway obstruction
  - • Urea cycle abnormalities—present with tachypnea, alkalosis on day 1–2 but without cyanosis or desaturation

- ■ Treatment
  - • Secure the airway and listen for breath sounds over all lung fields
  - • Obtain chest x-ray
  - • Give supplemental oxygen
  - • Intubation and ventilation for respiratory failure (arterial oxygen <60 mm Hg with inspired oxygen concentration of >60%) or apnea
  - • Umbilical artery catheterization allows repeated evaluations of Pa_{O_2}
  - • Give ampicillin and gentamycin IV for presumed pneumonia/sepsis until diagnosis is clarified

- ■ Pearl

20

Complications of meconium aspiration (edema, surfactant deficiency, pulmonary hypertension, decreased cardiac output) are caused by hypoxic-ischemic injury to the lungs, not to airway obstruction from meconium.

Hyaline Membrane Disease/
Respiratory Distress Syndrome (RDS)

- ■ Essentials of Diagnosis
  - Most common cause of respiratory distress in preterm infants
  - Caused by insufficient pulmonary surfactant which results in atelectasis and ↓lung compliance
  - Symptoms—tachypnea (>60 breaths/min), cyanosis, expiratory grunting, poor air movement at auscultation, inspiratory retractions
  - Chest x-ray shows hypoexpansion, generalized "ground glass" opacity, and air bronchograms
  - Proteinaceous membranes in the alveoli at autopsy

- ■ Differential Diagnosis
  - Congenital or acquired pneumonia
  - Congestive heart failure
  - Other causes of newborn respiratory distress (See Respiratory Distress in term and preterm infants)

- ■ Treatment
  - Antenatal betamethasone administered to mother in premature labor improves lung maturity
  - Early airway insufflation with artificial surfactant via endotracheal tube
  - Nasal CPAP of 5–6 cm H_2O with inspired oxygen titrated to arterial oxygen saturation
  - Intubation and mechanical ventilation for severe cases

- ■ Pearl

20

Extubation as early as possible with institution of CPAP minimizes lung injury from barotrauma and oxygen toxicity and reduces the risk of chronic lung disease.

Bronchopulmonary Dysplasia

- ■ Essentials of Diagnosis
  - Acute respiratory distress starting in the first week of life, usually in premature infants who require positive pressure ventilation
  - Affects 30% of infants <1000 g birth weight
  - Initial stage is hyaline membrane disease (lack of pulmonary surfactant) and vascular congestion (patent ductus arteriosus)
  - Barotrauma, oxygen toxicity, and inflammation all play a role in pathogenesis
  - Pulmonary histology includes decreased numbers of alveoli and fibrovascular changes in small airways

- ■ Differential Diagnosis
  - Meconium aspiration syndrome with pulmonary hypertension
  - Congenital pulmonary infections—cytomegalovirus (CMV) or ureaplasma
  - Cystic adenomatoid malformation
  - Recurrent pulmonary aspiration
  - Total anomalous pulmonary venous return
  - Idiopathic pulmonary fibrosis

- ■ Treatment
  - Careful attention to growth, nutrition, infection prevention/ treatment (especially respiratory syncytial virus [RSV])
  - Prenatal steroids and immediate postnatal surfactant therapy
  - Short course of postnatal glucocorticoid therapy increases success of weaning from ventilator
  - Bronchodilators (β-adrenergic agonists) and careful pulmonary toilet
  - Inhaled oxygen to keep saturation ~93% (avoiding retinal toxicity while preventing development of pulmonary hypertension)
  - Long-term sequelae—reactive airways, pulmonary hypertension, chronic obstructive lung disease, abnormal lung growth

20

- ■ Pearl

Immediate treatment of premature infants with inhaled surfactant, improved ventilation strategies, prenatal glucocorticoids, effective therapies for patent ductus arteriosus, and aggressive antibiotic therapy have not changed the frequency of BPD but have greatly improved outcome.

Intrauterine Drug Exposure

- ■ Essentials of Diagnosis
  - • History is often unreliable
  - • Look for telltale signs of neuromuscular disease with alternating somnolence and irritability, hypo- and hypertonia, and poor feeding

- ■ Differential Diagnosis
  - • *Cocaine* causes maternal hypertension, decreased uterine blood flow, fetal hypoxemia, ↑rate of stillbirths, placental abruption, and premature delivery. Infants have ↑risk for SIDS
  - • *Opioids* cause irritability, hyperactivity, incessant hunger, salivation, emesis, diarrhea, weight loss, tremors, seizures, nasal stuffiness, intrauterine growth retardation
  - • *Alcohol* is teratogenic. Causes fetal alcohol syndrome (see Child Development and Behavior) and withdrawal symptoms similar to opioids
  - • *Tobacco*—intrauterine growth retardation increases in proportion to extent of maternal smoking, mild neurodevelopmental handicaps

- ■ Treatment
  - • Treatment of withdrawal symptoms may include—decreased environmental stimulation, swaddling, phenobarbital, methadone
  - • Social service involvement and sometime child protective services
  - • Avoid use of any unnecessary medications during pregnancy
  - • Parent education about the use of supine sleeping position to reduce the risk of SIDS

- ■ Pearl

20

Drugs with potential fetal toxicity include antineoplastics, antithyroid, benzodiazepines, warfarin, lithium, angiotensin-converting enzyme (ACE) inhibitors, immunosuppressants, thalidomide.

Neonatal Hypoglycemia

- ■ Essentials of Diagnosis
  - Blood glucose <40 mg/dL regardless of gestational age or clinical condition is too low
  - Neonates with hypoglycemia often display no symptoms
  - Symptoms—lethargy, irritability, jitteriness, poor feeding, seizures, ↓level of consciousness, coma
  - Increased risk—infants of diabetic mothers, infants with intrauterine growth retardation, stressed infants, preterm infants

- ■ Differential Diagnosis
  - Islet cell hyperplasia—Beckwith-Wiedemann syndrome, erythroblastosis
  - Genetic hyperinsulinism
  - Inborn errors—galactosemia, glycogen storage diseases
  - Endocrine—hypopituitarism
  - Complication of birth asphyxia
  - Complication of sepsis

- ■ Treatment
  - Blood sugar <40 mg/dL without symptoms—feed and repeat glucose
  - Blood sugar <40 mg/dL with symptoms—start IV within 10 minutes and give 2 mL/kg of 10% dextrose bolus followed by 3.6 mL/kg/h constant infusion. Monitor glucose within 30 minutes
  - Blood sugar <20 mg/dL with/without symptoms—start IV within 10 minutes and give 2 mL/kg 10% dextrose bolus followed by 3.6 mL/kg/h constant infusion. Monitor glucose within 30 minutes

- ■ Pearl

20

The principal causes of morbidity from neonatal hypoglycemia are failure to anticipate, failure to treat promptly and effectively, and failure to make sure hypoglycemia does not recur when treatment is stopped.

Neonatal Jaundice

- **Essentials of Diagnosis**
  - Jaundice (yellow color) of the skin with clear urine and yellow stools caused by unconjugated hyperbilirubinemia
  - Common in preterm and breast-fed infants
  - Bilirubin encephalopathy (kernicterus) occurs when unconjugated bilirubin deposits in basal ganglia. Rarely occurs in term neonates unless unconjugated bilirubin concentration is >25 mg/dL
  - Very low birth weight and very premature infants have risk of kernicterus at lower unconjugated bilirubin concentrations

- **Differential Diagnosis**
  - Physiological jaundice—occurs with normal red cell breakdown after birth. Unconjugated bilirubin usually <20 mg/dL. Spontaneous resolution in 1–12 weeks
  - Immune hemolysis—ABO and Rh incompatibility
  - Nonimmune hemolysis—hereditary spherocytosis, glucose-6-phosphate dehydrogenase deficiency
  - Enclosed hemorrhage—cephalhematoma, extensive bruising, intracranial bleed
  - Increased enterohepatic circulation of bilirubin—intestinal obstruction, constipation
  - Polycythemia
  - Infants of diabetic mothers
  - Genetic syndromes with ↑bilirubin—Crigler-Najjar syndrome, Gilbert syndrome, hypothyroidism

- **Treatment**
  - Increased fluid intake stimulates perfusion of liver and bilirubin clearance
  - Increased calories improves hepatic conjugation
  - Phototherapy promotes conjugation of bilirubin in skin with renal excretion
  - Exchange transfusion for severe hyperbilirubinemia
  - Intravenous immunoglobulin (IVIG) for severe antibody-mediated hemolysis

- **Pearl**

"Breast milk jaundice" is most often caused by poor enteral intake and increased enterohepatic circulation of bilirubin, not to any specific inhibitors of conjugation in breast milk.

Retinopathy of Prematurity (ROP)

- ## Essentials of Diagnosis
  - Risk factors—birth at <28 weeks' gestation, birth weight <1250 g
  - The role of oxygen in causing or preventing ROP is still unclear
  - Abnormal peripheral retinal vascularization progresses from stage I (incomplete vascularization) to stage V (severe vascular proliferation with retinal detachment and blindness)
  - Regular ophthalmologic examination of at-risk infants to identify distribution (zones) and severity of vascular changes
  - Retinopathy in zone 1 (directly around the optic nerve) carries highest risk of blindness

- ## Differential Diagnosis
  - Retinal hemorrhage
  - Incomplete retinal vascularization—a normal finding in premature infants
  - Rush disease—ROP which progresses very rapidly to retinal detachment

- ## Treatment
  - Most acute phase ROP begins spontaneous involution at 38.6 weeks mean postmenstrual age
  - Treatment is required for 5 contiguous or 8 noncontiguous 30° retinal wedges with stage III vascular changes around the optic nerve
  - Diode laser therapy causes less inflammation and is replacing cryotherapy
  - Surgical therapy for retinal detachment
  - Early treatment of smaller, sicker neonates may reduce unfavorable outcome

20

- ## Pearl
  Children with a history of ROP need lifelong monitoring for later development of strabismus, amblyopia, myopia, and glaucoma.

Intraventricular Hemorrhage

- **Essentials of Diagnosis**
  - Hemorrhage in the ependymal germinal matrix with extension into the ventricles caused by ischemia/reperfusion injury to the matrix capillaries
  - 50% occur before 24 hours of age
  - Incidence is 20–30% in infants born <31 weeks' gestation or <1500 g birth weight. ↑incidence with ↓gestational age and intrauterine infection
  - Small bleeds may cause no symptoms or gradual-onset symptoms
  - Large bleeds—hypotension, acidosis, irritability, decerebrate posturing, apnea, hypoventilation, fixed pupils, bulging anterior fontanel
  - Routine cranial ultrasound is performed in all infants <32 weeks' gestational age. Follow-up ultrasounds will monitor progression or resolution
  - Prognosis good in small hemorrhage—cerebrospinal fluid (CSF) shunting rarely needed, development equal to nonbleeding infants of the same size
  - Large hemorrhage carries mortality of 10–20% and high risk of cerebral palsy and cognitive delays

- **Differential Diagnosis**
  - Routine screening in the intensive care nursery usually leaves little doubt about whether a bleed has occurred
  - Other causes of neurologic symptoms in neonates—brain malformation, meningitis, birth asphyxia, metabolic disease, sepsis

- **Treatment**
  - Supportive treatment—fluids, transfusion, oxygenation, and ventilatory support
  - Ventriculo-peritoneal shunting for postbleeding obstructive hydrocephaly
  - Antinatal corticosteroids to mother may decrease incidence of bleeding
  - Babies born by cesarean section have decreased rate of intracranial bleeding but guidelines on elective C-section are not specific
  - Early indomethacin administration may decrease frequency and severity of intraventricular hemorrhage possibly through prevention and/or treatment of PDA

- **Pearl**

Regardless of symptoms all infants born at 29–32 weeks' gestation should have an ultrasound at 4–6 weeks to look for consequences of an undetected intracranial hemorrhage—ventriculomegaly or periventricular leukomalacia.

Neonatal Seizures

■ Essentials of Diagnosis

- Usual onset 12–48 hours
- Typical neonatal seizures are not well-organized tonic-clonic
- Common signs—horizontal deviation of the eyes, eyelid blinking or fluttering, sucking, lip smacking, drooling, swimming, rowing or paddling movements, apnea spells
- Seizures from hypoglycemia, central nervous system (CNS) infection, inborn errors of metabolism and developmental defects, and poor-controlled seizures due to intracranial bleed or hypoxic-ischemic brain injury carry poor prognosis
- Investigations should screen for all diagnoses below

■ Causes of Neonatal Seizures

- Hypoxic-ischemic injury—causes 60% of seizures in neonates. Onset 24 hours
- Intracranial bleed—up to 15% of cases with underlying periventricular-intraventricular bleed, subdural-subarachnoid bleed, stroke
- Infection—12% of cases
- Hypoglycemia—small for dates, infants of diabetic mothers
- Hypocalcemia/hypomagnesemia—low birth weight, infants of diabetic mothers, hypoparathyroidism
- Hyponatremia—associated with inappropriate antidiuretic hormone (ADH) secretion
- Amino acid, organic acid, and urea cycle inborn errors of metabolism
- Pyridoxine dependency—seizures do not respond to routine medication
- Drug withdrawal
- Benign familial neonatal seizures
- Idiopathic—10% of cases

20

■ Treatment

- Ensure adequate ventilation and perfusion
- Give 2 mL/kg 10% dextrose solution to all infants
- Monitor and correct electrolyte abnormalities
- Give phenobarbital 20 mg/kg IV. Other therapy may include fos-phenytoin, valproate, lorazepam
- Specific diagnostic testing may include imaging, blood sugar, and electrolytes, metabolic evaluations, drug screen

■ Pearl

Although pyridoxine-dependent seizures are rare, a trial of pyridoxine is indicated in all refractory seizures.

Neonatal Bacterial Sepsis

- **Essentials of Diagnosis**
  - Early-onset sepsis (<5 days) occurs in 4–5/1000 live births. Rupture of membranes >24 hours before birth increases rate to 1/100. Maternal chorioamnionitis increases rate to 1/10 live births
  - Symptoms of early bacterial infection—respiratory distress due to pneumonia, low Apgar scores, poor perfusion, hypotension
  - Symptoms of late-onset bacterial infection (>5 days)—poor feeding, lethargy, hypotonia, temperature instability, altered perfusion, increased oxygen requirement, apnea
  - Late-onset infection more often associated with meningitis, urinary tract infection, umbilical stump, or other localized infection

- **Differential Diagnosis**
  - Most common cause of early-onset infection—group B β-hemolytic streptococci (GBS), gram-negative enterics (mostly *E coli, Haemophilus influenzae, Listeria monocytogenes*)
  - Most common cause of late-onset sepsis—coagulase negative staphylococci, *S aureus*, GBS, *Enterococcus,* and gram negatives

- **Treatment**
  - Prevent GBS infection by treating culture positive mother with penicillin given intrapartum >4 hours before delivery
  - Culture suspect infant's urine, blood, CSF, and obtain chest x-ray
  - Initiate treatment of suspected early sepsis before culture results are complete—ampicillin plus aminoglycoside or third-generation cephalosporin
  - Treat suspected late sepsis with coverage expanded to include staphylococci and pseudomonas—Ampicillin, vancomycin, and third-generation cephalosporin

20

- **Pearl**

Premature infants are at higher risk than term neonates for bacterial sepsis. Err on the side of aggressive culture and treatment in premature infants.

Necrotizing Enterocolitis (NEC)

■ Essentials of Diagnosis

- Most common acquired gastrointestinal (GI) emergency in the newborn. Affects 10% of preterm infants <1500 g birth weight
- Increased risk in term infants with polycythemia, congenital heart disease, birth asphyxia
- Pathogenesis multifactorial—previous intestinal ischemia, bacterial or viral infection, immunologic immaturity, prematurity
- Typical presentation—abdominal distention, gastric residual after feedings, heme-positive or bloody stool, poor perfusion, apnea spells
- Laboratory findings—↑WBC, ↓platelets, hyperglycemia, metabolic acidosis, disseminated intravascular coagulation (DIC)
- Plain abdominal films—ileus, bowel wall edema, pneumatosis (air in the bowel wall)

■ Differential Diagnosis

- Neonatal bacterial sepsis and cardiac decompensation—may have similar nonspecific presentation
- Benign pneumatosis—healthy infants may have striking bowel wall air during viral gastroenteritis or after abdominal surgery
- Older children with multiorgan-system failure, immunosupression, heart transplant, or leukemia develop pneumatosis as a preterminal event
- Pneumothorax may cause air to dissect into the bowel wall

■ Treatment

- Stop all enteral feedings
- Correct perfusion—give IV fluids to replace third-space GI losses
- Broad-spectrum antibiotic coverage—ampicillin, third-generation cephalosporin, and possibly coverage for anaerobes
- Surgery indicated for perforation, abdominal wall cellutitis, resistant acidemia suggesting dead bowel
- Infants with firm diagnosis of NEC should be NPO and receive antibiotics for 10–14 days

20

■ Pearl

Intestinal resection in patients with NEC is the most common cause of short bowel syndrome in children.

21

Adolescent Disorders

21

Substance Abuse

- ■ Essentials of Diagnosis
  - • Substances of abuse and/or dependency—alcohol, marijuana, opioids, cocaine, amphetamines, sedatives, hallucinogens, inhalants, nicotine, anabolic steroids, γ-hydroxy-butyrate, ecstasy
  - • Experimentation with substances of abuse is common in children as part of establishing independence and autonomy
  - • Progression and continuation of substance abuse has potentially severe consequences—chronic polysubstance abuse; addiction; compromised physical, cognitive, and psychosocial development

- ■ Differential Diagnosis
  - • Psychiatric emotional disorders
  - • Neurologic disease
  - • Overmedication—especially in chronic pain

- ■ Treatment
  - • No approach to prevention is uniformly effective
  - • Primary programs aim at education and awareness in families, elementary and middle school students
  - • Secondary programs aim at prevention in at-risk populations (children of alcoholics)
  - • Tertiary programs aim at decreasing abuse in known users and addiction prevention
  - • Recognize and treat toxic overdose (see Chap. 26, Poisoning)

- ■ Pearl

Problems associated with substance abuse—school dropout and failure, runaway, unexplained injury, new emotional and psychiatric problems, suicide attempt, motor vehicle accident, sexual promiscuity, sexually transmitted disease, illegal and high-risk behavior.

21

Vaginitis

- ■ **Essentials of Diagnosis**
  - Major presenting symptoms—vaginal discharge, itching, pain, rash
  - Vaginal wet prep and culture required to identify sources—candida, trichomonas, gonorrhea, herpes, chlamydia, *Streptococcus pneumoniae*, *Shigella*
  - Bacterial vaginosis more common in sexually active women and girls. Caused by indigenous species—*Gardnerella, Bacteroides, Peptococcus, Mycoplasma hominis,* lactobacilli, anaerobes
  - Addition of potassium hydroxide (KOH) to a vaginal smear releases a typical fishy odor (amines) in bacterial vaginosis

- ■ **Differential Diagnosis**
  - Physiologic leucorrhea of menarche is harmless
  - Sexual abuse
  - Recurrent or resistant candida infections suggest diabetes, pregnancy, overuse of antibiotics, oral contraceptives, immunodeficiency
  - Contact vaginitis (soaps, douches, bubble bath) or vaginal foreign body
  - Crohn disease, Behçet disease, vaginal or uterine rhabdomyosarcoma all may present with vaginal discharge ± vulvar ulcers

- ■ **Treatment**
  - Treat identified pathogens with specific antibiotics
  - Treat bacterial vaginosis with topical/systemic metronidazole or clindamycin
  - A pregnancy test should be performed in new-onset vaginitis
  - Experienced personnel essential in taking history and examining children and adolescents with vaginal discharge

21

- ■ **Pearl**

In a sexually active girl with vaginitis, specimens should be taken for other sexually transmitted disease, even if the wet prep suggests candida or bacterial vaginosis.

Breast Disease

- ■ Essentials of Diagnosis
  - Benign breast masses in girls—fibroadenoma (most common in upper outer breast quadrant), fibrocystic disease, cysts, abscess, mastitis, fat necrosis. Rarely lymphangioma, hemangioma, neurofibromatosis, nipple adenoma or keratoma, mammary duct ectasia, lipoma, hematoma
  - Galactorrhea (male and female) usually benign and transient. If persistent, look for prolactinoma, hypothalamic disease, chest wall herpes zoster or drugs in boys or girls. Hypothyroidism, pregnancy, recent abortion/parturition, or emotional distress in girls
  - Obstructed or ectatic ducts may cause mastitis or abscess in nonlactating girls or boys

- ■ Differential Diagnosis
  - Transient breast asymmetry is normal in pubertal girls. Also consider breast hypoplasia, amastia, absence of the pectoralis major muscle, unilateral virginal hypertrophy
  - Malignant masses are rare—hemangiosarcoma, rhabdomyosarcoma, ductal carcinoma, cystosarcoma phylloides, metastatic disease
  - Adolescent male gynecomastia is usually benign, may be unilateral. Type I—firm, tender, subareolar breast tissue due to transient testosterone/estrogen imbalance. Type II (pseudogynecomastia)—due to excess fat and prominent pectoralis major
  - In boys with pre- or postpubertal gynecomastia, consider drugs, malignancy (testicular, adrenal, pituitary), Klinefelter syndrome, hypogonadism, thyroid or hepatic dysfunction, malnutrition

- ■ Treatment
  - Benign hypertrophy or asymmetry requires education, reassurance, and monitoring in boys and girls
  - Fibroadenomata and cysts usually resolve after puberty but occasionally require biopsy, ultrasound
  - Oral contraceptives may relieve cyclic nodularity and tenderness of fibrocystic disease
  - Galactorrhea and pre- or postpubertal gynecomastia in boys should always be investigated for a pathologic cause
  - Biopsy is needed to determine therapy for malignant breast tumors

21

- ■ Pearl

Breast examination is part of the childhood physical examination as soon as breast buds appear. If the preadolescent views breast examination as routine it will facilitate communication among child, parents, and physician about breast health.

Eating Disorders

- ■ Essentials of Diagnosis
  - Anorexia nervosa (AN)—body weight <85% of expected from height, fear of weight gain, disturbed body image, denial, attempts to camouflage thinness, amenorrhea, bradycardia, hypothermia, lanugo, dry skin, hypokalemia, hyponatremia
  - Bulimia nervosa—episodic binge eating with inappropriate compensatory behavior (emesis, laxatives, enemas, diuretics, diet pills, fasting, excessive exercise), sense of being out of control during and after attacks, disturbed body image, body weight usually normal
  - Female predominance in both disorders. Prepubertal onset more common in anorexia

- ■ Differential Diagnosis
  - Eating disorder not otherwise specified—patients not fitting criteria for either diagnosis but with features of both. May be a precursor of AN or bulimia
  - Depression, anxiety disorder, sexual abuse
  - Inflammatory bowel disease, peptic ulcer or gastroesophageal (GE) reflux disease, celiac disease, diabetes, hyper/hypothyroidism, malignancy, adrenal insufficiency
  - Dental disease in bulimia

- ■ Treatment
  - Early intervention and education may prevent full-blown disease
  - Recognize the early signs of anorexia—sudden intense low fat, low carbohydrate diet, complaints of early satiety, failure to join family meals, intense concern over body image, unexplained weight loss, amenorrhea
  - Unexplained disappearance of groceries may alert parents to bulimia
  - Team approach to treatment is most successful with nutritional monitoring, education, family counseling, psychiatric evaluation and treatment, and medical subspecialists as needed
  - Hospitalization may be needed. Mortality in AN from suicide, electrolyte disturbance, or cardiac arrhythmia is up to 18% depending upon disease severity

- ■ Pearl

Every routine adolescent medical encounter must include appropriate questioning about body image and attitudes toward food or eating disorders will be missed.

22

Developmental and Behavioral Disorders

22

Colic

- ■ **Essentials of Diagnosis**
  - Severe continuous crying in infants 1–6 months of age with no obvious physical cause
  - Crying >3 h/day, >3 days/week for >3 weeks. Often in the late afternoon and evening
  - Child thriving with normal physical examination and development
  - Most likely cause is immaturity of self-settling and self-organizing behaviors in normal infant
  - Complete history, careful physical examination, screening urinalysis (UA), blood count, fecal occult test are all negative but are recommended to screen for organic disease

- ■ **Differential Diagnosis**
  - Normal variant—daily duration of crying increases after birth, peaks at 6 weeks, and tapers off by 12–16 weeks
  - Maternal anxiety, inexperience, or depression
  - Common organic conditions associated with crying—trauma (broken clavicle, neurologic birth injury, child abuse), corneal abrasion, urinary tract infection, peptic disease (especially gastroesophageal [GE] reflux), constipation, central nervous system disorder
  - Hunger—inadequate maternal milk supply or breast-feeding techniques
  - Milk protein intolerance is a rare cause of colic

- ■ **Treatment**
  - Education of parents about progression of normal crying behavior
  - Continued availability of medical personnel for interval evaluation
  - Elimination of unnecessary stimulation of child and organization of child's schedule
  - Medications rarely helpful. Acid blockers and milk protein-free diet are often tried

22

- ■ **Pearl**

Do not underestimate the devastating distress of parents of colicky infants. They feel exhausted, inadequate, and are worried that serious disease is being missed or ignored. They require education, support, respect, and sympathy.

Feeding Refusal

- **Essentials of Diagnosis**

  - Apparent inability or active refusal to eat in infants and toddlers
  - Organic causes in young infants—birth injury, renal tubular acidosis, exhaustion with eating secondary to congenital heart and lung disease
  - Motor weakness and incoordination—Zellweger syndrome, spinal muscular atrophy, cricopharyngeal achalasia
  - Pain or fear associated with eating may provoke refusal—peptic disease, esophagitis, food allergy, cleft palate, constipation, chronic aspiration
  - Medically necessary withholding of feeds in neonates prevents imprinting of normal behavior—esophageal atresia, catastrophic neonatal illness, neonatal surgery (especially gastrointestinal [GI] and cardiac), extreme prematurity
  - A 3-day record of intake is the first step in diagnosis and therapy. Other tests based upon symptoms—GI, x-rays, complete blood count (CBC), UA, serum HCO_3, thyroid panel, liver panel

- **Differential Diagnosis**

  - Abnormal parental expectations for intake
  - Normal toddler eating behavior is erratic with days of poor calorie intake separated by days of compensatory increased intake
  - Overzealous (force) feeding may lead to refusal behavior
  - Abnormal child rearing or neglect

- **Treatment**

  - Observation of behavior during feedings often identifies a cause
  - Establish consistent feeding routines—timing, place, amounts, textures, predictable positive and negative reinforcement, realistic goal setting
  - Occupational and physical therapy may be helpful in newborns in whom feedings were withheld for medical reasons
  - Children with profound motor, neurologic, cardiac, or GI-related food refusal may require gastrostomy
  - If food refusal leads to failure to gain, inpatient behavioral therapy in a multidisciplinary setting may be needed

- **Pearl**

The term "infant anorexia" sometimes applied to the infant with food refusal should be abandoned. It suggests a psychological problem akin to anorexia nervosa in older children which if not completely erroneous, is vanishingly rare.

Sleep Disorders

■ Essentials of Diagnosis

- Night terrors occur in 3% of children usually within 2 hours of falling asleep (deep non–rapid eye movement [REM] sleep)
- Night terrors last ~30 minutes with screaming, thrashing, tachypnea, tachycardia, sweating, incoherence, sleep walking. Child has no recall of event in the morning
- Obstructive sleep apnea—loud snoring, chest retraction, morning headache, dry mouth. Peak age 2–6 years. Associated with adenoid and tonsillar hypertrophy, obesity, jaw and other facial anomalies, hypotonia
- Dyssomnia—frequent night-time wakening or difficulty falling asleep with frequent demands for parental attention. Usually a learned behavior. Starts at ~9 months of age
- Careful physical examination, medical and psychosocial history clarifies diagnosis and establishes parental confidence

■ Differential Diagnosis

- Nightmares—frightening dreams during REM sleep. Child is fearful but oriented, seeks parental reassurance, and usually remembers the event the next morning
- Exaggerated periodic breathing—may resemble obstructive sleep apnea
- Psychiatric problems
- GE reflux—sometimes causes night-time wakening because of pain or choking
- Hunger—inadequate daytime food/fluid intake associated with night-time demands for food or bottle

■ Treatment

- *Night terrors*—parent education, protection of child during spell, regular sleep schedule, avoidance of sleep deprivation. Scheduled waking of child before spells if night terrors occur predictably
- *Nightmares*—reassurance, night light, establish a routine response to nightmares so child can calm himself/herself when they occur
- *Dyssomnia*—set developmentally appropriate limits on parental visits to the bedroom after child is put in bed, establish regular bedtime rituals with age-appropriate bedtimes, ensure adequate daytime calorie intake, avoid exhaustion
- Polysomnography may help clarify diagnosis of obstructive sleep apnea
- Treat physical causes of sleep apnea—adenoidectomy, weight reduction

■ Pearl

Keeping a tired child awake so he/she can have "quality time" with parents does the child no good and deprives parents of quality time with each other.

22

Temper Tantrums and Breath Holding

- **Essentials of Diagnosis**
  - 50–80% of 1–4 year olds have ≥ 1 temper tantrum per week usually provoked by frustration with loss of control
  - Behavior during tantrum—crying, throwing himself/herself on floor, kicking, screaming, striking people or objects, breath holding spell
  - Breath-holding spells are reflexive, involuntary, response to anger (child usually cyanotic), surprise, mild injury (child usually pallid). Onset is during expiration
  - Breath holding may resolve spontaneously or child may experience loss of consciousness, hypotonia, opisthotonos, body jerks, urinary incontinence, hypoxic seizure, or cardiac arrhythmia
  - Descriptive diagnosis
  - The prognosis for tantrums and breath holding is good

- **Differential Diagnosis**
  - Breath holding differential includes seizure, cardiac arrhythmia, orthostatic hypotension, iron deficiency anemia, Rett syndrome, familial dysautonomia, lung disease, laryngeal spasm, airway obstruction, tetany
  - Severe or very frequent temper tantrums suggest underlying developmental disorder, metabolic disease, psychiatric disorder, or autism

- **Treatment**
  - Behavioral treatment of temper tantrums—prevent frustration, use distraction when frustration occurs, stay nearby the child to prevent self-injury, avoid unnecessary conflict, offer choices rather than specific commands
  - Breath holding—evaluate child for possible organic disorders
  - If breath holding causes loss of consciousness, put child in lateral position to protect against aspiration and head injury
  - There are no prophylactic medications for breath holding. Subcutaneous atropine can be given if spells cause bradycardia

- **Pearl**

Rather than telling a child with temper tantrums that he/she must go to bed now, parents should offer reasonable choices that avoid conflict. "Would you like to read a story or play a game of cards with me before you go to bed?"

22

Attention-Deficit/Hyperactivity Disorder (ADHD)

- ■ Essentials of Diagnosis
  - Affects 2–10% of school-age children with a triad of symptoms—impulsivity, inattention, hyperactivity. Substantial genetic component
  - Hyperactive impulsive type—fidgetiness, difficulty remaining still, excessive running, climbing and talking, inability to engage in quiet activities, difficulty taking turns, interrupting others
  - Inattentive type—inattentive to detail, distractible and forgetful; fails to listen, follow instructions, organize tasks, and stay on task; reluctant to engage in tasks; loses utensils
  - Most children are combinations of the 2 major subtypes

- ■ Differential Diagnosis
  - ADHD often associated with/caused by other psychiatric problems—mood disorder, conduct disorder, oppositional defiant disorder, tics, Tourette syndrome
  - Genetic disorders—fragile X, Williams syndrome, Angelman syndrome, XXY syndrome, Turner syndrome
  - Brain injury—fetal alcohol syndrome (FAS), prematurity, trauma, hypoxia
  - Hyperthyroidism, drug abuse, alcohol abuse may resemble ADHD

- ■ Treatment
  - Most children improve by 10–25 years of age, though condition may persist into adulthood
  - Behavior modification usually helps the child with uncomplicated ADHD
  - Preferential classroom seating, positive reinforcement, consistent structure at home and school, repetition of information, instruction using both visual and auditory modalities
  - Commonly used medications—methylphenidate, dextroamphetamine, atomoxetine
  - Hyper-reactivity and motor tics—clonidine and guanfacine
  - Tricyclic antidepressants and bupropion sometimes used but the latter may lower seizure threshold

22

- ■ Pearl

There are many somewhat disobedient or immature school children in whom the diagnosis of ADHD has been made without adequate evaluation. Children should not receive powerful medications to eliminate minor behavioral immaturity.

Fetal Alcohol Spectrum Disorders

- **Essentials of Diagnosis**
  - FAS—dysmorphic facies (short palpebral fissures, thin upper lip, indistinct or smooth philtrum), growth deficiency and neurodevelopmental abnormalities resulting from intrauterine alcohol exposure
  - Partial FAS—neurodevelopmental problems without major dysmorphism
  - Alcohol is a teratogen and may cause congenital anomalies of the heart, skeleton, kidneys, eyes, and ears as well as FAS
  - The diagnosis rests on history of alcohol use (especially during first trimester) and typical clinical findings

- **Differential Diagnosis**
  - The FAS facies may suggest other syndromes—Williams syndrome
  - Consider FAS in children with ADHD
  - Consider FAS in children with failure to thrive, school failure, depression, panic attacks, anxiety, mood disorders, psychosis

- **Treatment**
  - Prevention of alcohol intake, especially in the first trimester
  - Methylphenidate for the associated ADHD
  - Selective serotonin reuptake inhibitors (SSRIs) can help with anxiety, panic attacks, and depression
  - Valproate or carbamazepine may be helpful as mood stabilizers
  - Psychotic features require evaluation and careful selection of therapy

- **Pearl**

There are no reliable data on exact amount or timing of alcohol consumption necessary for teratogenesis or fetal alcohol spectrum disorders. Strong evidence indicates that binge drinking during the first trimester is a major risk factor.

22

23

Psychiatric Disorders

23

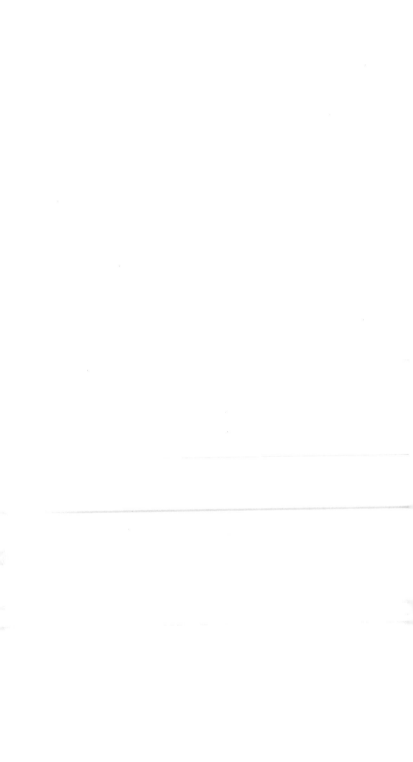

Autistic Disorder

■ Essentials of Diagnosis

- Severe deficits in social responsiveness and interpersonal relationships
- Abnormal speech and language development
- Behavioral peculiarities—ritualized, repetitive, stereotyped behaviors; rigidity; poverty of age-typical interests and activities
- Onset before age 3 years; male predominance (3:1)
- Incidence 16–40/10,000 school-age children
- Seizures occur in 30%

■ Differential Diagnosis

- Primary associated diseases are—prenatal rubella, phenylketonuria, tuberous sclerosis, infantile spasms, postnatal central nervous system (CNS) infections, fragile X syndrome, other metabolic disorders
- Hearing or visual impairment may mimic autism
- Global developmental delay

■ Treatment

- No uniformly effective therapy
- Early intervention to facilitate development of reciprocal, interactive, language and social skills
- Occupational therapy for sensory integration
- Behaviorally oriented special education
- Medications to reduce target symptoms—hyperactivity, aggressiveness, inattention, depression, obsessive behavior, mood swings, self-destructive behavior, stereotypy

■ Pearl

The best outcomes occur in children with normal intelligence who have acquired symbolic language skills by age 5 years. One-sixth of autistic children are gainfully employed as adults and one-sixth function in sheltered environments.

23

Nonautistic Pervasive Developmental Disorders

- ■ Essentials of Diagnosis
  - • Substantial social impairment, either primary or representing loss of previous social skills
  - • Abnormalities of speech and language development or behaviors resembling autism
  - • Milder, more common, and later onset than autism without the complete set of autistic diagnostic criteria
  - • Most Rett syndrome cases are girls with mutation of the *MECP2* gene
  - • Childhood disintegrative disorder may start up to age 9 years

- ■ Differential Diagnosis
  - • Asperger syndrome (male predominance) and Rett syndrome (female predominance) are common primary causes
  - • Developmental speech and language disorders
  - • Hearing impairment
  - • Global developmental delay
  - • Other psychiatric disorders

- ■ Treatment
  - • Cognitive behavioral therapy to reinforce appropriate social and language skills and behavior
  - • Rett syndrome and childhood disintegrative disorder have worse prognosis than Asperger syndrome
  - • Test and treat for other psychiatric conditions

- ■ Pearl

If a school boy of normal intelligence is socially naive and inept, is picked on by other class members, seems to "walk to a different drummer" and has rigidly limited but intense interests, consider Asperger syndrome. These boys can be helped with accurate diagnosis and social skill therapy.

23

Depression

■ Essentials of Diagnosis

- Persistent dysphoric mood, mood lability, irritability, or depressed appearance
- Neurovegetative signs and symptoms—changes in sleep, appetite, concentration, and activity patterns
- Suicidal ideation and feelings of hopelessness
- 1–3% incidence before puberty and ~8% in adolescence
- Female:Male ratio is equal in preadolescence and increases to 5:1 in adolescence
- Patients feel bored, friendless, and isolated. School work may deteriorate
- Nonorganic headache, fatigue, abdominal pain, insomnia

■ Differential Diagnosis

- Dysthymic disorder has less severe but equally chronic symptoms
- Adjustment disorder with depressed mood is a reaction to stress
- Hypothyroidism
- Substance abuse
- Other organic disorders—brain tumor, inflammatory bowel disease, Wilson disease

■ Treatment

- Comprehensive care includes immediate therapy of depressive episode, education, and individual and family therapy
- Cognitive behavioral therapy may be effective
- Medications may be indicated for moderate to severe depression

■ Pearl

The adolescent with depression must be monitored long term to identify complications of medication, new life stresses that might precipitate acute deterioration, and additional psychiatric diagnoses especially bipolar disorder.

23

Bipolar Affective Disorder

- ■ Essentials of Diagnosis
  - • Periods of abnormally, persistently elevated expansive or irritable mood, and heightened levels of energy and activity
  - • Associated symptoms—grandiosity, diminished need for sleep, pressured speech, racing thoughts, impaired judgment
  - • No history of prescribed or illicit drug use
  - • Onset before puberty uncommon; 1% prevalence after puberty; cyclic pattern less prominent than in adults
  - • In 70%, presentation is with depressive symptoms

- ■ Differential Diagnosis
  - • Attention-deficit/hyperactivity disorder(ADHD) is highly associated
  - • Drug-induced mania or depression
  - • Agitated major depressive disorder
  - • Mood disorder
  - • Physical/sexual abuse or exposure to domestic violence may produce similar symptoms
  - • Hyperthyroidism

- ■ Treatment
  - • Medical therapy usually necessary—lithium, carbamazepine, valproate, olanzapine, risperidone are approved drugs
  - • Supportive psychotherapy for patient and family is critical

- ■ Pearl

Although it may be possible to discontinue neuroleptic medication after the acute episode passes, it is usually necessary to continue mood stabilizers for a year or even for life.

23

Suicide

- ## Essentials of Diagnosis
  - Third leading cause of death between 10 and 24 years
  - 2 million suicide attempts per year in United States
  - Adolescent female suicide attempt rate three to four times greater than males
  - The number of completed suicides is 3–4 times greater in males than females
  - Suicide risk is increased by mood disorder, severe depressive episode, mood disorder, conduct disorder, psychotic delusions
  - Clues to suicidal intent include—verbally wishing to be "dead," dysphoria, social crisis (loss of girl or boyfriend), previous attempt

- ## Differential Diagnosis
  - Substance abuse
  - Conduct disorder
  - Depression
  - Accidental injury

- ## Treatment
  - Patients attempting suicide must be monitored and counseled
  - Hospitalization for evaluation and therapy is appropriate
  - Awareness of problem must be increased in schools and community
  - Copycat behavior should be addressed in schools

- ## Pearl

A frank discussion of suicidal ideation does not increase the risk of suicide. It may decrease it.

23

Schizophrenia

- ■ Essentials of Diagnosis
  - Delusional, bizarre, morbid thoughts
  - Disorganized, rambling, illogical speech patterns
  - Disorganized or bizarre behavior
  - Hallucinations
  - Paranoia or ideas of reference
  - Negative symptoms include flat affect, avolition, alogia
  - Usually preceded by school deterioration, loss of peer relationships, depression, or nonspecific psychiatric symptoms
  - Family history is sometimes positive

- ■ Differential Diagnosis
  - Some fantastic thinking in childhood is developmentally appropriate—imaginary friends
  - ADHD, learning disabilities
  - Consider child abuse
  - Substance abuse
  - Metabolic diseases, endocrinopathies, Wilson disease, CNS infection

- ■ Treatment
  - Decrease active psychotic symptoms with neuroleptic medication and environmental modification. Hospitalization may be appropriate
  - Support the development of social and cognitive skills
  - Reduce the risk of relapse with maintenance medication and psychotherapy
  - Provide support and education to family and patient

- ■ Pearl

Onset prior to age 13 years, poor premorbid functioning (oddness or eccentricity), and predominance of negative symptoms (withdrawal, apathy, flat affect) over positive symptoms (hallucinations, paranoia) are associated with more severe disability.

23

Conduct Disorders

- ■ Essentials of Diagnosis
  - • Defiance of authority
  - • Violating the rights of others or norms of society
  - • Aggressive behavior toward persons, animals, and/or property
  - • Affects 9% of males and 2% of females <18 years
  - • Environmental associations—domestic violence, child abuse, drug abuse, shifting parental figures, poverty
  - • Common symptoms—running away, academic failure, fighting, defiance, tantrums, vandalism, promiscuity, sexual perpetration, criminal behavior, drug abuse, hyperactivity

- ■ Differential Diagnosis
  - • ADHD
  - • Mood disorders
  - • Psychomotor seizures
  - • Learning disorders

- ■ Treatment
  - • Treatment complicated by the common environmental psychosocial problems
  - • Stabilize the environment
  - • Residential treatment may be effective
  - • Mood stabilizers, neuroleptics, stimulants, and antidepressants often used, not proven effective universally

- ■ Pearl

The prognosis of this disorder depends upon the ability of the child's support system to mount an effective treatment intervention consistently. It is worse for children who present before age 10 years.

23

Anxiety Disorders

- **Essentials of Diagnosis**
  - *School refusal*—persistent school avoidance related to symptoms of anxiety
  - *Generalized anxiety disorder*—intense, exaggerated, or irrational worry often about future events
  - *Panic disorder*—unprovoked fear with sympathetic hyperarousal often with hyperventilation and palpitations
  - *Post-traumatic stress disorder (PTSD)*—fear or actual re-experiencing a past traumatic event with intense sympathetic hyperarousal
  - *Separation anxiety*—developmentally inappropriate wish to maintain proximity of caregiver. Unreasonable fears about family or personal integrity
  - *Phobia*—intense unreasonable fear of a specific stimulus (school, heights, open space)

- **Differential Diagnosis**
  - Learning disabilities
  - Onset of schizophrenia, depression
  - Bullying at school may produce school refusal
  - Consider pregnancy in the adolescent female

- **Treatment**
  - Diagnose comorbid diseases and situations
  - Medication may be required to reduce anxiety
  - Education of child and family and reassurance about organic diseases is critical

- **Pearl**

Returning to school is the therapy of choice for school refusal. The plan for returning should be developed with parents, child, and school personnel and then instituted with sympathetic firmness. Further school avoidance only reinforces the problem.

23

Obsessive-Compulsive Disorder (OCD)

- ■ Essentials of Diagnosis
  - Recurrent obsessive unrealistic thoughts, impulses, or images that cause marked anxiety or distress (contamination, cleanliness)
  - Attempts to ignore or suppress such irrational thoughts or impulses
  - Repetitive compulsive behaviors or mental acts in response to irrational thoughts in an attempt to prevent or reduce the distress they cause (hand washing, counting, putting objects in order)
  - Obsessions and compulsions produce significant disruption of normal activities

- ■ Differential Diagnosis
  - Trichotillomania is a form of OCD
  - Strong genetic familial component
  - Questionable association with group B streptococcus infection and subsequent autoimmune disorder
  - May be associated with Down syndrome

- ■ Treatment
  - Best treated with combination of cognitive behavioral therapy and medication (fluvoxamine and sertraline are approved for OCD in children)
  - Tricyclic antidepressant clomipramine approved for use in adults

- ■ Pearl

OCD is lifelong but therapy is associated with improved control and remissions in most patients.

23

Post-Traumatic Stress Disorder (PTSD)

- **Essentials of Diagnosis**
  - Symptoms follow a traumatic event(s) such as observation of violence, physical or sexual abuse, natural disaster, accidents (dog bites, car accident), unexpected personal tragedy
  - Autonomic hyperarousal symptoms—easy startle, increased heart rate, hypervigilance, sweating, nausea, hyperventilation
  - Avoidant behaviors, fear of strangers, fear of the dark, fear of being alone, and numbing of responsiveness
  - Flashbacks to a traumatic in the form of nightmares or intrusive thoughts
  - Risk increases in individuals with previous history or trauma or unstable social situation

- **Differential Diagnosis**
  - Reactive attachment disorder may follow infant trauma or neglect
  - OCD
  - Anxiety disorder

- **Treatment**
  - Education of child and family as to source of disorder
  - In children, reassurance, repeated explanation, occupational therapy to decrease reactivity and improve self-soothing skills
  - Establishment of daily safe routines
  - Sertraline is approved for severe PTSD in adults
  - Specific therapy for depression, anxiety, nightmares, and aggression
  - Frequently used drugs in children include clonidine, guanfacine, mood stabilizers, antidepressants, and neuroleptics

- **Pearl**

As many as 25% of young people exposed to violence develop some symptoms of PTSD.

23

Somatoform Disorders

- **Essentials of Diagnosis**
  - Symptoms suggest a physical disorder
  - No physical disorder accounts for symptoms after evaluation
  - Symptoms cause distress, dysfunction, or both
  - Symptoms are not caused by malingering

- **Differential Diagnosis**
  - Hypochondriasis—generalized worry about health and diseases impacting it
  - Malingering—conscious creation of symptoms
  - Munchausen syndrome—conscious creation of symptoms to obtain medical interventions (usually surgery)
  - Conversion disorder—symptoms precipitated by stressful event that result in secondary gain
  - Somatization disorder—preoccupation with somatic symptoms to the exclusion of other interests
  - Body dysmorphic disorder—preoccupation with an imagined defect in personal appearance
  - Somatoform pain disorder—preoccupation with pain resulting in distress beyond that expected from physical findings
  - True organic disease, anxiety, psychosis, depression

- **Treatment**
  - Generally responds to careful evaluation, education, and reassurance
  - Psychiatric consultation helpful for incapacitated patients
  - Regular, short, focused medical evaluation to address current complaints
  - Avoid invasive procedures

- **Pearl**

Do not abandon the patient with somatoform disorder. Their continued functioning may be a direct result of consistent, repeated, sympathetic evaluation of their concerns.

23

24

Child Abuse

24

Physical Abuse

- ■ Essentials of Diagnosis
  - Intentional injury to child, often inflicted by caregiver or family member
  - Common signs—bruises, burns, retinal hemorrhages, fractures, head and abdominal trauma
  - Historians give discrepant, evolving, improbable, or no explanation for injury. Delay in seeking care. Inappropriate affect in caregiver
  - Escalating severity or number of injuries over time without intervention
  - Caregiver often isolated socially with unrealistic expectations for the child's behavior and level of maturity
  - Bruise shapes may suggest mode of injury—slap, strap, pinch
  - Hot water scalding gives stocking/glove extremity burns, "doughnut hole" buttock burns
  - Branding burns from cigarettes, curling irons, lighters, irons, barbeque grills are often easily recognizable

- ■ Differential Diagnosis
  - Bone disease—osteogenesis imperfecta
  - Acquired or genetic bleeding disorders and coagulopathies
  - Metabolic diseases—especially glutaric acidemia which may present with retinal and intracranial hemorrhage
  - Neurologic or muscle disease producing abnormal respiratory control, seizures, lethargy, hypotonia

- ■ Treatment
  - Suspected child abuse must be reported. Physicians are legally protected in most states when reporting suspected abuse
  - Document physical injuries with photographs
  - Document skeletal survey, coagulation studies, and any tests done to find a potential unifying alternative diagnosis
  - Consult child advocacy team, social services and, if necessary, hospital security or law enforcement at presentation
  - Separate child from suspected perpetrator either by hospitalization or by foster placement until situation clarified

24

- ■ Pearl

Studies have shown that rolling off the bed or the couch does not cause skull or long bone fractures in infants and children.

Sexual Abuse

- **Essentials of Diagnosis**
  - Majority of sexual abuse victims have nonspecific physical findings
  - Most offenders are male and are friends or relatives of the victim
  - Patient may display—age-inappropriate sexual knowledge or play, sexual abuse of other children, sleep disturbance, eating disorder, depression, anxiety, phobia, aggression, low self-esteem, conversion reaction, suicide attempt, excessive masturbation
  - Medical presentations—recurrent urinary tract infections (UTI), genital, anal or urethral trauma, vaginitis, encopresis, enuresis, sexually transmitted diseases, pregnancy, depression, suicide attempt
  - Sympathetic questioning during routine health maintenance visits of teenagers may reveal sexual abuse
  - All teenagers should be asked about solicitation for illegal sexual activity over the Internet

- **Differential Diagnosis**
  - Recurrent UTI, anal and urethral trauma, vaginitis, encopresis, enuresis, emotional problems can all occur in the absence of sexual abuse
  - Condylomata acuminata may occur in the absence of sexual abuse especially in the infants of mothers with condylomata
  - False allegations of sexual abuse are sometimes made during parental marital discord or custody disputes
  - Perianal rashes (perianal strep, plexiform neurofibroma, poor hygiene, candida, psoriasis) may be mistaken for sexual abuse

- **Treatment**
  - Violent sexual abuse requires multidisciplinary evaluation in the hospital—surgery, obstetrics, urology, psychiatry, social services
  - Nonviolent sexual abuse leaves emotional scars which require support, counseling, and specific steps to stop the abuse
  - For sexual contact within 72 hours—check fluids on patient or clothing for semen or acid phosphatase. Document results
  - Suspected chronic sexual contact—obtain specimens for sexually transmitted diseases and pregnancy

24

- **Pearl**

See the American Academy of Pediatrics Web site for guidelines on evaluation of sexual abuse.

Neglect

■ **Essentials of Diagnosis**

- Neglect is harder to document than abuse and requires long-term acquaintance with patient and family
- Neglectful parents fail to recognize the physical or emotional states of their children
- Failure to gain weight at a rate appropriate to size and age may be a sign of neglect
- The child disabled by birth defects or chronic organic disease is at higher risk for physical, emotional, and medical neglect
- The flattened, hairless occiput, formerly a sign of neglect, is now common with the routine supine sleep positioning to reduce sudden infant death syndrome (SIDS) risk

■ **Differential Diagnosis**

- Organic causes of failure to thrive
- Organic causes of emotional, cognitive, and behavioral problems
- Deprivation secondary to poverty

■ **Treatment**

- Like child abuse, child neglect must be reported
- Meticulous, long-term social service evaluation of family to identify remediable problems
- Documentation of weight gain and calorie intake with nutrition counseling and follow-up
- Family support utilizing in resources such as visiting nurses or paraprofessionals

■ **Pearl**

The use of home visitors to support and educate parents and caregivers can prevent child neglect and abuse. Such services prevent parental isolation and provide them with a connection to support services in times of crisis.

24

Munchausen Syndrome by Proxy

- **Essentials of Diagnosis**
  - Syndrome in which caregiver simulates or creates symptoms in a child in order to obtain medical attention
  - Worrisome symptoms reported or present—apnea, dehydration, emesis, diarrhea, sepsis often with multiple organisms, change in mental status, fever, seizure, gastrointestinal (GI) bleeding, allergies
  - Symptoms are often only observed by perpetrator
  - Perpetrator often has some medical training
  - Perpetrator is cooperative with evaluation until challenged by suspected diagnosis. May threaten legal action
  - Perpetrator cannot be reassured that patient is normal. Doctor shopping common. The child is kept out of normal activities
  - Testing may include urine, blood and stool toxicology, coagulation studies, head computed tomography (CT), echocardiogram (ECG), metabolic screen

- **Differential Diagnosis**
  - Munchausen by proxy mimics many organic diseases
  - Seizure or other neurologic disorder
  - Gastroesophageal (GE) reflux, peptic ulcer, food allergy
  - Immune deficiency with recurrent sepsis, diarrhea, or other infections
  - Bleeding disorder
  - Metabolic diseases especially glutaric acidemia
  - Autoimmune disease

- **Treatment**
  - Some evaluation for organic disease is mandatory, but resist caregiver demands for invasive tests or therapies if they are not medically indicated
  - Involve social services or child advocacy team as soon as diagnosis is suspected
  - Observation of the child in absence of suspected perpetrator may be needed
  - The perpetrator may be depressed, may have organic brain disease and may require therapy

24

- **Pearl**

Confirmation of this diagnosis usually requires an in-patient evaluation. In the majority of cases, the mother is the perpetrator.

25

Emergencies and Injuries

25

Acute Intracranial Hypertension

- **Essentials of Diagnosis**
  - Altered behavior, decreased level of consciousness, headache, vomiting, blurred vision, double vision, seizures, decerebrate posturing, abnormal respiration, coma
  - Optic disc swelling, cranial nerve palsies (especially abducens), systemic hypertension, bradycardia
  - Imaging with magnetic resonance imaging (MRI) and computed tomography (CT) essential to diagnosis

- **Causes of Intracranial Hypertension**
  - Obstruction of cerebrospinal flow (CSF)—brain tumor, infection, hematoma
  - Vasogenic and cytotoxic edema—head trauma, tumor, abscess, infarct, hypoxic/ischemic injury, cardiac arrest, metabolic disease, dural sinus thrombosis
  - Pseudotumor cerebri—hyper- or hypovitaminosis A, corticosteroid use, corticosteroid withdrawal, tetracycline, nalidixic acid, lead poisoning, hypocalcemia, hyperparathyroidism, adrenal insufficiency, systemic lupus erythematosus (SLE), Guillain-Barré syndrome, CO_2 retention, idiopathic

- **Treatment**
  - Intracranial pressure >15–20 cm water should be treated if it is causing symptoms. Object of treatment is to preservation of cerebral blood flow
  - Treat primary cause
  - Intensive support of cardiac and respiratory function
  - Moderate hypothermia to reduce metabolic needs
  - Osmotic diuresis with mannitol
  - Barbiturate sedation
  - Hyperventilation to reduce CO_2 may be effective
  - Vasogenic intracranial hypertension may respond to corticosteroids
  - CSF drainage for obstructing lesions

- **Pearl**

The classic Cushing's triad of bradycardia, hypertension, and apnea associated with acute intracranial hypertension may not occur until late in the course and is often incomplete in children. Don't depend on it.

25

Burns

- ■ Essentials of Diagnosis
  - First degree—injury of superficial epidermal layers is painful, dry, red, hypersensitive, heals with minimal scarring
  - Second degree—superficial partial-thickness injury is red, blistered, painful; deep partial-thickness injury is white, dry, blanches with pressure, decreased sensitivity to pain
  - Third degree—injury to all epidermal and dermal elements; skin is devascularized; no pain; scarring expected
  - Minor burn defined as <10% of body surface for first- and second-degree burns or <2% for third-degree burns
  - Burns of the hands, feet, face, eyes, ears, and perineum are major burns
  - Secondary infection worsens the prognosis of all burns

- ■ Causes
  - Thermal burns—hot water or food, appliances, flames, grills, vehicle related, curling irons
  - Electrical burns—may cause deep tissue injury and necrosis, mental confusion, peripheral nerve injury, cardiac arrhythmia
  - Inhalation burns may cause severe respiratory injury

- ■ Treatment
  - First- and second-degree burn—debridement, cleansing, topical antibiotic, analgesics
  - Third-degree burns >2% of body surface may require intensive care for debridement, antibiotics, fluid and electrolyte management, nutrition, and grafting
  - Team of subspecialists (surgery, plastic surgery, rehabilitative medicine, infectious disease, social service) should be involved in all major burns

- ■ Pearl

The pain, morbidity, and mortality of burn injury; its association with child abuse; and its preventable nature in most situations make this injury a major concern in pediatrics.

25

Head Injury/Concussion

- **Essentials of Diagnosis**
  - Essential elements of history—time and mechanism of injury, how far and onto what surface did the child fall, loss of consciousness, antegrade or retrograde amnesia, emesis, headache ataxia, seizure visual disturbance
  - Essential elements of physical examination—level of consciousness, associated injuries, presence of CSF leak from ears or nose, periorbital hematoma (possible basilar skull fracture), full neurologic and funduscopic examination
  - Concussion diagnosed as brief loss/alteration of consciousness with rapid return to normal. No focal findings on examination. May be associated pallor, amnesia, emesis
  - Obtain head CT scan for major skull/scalp/face injury or hematoma, lateralizing findings, persistent vomiting, persistent altered mental status
  - A normal neurologic examination in infants does not rule out significant intracranial hemorrhage

- **Causes**
  - Trauma
  - Child abuse, shaken baby syndrome
  - Drug toxicity or overdose may precipitate head injury but may also mimic it

- **Treatment**
  - Discharge patients with mild injury from the emergency department after short observation if the examination is normal and caregivers understand the indications for re-evaluation
  - Persistent neurologic deficits after head injury require in-hospital monitoring or prolonged emergency department observation
  - Deteriorating mental status requires urgent evaluation—CT of the head and neurosurgical consultation

- **Pearl**

Skull x-rays an insensitive examination for head injury. They are only helpful in evaluating penetrating head trauma, depressed skull fracture, or foreign body.

25

Hyperthermia

- **Essentials of Diagnosis**
  - Mild—core body temperature normal or slightly elevated, relative sodium deficiency, muscle cramps on exertion
  - Heat exhaustion—core temperature normal or slightly increased, sweating prominent, salt and water depletion, weakness, headache, disorientation, pallor, thirst, nausea, muscle cramps
  - Heat stroke—life-threatening failure of thermoregulation, rectal temperature >40°C
  - Patient with heat stroke is incoherent, combative, vomiting, shivering, comatose. May have seizures, nuchal rigidity decerebrate posturing, multiple organ system failure

- **Causes of Hyperthermia**
  - Sudden endo- and exotoxin release during treatment of infection
  - Malignant hyperthermia—during anesthesia with halothane and succinylcholine derivatives in genetically sensitive individuals
  - Drug induced—Ecstasy, methamphetamine
  - Neuroleptic malignant syndrome
  - External heating—child left in closed automobile

- **Treatment**
  - Cool patient with cool mist, ice, fans
  - Administer 100% oxygen. Secure the airway
  - Administer intravenous (IV) fluids
  - Admit to intensive care for monitoring

- **Pearl**

The temperature in a closed automobile rises very quickly. Fatal heat stroke has occurred in children left in a closed automobile when the outside temperature was as low as 70°F.

Drowning

- ■ Essentials of Diagnosis
  - Second leading cause of death by unintentional injury in children
  - Risk factors—alcohol, swimming without supervision, epilepsy
  - Morbidity and mortality stem from central nervous system (CNS) and pulmonary insult
  - Dry drowning—laryngospasm upon immersion in water leads to loss of consciousness and cardiovascular collapse before aspiration of water
  - Irreversible CNS damage occurs after 4–6 minutes of submersion. Submersion directly in ice cold water may depress cerebral metabolism and carry less severe prognosis

- ■ Differential Diagnosis
  - Consider associated injuries—neck or head injury, drug usage

- ■ Treatment
  - Prevention of drowning is paramount
  - CPR should be started immediately upon discovery of non-breathing child
  - "Drown-proofing" a child does not replace adequate supervision

- ■ Pearl

Children <1 year are most likely to drown in the bathtub. Children 1–4 years old drown in home swimming pools. Adequate supervision can prevent these tragedies.

Bites

- **Essentials of Diagnosis**
  - Dog bites to head and neck occur in young children. Upper extremity bites more common in school-aged children
  - Most fatal bites in children are from dog attack with exsanguination
  - Take photographs of human bite wounds in children. They may be evidence of child abuse
  - Bites to the hand require expert care to prevent small joint and tendon sheath infections
  - Joint, periosteum, or neurovascular bundle may be damaged and contaminated in deep bites

- **Infectious Complications**
  - Infection is the major risk of nonfatal dog, cat, and human bites
  - Bacterial pathogens of human bites—streptococci, anaerobes, staphylococci, and *Eikenella corrodens*
  - Bacterial pathogens of dog and cat bites—*Pasturella multocida,* streptococci, staphylococci, and anaerobes. Cat bites can transmit cat scratch disease (*Bartonella henselae*)
  - Cat bites produce puncture wounds and carry higher risk of infection than dog bites

- **Treatment**
  - Rigorous cleansing of all bites with debridement of devitalized tissue
  - Suture facial bites for cosmetic reasons only. Other bites should not be sutured to reduce infection risk
  - Antibiotics—penicillin plus cephalexin or amoxicillin/clavulanic acid
  - Rabies is rare in developed countries but prophylaxis may be appropriate in some cases. Tetanus booster should be given

- **Pearl**

For reasons unclear, dog bites are more common in boys and cat bites more common in girls.

26

Poisoning

26

Acetaminophen

■ Essentials of Diagnosis

- Most common pediatric poisoning
- Emesis and ↑serum transaminases occur within hours followed within 24–72 hours by hepatic synthetic dysfunction, jaundice, and sometimes liver failure
- Acute single overdose and therapeutic doses repeated too frequently both cause toxicity
- Hepatotoxicity is ten times more common in adolescents and adults than children <5 years. Hepatotoxicity increases with acute and chronic alcohol use
- Cytochrome P-450 produces toxic intermediary of Tylenol, N-acetyl-p-benzoquinone imine (NAPQI) that is hepatotoxic
- Predict hepatic risk in acute ingestions by measuring serum acetaminophen and relating level on standard nomogram to number of hours since ingestion

■ Differential Diagnosis

- Toxic causes of liver failure—mushrooms, carbon tetrachloride
- Infectious causes—hepatitis A, B, C
- Reyes syndrome resembles the early phase of acetaminophen overdose
- First presentation of medium-chain acyl-CoA dehydrogenase (MCAD) and long-chain acyl-CoA dehydrogenase (LCAD) resemble acute acetaminophen overdose

■ Treatment

- Severity of suicidal ideation must be evaluated
- Consider other drug ingestion in patients with intentional overdose
- N-Acetylcysteine (NAC) can be given up to 24 hours after ingestion but is most effective within 8 hours
- Oral loading dose of NAC is 140 mg/kg with 70 mg/kg given every 4 hours thereafter for 72 hours
- Loading dose of intravenous (IV) NAC is 150 mg/kg over 15–60 minutes with second infusion of 50 mg/kg over 4 hours and 100 mg/kg over 16 hours

■ Pearl

Many over-the-counter medications contain acetaminophen. Inadvertent chronic overdose through use of multiple medications is common.

26

Alcohol

- **Essentials of Diagnosis**
  - Acute poisoning common in binge drinkers
  - Acute overdose—euphoria, lack of inhibition, incoordination, emesis, diuresis, dehydration, hypoglycemia, gastritis, seizure, retrograde amnesia, coma, death
  - Dehydration, acidosis, hypoglycemia, respiratory depression, and pulmonary aspiration are the critical issues to treat in acute poisoning
  - Measure blood alcohol level in suspect patients
  - Adult standards: Impaired faculties at .05–.08%. Intoxication .08–.1%. Coma and death .5%

- **Differential Diagnosis**
  - Other drug—stimulants, depressants, antidepressants, hallucinogens
  - Head injury, intracranial hemorrhage
  - Methanol intoxication

- **Treatment**
  - IV fluids and IV glucose
  - Treat acidosis
  - Dialysis indicated in life-threatening poisoning
  - Treat cerebral edema with dexamethasone .1 mg/kg every 4–6 hours

- **Pearl**

Binge drinking among high school and college students is a major health risk. Education of students, staff, law enforcement, and medical personnel is necessary to prevent mortality.

Amphetamine

- **Essentials of Diagnosis**
  - Widely available and easy to synthesize in home laboratories
  - Tolerance develops quickly
  - Many slang names include crank, meth, speed, crystal, ice
  - Central nervous system (CNS) stimulation, euphoria, anxiety, hyperactivity, hyperpyrexia, hypertension, abdominal cramps, vomiting, urinary retention, rhabdomyolysis, toxic psychosis, violent behavior
  - Suspect methamphetamine use in individuals with unexplained dental erosion of the incisors
  - Chronic use—insomnia, weakness, disorganized thoughts, visual hallucinations, irritability, tremor, depression, suicidal ideation
  - Risk to children of fire and toxic solvent exposure in the home as well as neglect and abuse

- **Differential Diagnosis**
  - Paranoid schizophrenia
  - Anxiety and panic attacks
  - Alcohol, stimulants, hallucinogens

- **Treatment**
  - In acute poisoning—empty the stomach, give activated charcoal
  - Diazepam titrated to effect
  - Extreme agitation—droperidol or haloperidol
  - Chronic users may be withdrawn rapidly

- **Pearl**

Many users take combinations of amphetamine and barbiturate. In toxic patients, measure barbiturate level and monitor for late appearing respiratory depression secondary to barbiturate.

26

Antihistamine

- Essentials of Diagnosis
  - CNS depression is most common. Children may have idiosyncratic agitation, hallucinations, delirium, ataxia, tremor, rhabdomyolysis, ventricular arrhythmia, and convulsions
  - Anticholinergic effects include dry mouth, dilated pupils, blurred vision, flushed face, fever, hallucinations, tachycardia, ventricular arrhythmia (inhibition of potassium rectifier current)
  - Nonsedating antihistamines (terfenadine and astemizole) may cause increased QT interval and torsades de pointes. Loratadine has prolonged half-life
  - Toxicity to be expected at doses above 10 mg/kg in most conventional antihistamines
  - Chronic poisoning occurs at low doses and may be inadvertent as many over-the-counter medications contain antihistamine

- Differential Diagnosis
  - Other sedative, stimulant, and psychotropic drugs
  - CNS trauma or encephalopathy
  - Psychiatric illness

- Treatment
  - Reduce drug absorption acutely with activated charcoal by mouth
  - Emetics usually not effective and may complicate management
  - Physostigmine 0.5–2 mg IV slowly reverses central and peripheral anticholinergic effects and is used for diagnosis not treatment
  - Diazepam 0.1–2 mg/kg IV for seizures
  - Supportive care and monitoring

- Pearl

Think antihistamine if the patient is mad as a hatter, red as a lobster, dry as a bone, blind as a bat, and hot as Hades (or some variant thereof).

Arsenic

- **Essentials of Diagnosis**
  - Used in insecticides, rodenticides, weed killers, and wood preservatives and kills by allosteric inhibition of multiple enzyme systems
  - Absorbed through GI and lungs with some absorption through skin
  - Industrial ground water and well water in areas with high soil arsenic are the most common causes of chronic arsenic poisoning worldwide
  - Sodium arsenite in liquid preparations is highly lethal. Organic arsenates in weed killer are less soluble and less toxic
  - Acute poisoning—abdominal pain, vomiting, bloody diarrhea, cardiovascular collapse, paresthesias, neck pain, garlic breath odor, convulsions, coma, anuria, exfoliative dermatitis
  - Chronic poisoning—anorexia, weakness, emotional lability, abdominal pain and cramps, dermatitis, nail changes, alopecia, anemia, diabetes
  - Long-term effects—diabetes, liver disease, vascular disease, Raynaud phenomenon, polyneuritis, malignancy, lower extremity gangrene
  - EPA water standards—10 ppb is highest acceptable arsenic level

- **Differential Diagnosis**
  - Heavy metal poisoning

- **Treatment**
  - Acute poisoning—activated charcoal with repeated intramuscular (IM) injections of dimercaprol (BAL)
  - Succimer and penicillamine used for chronic toxicity
  - Treat chronic poisoning until urine arsenic excretion is <50 mg/ 24 hours
  - Public health efforts to reduce drinking of contaminated ground water

- **Pearl**

If you don't see "alkyl methanearsonate" on the label of a liquid arsenical, be suspicious that you are dealing with the highly toxic sodium arsenite.

26

Belladonna Alkaloids

- **Essentials of Diagnosis**
  - Includes atropine, jimsonweed, potato leaves, scopolamine, stramonium
  - Anticholinergic effects—dry mouth, dry skin, flushing, thirst, decreased sweating and hyperpyrexia, tachycardia, dilated pupils, blurred vision, dysphagia, urinary retention, delirium, and coma

- **Differential Diagnosis**
  - Antihistamine toxicity
  - Psychiatric illness—panic, anxiety
  - Simple dehydration
  - Alcohol, methamphetamine, cocaine, hallucinogens

- **Treatment**
  - Emesis or lavage particularly useful because of delayed gastric emptying
  - Activated charcoal in acute ingestions
  - Physostigmine .5–2 mg by slow IV reverses symptoms and helps with diagnosis
  - Control hyperpyrexia
  - Cardiac monitoring
  - Urinary catheter

- **Pearl**

Children, especially those with Down syndrome, are often quite sensitive to normal doses of atropine used during surgery, sedation, or resuscitation to increase heart rate.

Carbon Monoxide (CO)

- ■ Essentials of Diagnosis
  - Toxicity correlates with carboxyhemoglobin level taken very soon after acute exposure but not after lapse of time and oxygen administration
  - Worse with high altitude, high respiratory rate (young infants), pregnancy, lung disease, heart failure
  - Symptoms—headache, confusion, unsteadiness, coma. In severe poisoning, renal, cardiac, vegetative state or lesser permanent CNS injury may result
  - Laboratory findings—proteinuria, glycosuria, increased transaminases, echocardiogram (ECG) changes
  - Typical red skin color suggests CO poisoning

- ■ Differential Diagnosis
  - Drug overdose
  - Depression or other neuro-psychiatric disorder

- ■ Treatment
  - The half-life of carboxyhemoglobin in room air is 200–300 minutes Hyperbaric oxygen (2–2.5 atm) shortens half-life to 30 minutes
  - Nonspecific therapy of anoxic tissue injury
  - Dexamethasone may be used if cerebral edema present

- ■ Pearl

The most common time to see accidental acute or chronic CO injury in temperate climates is the first cold snap. Poorly ventilated furnaces or space heaters are the culprits.

26

Caustic Acids

- **Essentials of Diagnosis**
  - Strong acids are found in metal cleaners, toilet bowl cleaners, and batteries. Hydrofluoric acid is the most caustic
  - Tissue injury results with acids stronger than 1 N
  - Oral mucosal, esophageal, and gastric injury with perforation may occur
  - Symptoms—dysphagia, drooling, bloody emesis, pain, respiratory distress, thirst, shock, renal failure, peritonitis
  - Long-term complications are esophageal, laryngeal, gastric, and pyloric strictures. Scarring of lips and mouth

- **Differential Diagnosis**
  - Strong alkali ingestion causes similar problems
  - Used in suicide attempts especially in developing countries where acid cleansers are more common than alkali cleansers

- **Treatment**
  - Emetics contraindicated
  - Water or milk may be used to dilute ingested acid
  - Lavage areas of external exposure with water
  - Obtain plain abdominal x-ray to look for perforation and chest x-ray to look for edema, collapse, aspiration
  - Esophagoscopy to assess extent of damage
  - HF may cause symptomatic hypocalcemia

- **Pearl**

Hydrofluoric acid dermal exposure creates penetrating burns that can progress for hours or days after exposure. Large dermal exposures can produce hypocalcemia.

Caustic Bases

- ■ Essentials of Diagnosis
  - Alkalis are more common in American households than strong acids and hence cause more injuries per year
  - Liquid or powdered drain cleaners and Clinitest tablets are the most common ingestants. pH >13 usually required to produce tissue necrosis
  - Chlorinated bleaches added to strong acids or ammonia may produce irritating chlorine or chloramine gas that may cause lung irritation
  - Symptoms of ingestion—oral injury, dysphagia, respiratory distress, pulmonary edema, mediastinitis secondary to esophageal perforation, peritonitis secondary to gastric perforation
  - The extent of oral injury is not a predictor of esophageal injury

- ■ Differential Diagnosis
  - Strong acid ingestion
  - Other causes of acute mediastinitis or peritonitis
  - Suicide attempt

- ■ Treatment
  - Clean skin and mucous membranes with water
  - Water may be used as diluent
  - Esophagoscopy should be performed in the first 24 hours to evaluate for third-degree injury to the esophagus (circumferential full thickness burn) which may lead to stricture. Delay after 24 hours associated with ↑risk of esophageal perforation due to extensive tissue necrosis
  - If third-degree burns are present, consider gastrostomy and esophageal string to facilitate later dilations
  - Supportive treatment of shock, fever. Use of corticosteroids is controversial

- ■ Pearl

Household bleach is a 3–6% solution of sodium hypochlorite. It may cause a little oral irritation but does not cause significant esophageal or gastric injury.

26

Cocaine

- **Essentials of Diagnosis**
  - Absorbed after nasal, respiratory, GI, or IV administration
  - Prevents reuptake of endogenous catecholamine causing initial sympathetic discharge followed by catechol depletion with chronic use
  - Tachycardia, hyperpnea, hypertension, euphoria
  - Large IV exposure may produce seizures, hypotension, respiratory depression, rhabdomyolysis, hyperthermia cardiac arrhythmia, coma, and death from dysrhythmia
  - Look for nasal erosions in sniffers and skin ulcers caused by subcutaneous injection
  - Qualitative (spot urine) better than plasma level for diagnosis

- **Differential Diagnosis**
  - Amphetamine use
  - Alcohol use
  - Anxiety, panic, psychosis

- **Treatment**
  - Supportive treatment of catechol excess or catechol depletion
  - Consider simultaneous use of other drugs
  - Because of norepinephrine depletion, dopamine may be less effective in treating hypotension
  - Benzodiazepines for agitation

- **Pearl**

Body stuffing (sudden ingestion of a large dose to avoid discovery) or body packing (smuggling packets in body cavities) may produce sudden massive toxicity. Patient may be unable to give a history and treatment may be delayed. Plain abdominal x-rays may reveal packets in body packers.

Cyclic Antidepressants

■ **Essentials of Diagnosis**

- Low toxic threshold—1 of the top 3 fatal overdoses in the United States
- Symptom onset usually within 2 hours of ingestion with peak toxicity at 6 hours
- 4 mechanisms for toxicity—anticholinergic, α-adrenergic block-ade, norepinephrine and serotonin reuptake inhibition, myocardial fast sodium channel blockade (guanidine-like effect)
- Associated toxicities—mental depression and anticholinergic symptoms appear first, vasodilatation and resistant hypotension, seizures and cardiac arrhythmias (sinus tachycardia, heart block, and ventricular arrhythmia)
- High protein binding and high volume of distribution cause pro-longed toxicity and make hemodialysis ineffective
- Plasma and urine tests usually not helpful
- Amoxapine has fewer cardiovascular complications than other tricycles but a higher incidence of seizures

■ **Differential Diagnosis**

- Cardiac disease
- Psychiatric disease
- Antihistamine or anticholinergic overdose
- Guanidine
- Intracranial disease, trauma, seizure disorder

■ **Treatment**

- Gastric lavage within 2 hours of overdose
- Give activated charcoal by nasogastric tube
- Intubation and intensive support of vital signs indicated
- Norepinephrine or dopamine are most effective for hypotension
- Monitor ECG for prolongation of PR, QRS (>100 msec) and QT intervals
- Alkalinization and lidocaine reduce ventricular arrhythmia
- Adrenergics and dopamine are often ineffective for hypotension because of adrenergic blockade. Norepinephrine
- Physostigmine contraindicated

■ **Pearl**

Amitriptyline and nortriptyline are widely used in pediatrics either alone or in combination with other drugs for depression, chronic pain, migraine prophylaxis, enuresis, obsessive-compulsive disorder (OCD), attention-deficit/hyperactivity disorder (ADHD), school phobia, and separation anxiety. Toddlers and teenaged girls are at greatest risk for overdose. Warn parents how dangerous a single pill can be in a small child.

26

Hydrocarbons

- **Essentials of Diagnosis**
  - Symptoms—irritation of mucous membranes, emesis, bloody diarrhea, respiratory distress, cyanosis, tachycardia, fever, cardiac dilation, dysrhythmias, hepatosplenomegaly, hematuria, proteinuria
  - Huffing or sniffing hydrocarbon for recreation is common in teenagers and causes acute respiratory distress. Chronic abuse causes liver disease, leukoencephalopathy, peripheral neuropathy, and aplastic anemia depending on the hydrocarbon
  - Large oral ingestions more likely to cause renal and cardiac disease
  - Aromatic, low viscosity fluids most toxic—1 mL/kg of benzene, gasoline, kerosene, or red seal furniture polish may produce CNS depression
  - Aspiration either direct or from the circulation causes a necrotizing hydrocarbon pneumonia and pulmonary edema

- **Differential Diagnosis**
  - Acute pulmonary infection
  - Acute gastrointestinal (GI) infection
  - Other disorders causing CNS depression
  - Other disorders causing hematuria and proteinuria

- **Treatment**
  - Emetics and lavage contraindicated
  - Epinephrine should not be used with halogenated hydrocarbons because of cardiac irritability
  - Supportive care for respiratory symptoms with antibiotics for secondary infection

- **Pearl**

Kerosene ingestion is a common toddler accident. The smell of the breath usually gives you a clue to diagnosis. The intensity of smell does not tell you how much the child drank.

Insecticides

- **Essentials of Diagnosis**
  - Toxicity is due to chlorinated hydrocarbons (aldrin, chlordane, DDT, dieldrin), organophosphates (chlorothion, malathion, thio-TEPP) or their organic solvents
  - Chlorinated hydrocarbons—salivation, cramps, diarrhea, vomiting, CNS depression or irritability, paresthesias, seizures, local irritation to eyes, nose, throat, and skin. Very lipophilic
  - Organophosphates cause cholinesterase inhibition—dizziness, headache, blurred vision, miosis, tearing, salivation, nausea, vomiting, diarrhea, hyperglycemia, cyanosis, dyspnea, sweating, weakness, muscular twitching, convulsions, loss of reflexes, incontinence, coma
  - Repeated low-grade exposure to organophosphates (household spraying) may result in sudden toxic symptoms
  - Red cell cholinesterase <25% of normal indicates significant exposure

- **Differential Diagnosis**
  - Other hydrocarbon ingestions
  - Other anticholinergics

- **Treatment**
  - Decontaminate skin, nails, hair with soapy water and discard or wash clothing
  - Gastric lavage for recent ingestion of chlorinated hydrocarbons
  - Avoid fatty foods or medications by mouth. They increase the absorption of chlorinated hydrocarbons
  - Use atropine plus cholinesterase reactivator (pralidoxime) for organophosphate
  - Morphine, theophylline, aminophylline, succinylcholine, phenothiazines, and reserpine are contraindicated in organophosphate poisoning
  - Supportive treatment of seizures with benzodiazepines
  - Epinephrine may cause cardiac arrhythmias in chlorinated hydrocarbon ingestion

- **Pearl**

Use of chlorinated hydrocarbons has been curtailed because of environmental contamination. Lindane, a chlorinated hydrocarbon used for lice, is absorbed through the skin and causes toxicity if used in excess.

26

Iron

- ■ **Essentials of Diagnosis**
  - Injury results from local irritation and from overwhelming oxidant injury
  - 5 stages of toxicity:
    - hemorrhagic gastroenteritis within 30–60 minutes with shock, acidosis, coagulopathy, and coma
    - apparent improvement lasting 2–12 hours
    - delayed shock, acidosis, fever, coma
    - hepatic failure
    - late-onset pyloric stenosis due to local scarring
  - Serum iron >400 µg/dL requires therapy
  - Abdominal x-ray may demonstrate pills in the GI tract and help in estimating number ingested and planning therapy
  - Elemental iron intake in excess of 10 mg/kg (especially the ferrous salts) may produce significant toxicity

- ■ **Differential Diagnosis**
  - Other causes of acidosis, shock, and liver dysfunction
  - Chronic iron administration
  - Hemochromatosis may cause high serum iron levels

- ■ **Treatment**
  - Gastric lavage for liquid products. GI lavage with polyethylene glycol solution (Golytely) may hasten transit of pills and prevent absorption
  - Surgical removal of pills by gastrotomy is an option in massive pill overdose
  - Deferoxamine IV immediately to chelate absorbed iron. Contraindicated in renal failure
  - Hemodialysis, peritoneal dialysis, exchange transfusion may be used
  - Blood transfusion may be needed. Type and crossmatch patient
  - Monitor liver function and be prepared to treat

- ■ **Pearl**

It may take a while to get a serum iron level. Do not delay therapy in suspected ingestions while waiting for laboratory test result.

Lead

- ## Essentials of Diagnosis
  - Usually insidious with vague weakness, irritability, school failure, weight loss, vomiting, ataxia, constipation, headache, crampy abdominal pain
  - Sources include lead-based paint (>1% lead), artist's paints, fruit tree sprays, solder, brass alloys, home-glazed pottery, fumes from burning batteries
  - Blood lead screening identifies those at risk. >80 µgm/dL usually symptomatic
  - Blood smear shows hypochromia with basophilic stippling of red cells in chronic ingestion
  - Chronic lead poisoning produces encephalopathy—↑cerebrospinal fluid (CSF) opening pressure ↑CSF protein with white cell count <100 cells/mL

- ## Differential Diagnosis
  - Sideroblastic anemia
  - Psychogenic symptoms—depression, anxiety
  - GI disease, especially acid reflux and ulcer
  - Neurologic disorders
  - Attention-deficit hyperactivity or learning disability may be caused by lead poisoning or may mimic lead poisoning

- ## Treatment
  - Measure lead level at 6 months and yearly through childhood especially in endemic areas
  - Succimer chelation for levels >45 µgm/dL
  - Check environmental and remove sources of lead
  - Treatment guidelines for levels between 15 and 45 µgm not established
  - Dimercaprol and calcium EDTA are mainly used for encephalopathy
  - Acute encephalopathy may require anticonvulsants, mannitol, corticosteroids

- ## Pearl
  Ingested lead paint chips are the most common cause of poisoning in children. Fishermen may chew lead weights to soften them prior to attaching them to the fishing line. These and other lead sources are often apparent on abdominal plain films.

26

Mushrooms

- **Essentials of Diagnosis**
  - Symptoms vary with species, time of year, stage of maturity, quantity, method of preparation, and interval since ingestion
  - Muscarinic symptoms prominent—salivation, emesis, diarrhea, crampy abdominal pain, tenesmus, miosis, dyspnea
  - *Amanita phalloides* toxin responsible for 90% of deaths. Cooking does not destroy toxin
  - Symptom onset within 2 hours suggests muscarinic toxin. Onset 6–48 hours after ingestion suggests amanitin
  - Late symptoms—hypoglycemia, coma, convulsions, hallucinations, hemolysis, hepatic failure, renal failure

- **Differential Diagnosis**
  - Drug toxicity—hallucinogens, stimulants, muscarinics
  - Acute hepatic failure
  - Renal failure
  - CNS disease

- **Treatment**
  - Identify mushroom if possible and consult with mycology expert
  - Induce vomiting and follow with activated charcoal
  - Atropine for muscarinic symptoms and signs
  - Treat hypoglycemia
  - Penicillin, silibinin, or hemodialysis may be indicated in *Amanita* poisoning
  - Liver transplant may be required

- **Pearl**

Don't ever eat a mushroom picked by an amateur. It is too hard to tell the difference between harmful and harmless and a mistake could be fatal.

Opioids

- ## Essentials of Diagnosis
  - Opioid-related problems—drug addiction, acute drug overdose, infant withdrawal
  - Narcotic addicted adolescents—cellulitis, thrombophlebitis, endocarditis, human immunodeficiency virus (HIV), ob/gyn problems, peptic disease, other drugs of abuse, homelessness, depression, malnutrition, lawlessness
  - Fentanyl skin patches may cause toxicity and may also be abused
  - Acute overdose symptoms—respiratory depression, stridor, coma, ↑secretions, sinus bradycardia, urinary retention, constipation. Death is caused by aspiration, respiratory arrest, cerebral edema
  - Infants of addicted mothers—intrauterine growth retardation, postnatal yawning, sneezing, uncoordinated feeding, vomiting, diarrhea, irritability, tremor, restless movement, shrill cry, seizures, cardio-respiratory collapse with onset up to 8 days after birth
  - Easily detected in urine

- ## Differential Diagnosis
  - Other drug overdose with respiratory depression
  - CNS disorders, trauma, or infection in both overdose and infant withdrawal

- ## Treatment
  - Therapy for acute overdose—naloxone in dose sufficient to reverse symptoms (.01–.1 mg/kg to start) and subsequent doses as needed to treat immediate relapse of symptoms
  - For neonate withdrawal—barbiturates, methadone, supportive nutritional care. Therapy may be required for several weeks

- ## Pearl

Iatrogenic narcotic overdose can occur in postoperative patients with pain. It may be hard to determine whether depressed consciousness is an effect of anesthesia or of narcotic. Monitor vital signs and cumulative dose in hospitalized patients.

26

Phenothiazines

- **Essentials of Diagnosis**
  - Episodes of extrapyramidal symptoms lasting minutes to hours—torticollis, spasticity, poor speech, catatonia, inability to communicate, oculogyric crisis
  - Occasionally paradoxical hyperactivity, hyperglycemia, acetonemia, seizures, neuroleptic malignant syndrome
  - Appropriate therapeutic doses may cause symptoms
  - Symptoms most often associated with chlorpromazine, prochlorperazine, trifluoperazine, metaclopramide, promethazine
  - Long-term use or abuse may cause tardive dyskinesia

- **Differential Diagnosis**
  - Psychosis
  - Brain injury
  - Other drug overdose—antihistamines, sedatives, narcotics, hallucinogens

- **Treatment**
  - Extrapyramidal symptoms relieved with IV dephenhydramine or benztropine mesylate
  - Agitation may require diazepam
  - Supportive care for hypotension
  - Neuroleptic malignant syndrome treated with dantrolene or bromocriptine

- **Pearl**

Extrapyramidal syndrome is the reason many pediatricians do not use Reglan or Phenergan. Reversible or not, it is frightening to the affected patient. Deaths and delayed onset of symptoms have occurred with promethazine suppositories.

Salicylates

- ■ Essentials of Diagnosis
  - Uncoupling of oxidative phosphorylation causes hyperthermia, sweating, dehydration, decreased urine output, hypo- or hyperglycemia, respiratory stimulation with tachypnea, vomiting, respiratory alkalosis followed by acidosis in severe cases, hypokalemia, bleeding tendency
  - Intoxication is rarer because of public education and childproof containers
  - Serum salicylate level is readily available. Level reflects severity of acute but not of chronic overdose

- ■ Differential Diagnosis
  - Other causes of tachypnea and dehydration, especially diabetic ketoacidosis
  - Bacterial infections with acidosis, hyperpnea, and fever
  - Head trauma
  - Drug overdose especially stimulants, alcohol, methanol

- ■ Treatment
  - Gastric lavage and activated charcoal in severe recent ingestions
  - Fluid resuscitation and alkalinization of urine
  - Correct hypokalemia
  - Renal failure and pulmonary edema are indications for hemodialysis. Peritoneal dialysis relatively ineffective

- ■ Pearl

Oil of wintergreen contains methyl salicylate. It is very toxic yet is available over the counter for oral and topical use. Don't keep this drug around. It smells great and children may drink it.

Barbiturates

- **Essentials of Diagnosis**
  - Barbiturates open CNS chloride channels directly or by increasing γ-aminobutyric acid (GABA) activity, prolonging depolarization, and suppressing neurotransmission
  - Ingestion of >6 mg/kg long-acting or 3 mg/kg short-acting barbiturate is usually toxic
  - Overdose causes confusion, poor coordination, respiratory depression, pulmonary atelectasis, hypotension, miotic or fixed dilated pupils
  - Barbiturate urine and blood levels are available

- **Differential Diagnosis**
  - Other sedative drugs including narcotics, antihistamines, phenothiazines, alcohol, benzodiazepines
  - CNS injury producing depression
  - Propofol (ultrashort-acting anesthetic agent administered IV in a soy vehicle) may cause symptoms of soy allergy. Continuous infusion has been associated with myocardial failure

- **Treatment**
  - In acute ingestions activated charcoal
  - Careful respiratory monitoring and support with intubation if needed
  - Urinary alkalinization increases excretion
  - Hemodialysis not useful in short-acting barbiturate

- **Pearl**

Serum barbiturate level confirms that the drug has been ingested but does not correlate with level of intoxication because of variability of CNS binding, metabolism and tolerance. A level ~90 mg/L of a long-acting barbiturate is likely to cause significant morbidity.

Digitalis

- ■ Essentials of Diagnosis
  - Chronic toxicity from prescribed digoxin is the most common toxicity. Accidental acute overdose in children occurs in homes where patients are using digoxin
  - Nausea, vomiting, diarrhea, headache, delirium, confusion, visual problems (scotoma, halos) cardiac arrhythmias (PVC is most common also bradydysrhythmias, atrial fibrillation, paroxysmal atrial tachycardia, atrial flutter, heart block, ventricular tachycardia, ventricular fibrillation)
  - Arrhythmias are often the key to diagnosis in a child with nonspecific symptoms
  - Hyperkalemia may occur during acute overdose
  - Transplacental intoxication reported
  - Serum digoxin concentration is helpful in titrating therapy in cardiac patients but it takes time to evaluate
  - In suspected cases, start treatment before laboratory tests are available

- ■ Differential Diagnosis
  - GI disease
  - Neurologic disease
  - Psychiatric disease
  - Other drug overdose

- ■ Treatment
  - Correct acidosis
  - Treat bradycardia with atropine
  - Phenytoin, lidocaine, magnesium salts, amiodarone, bretylium may be required for arrhythmia
  - Definitive treatment is with digoxin immune Fab. Indications include hypotension, ventricular dysrhythmia, progressive bradydysrhythmia, elevated T waves and hyperkalemia

- ■ Pearl

The most common cause of chronic digoxin toxicity is not an inappropriately high prescribed dose, but decreased renal function, dehydration, electrolyte disturbance (especially hypokalemia), and drug interactions.

26

γ-Hydroxybutyrate

- **Essentials of Diagnosis**
    - Recent increase in recreational use—date rape drug
    - CNS depressant causing GABA-like effects
    - Produces deep, short-lived coma with respiratory depression lasting 1–4 hours. Depressed gag increases aspiration risk. Bradycardia
    - Withdrawal from chronic use associated with agitation, hallucination, tachycardia
    - No adequate blood or urine tests available

- **Differential Diagnosis**
    - Other sedative, narcotic, hallucinogen, alcohol
    - CNS infection or trauma
    - Psychiatric disease

- **Treatment**
    - Supportive care with close attention to airway management. Intubation may be necessary briefly
    - Sexual abuse occurs during surreptitious administration and should be evaluated. Check pregnancy test
    - Atropine may be used for symptomatic bradycardia
    - Associated alcohol poisoning is common
    - Withdrawal symptoms may require benzodiazepines, butyrophenones, or barbiturates for several days

- **Pearl**

The drug is tasteless allowing it to be administered to a victim without their knowledge or consent. The victim may not realize that their symptoms are drug related.

27

Bacterial and Spirochetal Infections

27

Group A Streptococcal (GAS) Cellulitis/ Necrotizing Fasciitis

- **Essentials of Diagnosis**
  - Site of entry for GAS cellulitis—superficial abrasion, insect bite, chicken pox, eczema, surgery
  - Cellulitis is tender, red, slightly raised (erysipelas), and spreads rapidly in subcutaneous tissue with minimal suppuration. Lymphatic spread causes adenopathy and septicemia
  - Necrotizing fasciitis may arise from major or minor skin trauma; 20–40% caused by GAS. GAS exotoxin is the cause of tissue necrosis
  - In necrotizing fasciitis skin at entry site may be very tender, pale, or red (resembling GAS cellulitis). Blistering may occur. Deep, woody edema develops. Skin becomes violaceous with rapidly progressive deep tissue necrosis
  - In both cellulitis and fasciitis—culture organism from pus, blood, deep tissues

- **Differential Diagnosis**
  - Necrotizing fascitis caused by *Staphylococcus aureus* (up to 30–40% of cases), *Clostridium perfringens, Bacteroides fragilis*. All organisms produce exotoxins
  - Cellulitis caused by other organisms—*Streptococcus pyogenes, S aureus*
  - Scarlet fever, toxic shock syndrome (TSS), underlying osteomyelitis, deep vein thrombosis, contact dermatitis may resemble either cellulitis or necrotizing fasciitis

- **Treatment**
  - Immediate antibiotic therapy crucial for control of cellulitis and fasciitis. Do not wait for culture results before treating
  - Initial therapy with penicillin, vancomycin, and clindamycin needed because of possible methicillin-resistant *S aureus*
  - Wide debridement of necrotic tissue, including amputation, may be required to control fasciitis
  - Hyperbaric oxygen may be of benefit in treating fascitis

- **Pearl**

The rapidity with which erysipelas and necrotizing fasciitis progress is terrifying. High index of suspicion and immediate empiric antibiotic treatment is critical to prevent severe complications or death.

Note: For other GAS infections see Pharyngitis (Chap. 16), Impetigo (Chap. 13), Rheumatic Fever (Chap. 2), Glomerulonephritis (Chap. 5), Toxic Shock syndrome (Chap. 27), Perianal Strep

27

Group B Streptococcal Infection (GBS)

- ■ Essentials of Diagnosis
  - • Risk factors for early-onset neonatal infection—age <7 days, untreated maternal vaginal GBS, gestational age <37 weeks, ruptured membranes >18 hours, young maternal age, low maternal GBS anticapsular antibodies
  - • *Early-onset GBS*—ill newborn often presents first with apnea then sepsis, meningitis, and/or pneumonia
  - • *Late-onset GBS*—age 1–16 weeks (median 4 weeks), 46% have sepsis, 37% have meningitis, others present with arthritis, osteomyelitis, otitis, ethmoiditis, conjunctivitis, facial/submandibular cellulitis, lymphadenitis, breast abscess, empyema, impetigo
  - • Beyond early infancy, GBS infection rare. May occur in immunocompromised children
  - • Diagnosis requires positive culture (blood, pleural fluid, cerebrospinal fluid [CSF], urine)

- ■ Differential Diagnosis
  - • Other acquired bacterial and viral infections of the newborn and young infant
  - • Intrauterine viral infection

- ■ Treatment
  - • Screen pregnant women at 35–37 weeks' gestation with vaginal and rectal culture, and give intrapartum chemoprophylaxis
  - • Intrapartum prophylaxis for women with GBS bacteriuria during pregnancy, previous GBS infant, and women with fever, premature rupture of the membranes (PROM) or gestation <37 weeks with unknown GBS status
  - • Intravenous (IV) ampicillin and an aminoglycoside is initial regimen for newborns with presumptive GBS
  - • Ceftriaxone is effective but may cause cholestasis in newborns

- ■ Pearl

The mode of acquisition of late-onset GBS is still poorly defined. It may be community acquired, not maternally acquired.

Gas Gangrene—*Clostridium perfringens*

- **Essentials of Diagnosis**
  - Fecal or soil contamination of wounds by spores of *C perfringens* (80%) or other clostridial species (20%)
  - In 1–20 days, tissue around wound develops hemorrhagic bullae, intense painful edema, muscle necrosis, serosanguineous exudate, crepitation
  - Rapid progression to—low-grade fever, intravascular hemolysis, jaundice, shock, delirium, renal failure, and death if untreated
  - Immediate antibiotics and surgery can reduce mortality to 20–60%
  - Prognosis poor with abdominal wall involvement, leucopenia, intravascular hemolysis, renal failure, and shock
  - Neutropenic patients at risk of muscle necrosis and sepsis from *Clostridium septicum*
  - Isolation of organisms requires anaerobic culture. Gram-stained blood smears may show gram-positive rods

- **Differential Diagnosis**
  - Gangrene and cellulitis caused by other organisms
  - Necrotizing fasciitis (group A β-hemolytic streptococcus and staphylococcus)

- **Treatment**
  - Prevent disease by wound cleansing to remove the anaerobic environment
  - Treat disease with aggressive debridement and removal of foreign bodies
  - Penicillin G combined with clindamycin or metronidazole
  - Clindamycin, metronidazole, meropenem, or imipenem for penicillin-allergic patients
  - Hyperbaric oxygen therapy is a potential adjunct but is not adequate as sole therapy

- **Pearl**

The x-ray finding of gas in the subcutaneous tissues is a late finding of gas gangrene and is not diagnostic. Other organisms as well as trauma and surgical procedures produce gas in the tissues.

27

Botulism—*Clostridium botulinum*

- **Essentials of Diagnosis**
  - Anaerobic, gram-positive, spore-forming soil bacillus produces powerful neurotoxin that prevents acetylcholine release at myoneural junctions
  - Disease results from ingestion of tasteless toxin often in home-canned food that has been prepared at temperature insufficient to kill spores (115°C) and then stored at room temperature
  - Lethargy, headache, double vision, dilated pupils, ptosis, dysphagia, dysarthria, descending skeletal paralysis, death from respiratory failure
  - Classic triad important for diagnosis—(a) afebrile, (b) symmetrical descending paralysis with bulbar palsies, (c) clear sensorium
  - Toxin can be identified in stool, gastric aspirate, serum or suspect food. Most laboratory tests including CSF are normal
  - Infant botulism—constipation, generalized hypotonia, progressing to respiratory failure in infants caused by *Clostridium botulinum* toxin secreted by organisms in the gut

- **Differential Diagnosis**
  - Guillain-Barré—ascending paralysis, sensory deficits, elevated CSF protein
  - Poliomyelitis, diphtheritic polyneuritis, both have ↑CSF protein
  - Tick paralysis—ascending motor paralysis
  - Myasthenia gravis—adolescent girls, ocular and bulbar symptoms, normal pupils, fluctuating weakness

- **Treatment**
  - Give trivalent equine antitoxin for food-borne botulism
  - Human botulinum-immune globulin for infant botulism decreases hospital stay and duration of assisted ventilation
  - Mortality rate ~6%
  - Symptoms subside over 2–3 months with complete recovery expected in both diseases

Pearl

The clostridia producing infant botulism have been isolated from honey used to sweeten an infant's pacifier. There is some suspicion that spores in dust from nearby construction sites may contaminate household utensils and cause infection.

27

Tetanus—*Clostridium tetani*

- ■ Essentials of Diagnosis
  - Wound contamination (often puncture wound) by soil containing *Clostridium tetani* spores. Incubation period 4–14 days
  - *C tetani* produces neurotoxin that reaches CNS by retrograde axon transport. Toxin binds to gangliosides, blocking inhibitory synapses, and increasing reflex excitability
  - Intense muscle spasms near wound site followed by trismus, dysphagia, hyperreflexia, opisthotonos, and facial grimacing. Seizures precipitated by minimal stimuli. Pneumonitis secondary to aspiration
  - Autonomic syndrome may occur—hypertension, ↑cardiac output, tachycardia, and arrhythmia
  - At risk—infants with soil contamination of umbilical stump, immunocompromised patients, IV drug users, and underimmunized normal people
  - This is a clinical diagnosis. CSF is normal. Muscle enzymes high. Organisms hard to grow

- ■ Differential Diagnosis
  - Poliomyelitis—asymmetrical paralysis
  - Rabies—trismus usually absent
  - Bacterial pharyngitis with dysphagia
  - Bacterial meningitis or head injury with decerebrate posturing
  - Phenothiazine reaction, narcotic withdrawal
  - Hypocalcemic tetany

- ■ Treatment
  - Prevent tetanus with series of 3 tetanus toxoid injections
  - Give booster at the time of injury if none received in 5–10 years
  - Surgical debridement of wounds to remove anaerobic environment
  - Tetanus-immune globulin prophylaxis for high-risk wounds and in human immunodeficiency virus (HIV) patients
  - Treat diagnosed cases with 3000–6000 U human tetanus immunoglobulin intramuscularly (500 U for infants)
  - Metronidazole decreases number of vegetative forms and decreases toxin production
  - Sedate with diazepam or other anxiolytic to prevent spasms and hypoxic episodes

- ■ Pearl

27

99% of tetanus cases in the United States are in nonimmunized or incompletely immunized individuals.

Diphtheria—*Corynebacterium diphtheriae*

- Essentials of Diagnosis
  - Pharyngitis, fever, and malaise followed rapidly by prostration and vascular collapse
  - Exotoxin produced by bacteriophage is absorbed on mucous membranes causing hemorrhagic, epithelial necrosis with thick, fibrinous, gray pseudomembrane over tonsils, pharynx, or larynx
  - Cervical adenopathy and edema causes "bull neck"
  - Stridor can progress to airway obstruction
  - Cutaneous, vaginal, and wound diphtheria show ulcerative lesions with pseudomembrane formation
  - Myocarditis 2–40 days after infection causes ST-T wave changes, dysrhythmia, and cardiac failure
  - Neuritis 2–4 weeks after infection causes pharyngo-palatal weakness, nasal speech and regurgitation, diplopia, strabismus, intercostal, diaphragmatic, or generalized paralysis
  - Diagnosis is clinical. Smear unreliable and culture difficult

- Differential Diagnosis
  - Other causes of pharyngitis—β-hemolytic streptococcus, Epstein-Barr virus (EBV), viral respiratory pathogens
  - Severe oral thrush, herpetic gingivostomatitis
  - Nasal foreign body or purulent sinusitis mimics nasal diphtheria
  - Epiglottitis and viral croup
  - Guillain-Barré syndrome, poliomyelitis, and acute poisoning mimic diphtheritic neuropathy
  - Viral myocarditis

- Treatment
  - Prevent infection by immunization with diphtheria toxoid
  - Treat patients with bed rest, strict isolation until respiratory secretions are noncontagious (7 days)
  - Administer diphtheria antitoxin within 48 hours of diagnosing pharyngitis
  - Penicillin G or erythromycin for 10 days
  - Immunize nonimmune contacts and treat with erythromycin for 7 days or IM benzathine penicillin G

- Pearl

Diphtheria is rare in the United States, but mortality can be as high as 25% especially with myocarditis. Neuritis is reversible, but occasionally cardiac disease persists.

27

Cat Scratch Disease—*Bartonella henselae*

- ## Essentials of Diagnosis
  - Scratch or contact with healthy cat causes papule or pustule at site of injury (may be conjunctival). Regional lymphadenopathy, lethargy, headache, and fever occur 10–50 days later
  - Other manifestations—erythema nodosum, thrombocytopenic purpura, conjunctivitis, parotitis, pneumonia, osteolytic lesions, retinitis, peripheral neuritis, hepatitis, and encephalitis
  - Immunocompromised individuals prone to bacillary angiomatosis, vascular tumors of skin and subcutaneous tissue, sepsis, peliosis hepatis
  - Indirect fluorescent antibody or enzyme-linked immunosorbent assay (ELISA) titer >1:64 supports diagnosis. Polymerase chain reaction (PCR) available, tissue biopsy may show gram-negative bacillary forms

- ## Differential Diagnosis
  - Bacterial lymphadenitis
  - Tuberculous or atypical tubercular adenitis
  - Other adenopathy associated with tularemia, plague, brucellosis, infectious mononucleosis, toxoplasmosis, lymphogranuloma venereum
  - Lymphoma, leukemia

- ## Treatment
  - Disease usually resolves without therapy and patient is typically not very sick
  - Reassurance and education are important
  - 5-day course of azithromycin speeds symptom resolution in some patients
  - Node aspiration relieves pain, but since pus is usually sterile it is not helpful in diagnosis
  - Treat immunocompromised patients with azithromycin, erythromycin, or doxycycline. Long-term treatment may be required to prevent relapses

- ## Pearl

It's amazing how often the contact with the cat is not mentioned or has been forgotten by the patient. You may have to ask both the patient and his/her mother several times.

27

Salmonella Enteritis—*Salmonella enteritidis, Salmonella typhimurium, Salmonella choleraesuis, Salmonella paratyphi*

- **Essentials of Diagnosis**
  - Gram-negative organisms with many serotypes (*Salmonella enteritidis*) penetrate small bowel; multiply in submucosal layers causing fever, emesis, diarrhea, white blood cells (WBCs) in stool, and occasionally bloody mucoid diarrhea (*Salmonella typhimurium*)
  - Fecal contamination especially of meats, milk, cheese, ice cream, eggs, and chocolate result in oral ingestion of organisms
  - Infants <2 years especially susceptible to systemic sepsis, meningitis, endocarditis, osteomyelitis cholecystitis, pyelonephritis, arthritis especially with *Salmonella choleraesuis, S typhimurium, Salmonella paratyphi*
  - Patients with sickle cell anemia or other hemoglobinopathies at risk for osteomyelitis
  - Diagnosis by stool culture

- **Differential Diagnosis**
  - Shigella, *Escherichia coli H0157*, *Campylobacter jejuni*—colitic infections with more bloody diarrhea
  - Yersinia enterocolitica infection may require stool culture to distinguish
  - Viral gastroenteritis—diarrhea more voluminous, no WBC in stool
  - Staphylococcal food poisoning has more rapid onset and vomiting is major symptom
  - Occasionally there may be confusion between secretory diarrhea (toxigenic *E coli*) and salmonella gastroenteritis

- **Treatment**
  - In uncomplicated gastroenteritis, antibiotics do not shorten the course of illness and may prolong fecal carriage
  - Antibiotics recommended in children <3 months, in chronically ill children including sickle cell, liver disease, recent gastrointestinal (GI) surgery, cancer, chronic renal or cardiac disease, depressed immunity
  - Admit children <3 months to hospital for evaluation and observation
  - Many strains resistant to ampicillin and to trimethoprim-sulfamethoxazole. Third-generation cephalosporins effective. Fluoroquinolones only used for multiple resistant organisms
  - Antibiotic treatment of asymptomatic carriers is not effective

- **Pearl**

Even carefully washed eggs can cause enteritis. S enteritidis can infect the ovaries of healthy hens some of whose eggs will be contaminated before the shell is applied. Although the phenomenon is rare, I'd recommend passing on the raw eggs!

Typhoid and Paratyphoid Fever—*Salmonella typhi, Salmonella paratyphi A, Salmonella schottmulleri, Salmonella hirschfeldii*

- ■ Essentials of Diagnosis
  - Typhoid fever (*Salmonella typhi*) and paratyphoid fevers often indistinguishable
  - Fecal-oral spread. Organisms penetrate GI tract causing transient bacteremia. Proliferate in RE cells of liver and spleen causing bacteremia
  - Prodrome—headache malaise, abdominal pain and distension, constipation followed by diarrhea (2–4 days in children)
  - Toxic stage—high fever, relative bradycardia, abdominal distension, dermal rose spots (bacterial emboli), splenomegaly, toxicity, encephalopathy, meningismus (2–4 days in children)
  - Diagnostic tests—culture typhoid and paratyphoid bacilli from blood, stool, urine, and bone marrow; leukopenia in prodrome, ↑liver enzymes, disseminated intravascular coagulation (DIC)
  - Complications—GI hemorrhage, GI perforation, pneumonia, meningitis, septic arthritis, abscesses, osteomyelitis, dehydration
  - Recovery stage lasts 2–3 weeks. 1–3% becomes chronic intestinal carriers

- ■ Differential Diagnosis
  - Other infections—typhus, brucellosis, malaria, tuberculosis, psittacosis, EBV
  - Kawasaki disease
  - Lymphoma
  - Perforation is usually cecal or terminal ileal and may mimic acute appendicitis

- ■ Treatment
  - Active immunization during epidemics and for travelers to endemic areas
  - Antibiotic susceptibility and local experience should guide therapy
  - Trimethoprim-sulfamethoxazole, amoxicillin, ampicillin, aminoglycosides, cephalosporins are effective. Ciprofloxacin or chloramphenicol sometimes required for multiple resistant organisms
  - Treat for 14–21 days
  - Patience, nutrition, support, and careful observation during convalescent phase. Relapses occur despite appropriate therapy

- ■ Pearl

27

Abdominal distension, tenderness, and ileus are dramatic and require experienced surgical evaluation. Since laparotomy in typhoid fever is, in the words of a surgical colleague, "like operating on wet Kleenex" it should be performed only if perforation has occurred or is imminent.

Shigellosis—*Shigella dysenteriae, Shigella flexneri, Shigella boydii, Shigella sonnei* (groups A, B, C, D)

- ■ Essentials of Diagnosis
  - Superficially invasive gram-negative rod. Enterotoxin produced by plasmid causes hemorrhagic colitis. Group A most severe. Group D most common
  - Incubation 2–4 days, cramps, bloody diarrhea, high fever, hallucinations, seizures
  - Disease most severe in infants. May be mild, self-limited in children
  - Fulminant dysentery with hemolytic uremic syndrome is a rare complication
  - Stool culture usually positive; dramatic left-shifted white count

- ■ Differential Diagnosis
  - *Salmonella, Campylobacter, E coli 0157:H7, Entamoeba histolytica*
  - Pseudomembranous colitis
  - Intussusception
  - Acute-onset ulcerative colitis
  - Infectious viral diarrhea—rarely bloody

- ■ Treatment
  - Supportive care with IV fluids and antipyretics; Benadryl sometimes relieves severe tenesmus. Do not use Imodium or Lomotil
  - Organisms often resistant to trimethoprim-sulfamethoxazole and amoxicillin
  - Organism may be sensitive to ampicillin, ceftriaxone, azithromycin, ciprofloxacin (in adults)
  - Tetracycline and chloramphenicol sometimes used
  - Long-term fecal carriage rare

- ■ Pearl

Hallucinations or seizures are probably the result of absorbed neurotoxin. They may precede the onset of GI symptoms.

Listeriosis—*Listeria monocytogenes*

- ■ Essentials of Diagnosis
  - Gram-positive aerobic rod. Contact with animals, contaminated food, and milk increases infection risk. One-fourth cases occur in pregnant women
  - Pregnant woman has mild fever, aches, and chills. Intrauterine or perinatal infection causes still birth or neonatal death in 20% of cases
  - Early neonatal infection (1–3 days)—fetal distress, respiratory distress; papular rash; diarrhea; fever; meningitis; hepatosplenomegaly; sepsis with miliary micro abscesses in liver, spleen, CNS, lung, and bowel
  - Late neonatal form (1–5 weeks)—meningitis and sepsis
  - Older children—infection rare, associated with immunodeficiency
  - ↑WBC with 10–20% monocytes, CSF cell count >500/µL with monocytosis in one-third of cases, positive maternal and infant blood culture

- ■ Differential Diagnosis
  - Hemolytic disease of the newborn
  - Group B streptococcal sepias
  - Intrauterine infection with cytomegalovirus (CMV), rubella, toxoplasmosis
  - Meningitis from echovirus, coxsackievirus, group B streptococcus, or gram-negative bacteria may mimic late neonatal listeriosis

- ■ Treatment
  - Avoid soft cheeses, raw meat, ready-to-eat foods, unpasteurized milk or cheese during pregnancy

- ■ Pearl

Despite aggressive antibiotic therapy, the mortality of early neonatal infection is as high as 27%.

Leptospirosis—*Leptospira icterohaemorrhagiae*

- **Essentials of diagnosis**
  - Spirochete found in urine of rats, dogs, cattle, pigs. Entry via skin or respiratory tract. Incubation 4–19 days
  - Initial phase 3–7 days' chills, fever, headache, myalgia, episcleritis, photophobia, cervical adenopathy, pharyngitis
  - Symptoms may resolve for 1–2 days and then reappear
  - Vasculitis causes muscle pain, back pain, abdominal pain and vomiting, encephalitis with headache, focal neurologic signs, and coma
  - Vasculitis also causes glomerulonephritis and hematuria, encephalitis, hepatitis and direct jaundice, acalculous cholecystitis, DIC with petechiae, bruising, GI bleed, and purpuric rash sometime with gangrene of extremities
  - Leptospires recoverable in blood and CSF in first 10 days of illness, in urine from week 2 to 4. Leptospiral agglutinins peak at 3–4 weeks. PCR available in some laboratories

- **Differential Diagnosis**
  - During prodrome, consider typhoid, typhus, rheumatoid arthritis, brucellosis, influenza
  - Later phase rule out hepatitis, encephalitis, glomerulonephritis, pneumonitis, endocarditis, Kawasaki disease, acute surgical abdomen, bacterial sepsis with DIC

- **Treatment**
  - Good sanitation, avoid contaminated water and soil, rodent control, immunize dogs
  - Immunization or antimicrobial prophylaxis with doxycycline in high-risk occupational exposure
  - Disease usually self-limited in 1–3 weeks and not associated with jaundice
  - Penicillin G as soon as diagnosis suspected. Oral doxycycline for mild illness

- **Pearl**

Mortality in this disorder is mostly in the elderly due to renal and hepatic failure (5%). Relapses may occur. Although there are usually no CNS sequelae, headache may persist.

27

Toxic Shock Syndrome (TSS) *Staphylococcus aureus*

- **Essentials of Diagnosis**
  - Staphylococcal TSS—sudden-onset fever, blanching erythroderma, diarrhea, emesis myalgia, prostration, hypotension, and multiorgan dysfunction
  - At risk—children with wounds infected with *S aureus*, young women using vaginal tampons
  - Other features—conjunctival suffusion; mucosal hyperemia; DIC; renal and hepatic dysfunction; myolysis; convalescent desquamation of palms, soles, fingers, and toes
  - Focal infection with *S aureus* without bacteremia. Organism produces toxic shock syndrome toxin 1 (TSST 1) or related enterotoxin
  - Positive culture in appropriate clinical setting is diagnostic

- **Differential Diagnosis**
  - Group A β-hemolytic streptococcus can produces a TSS with similar clinical features. Multiorgan system failure is more frequent feature
  - Kawasaki syndrome
  - Rocky Mountain spotted fever, leptospirosis
  - Drug reaction
  - Adenovirus, measles

- **Treatment**
  - Mortality ~2% with early recognition and treatment
  - Aggressively support vascular perfusion with IV fluid, colloid, inotropic agents
  - Removal of foreign bodies and drainage of local infections
  - IV vancomycin plus oxacillin, nafcillin, or clindamycin can be started empirically and reduced according to sensitivity testing.
  - Intravenous immunoglobulin (IVIG) and corticosteroids used in severe cases

- **Pearl**

Recurrences may occur in up to 15% of women with tampon-related TSS during subsequent menses, even those who have received appropriate antibiotics and who have stopped tampon use.

27

Lyme Disease—*Borrelia burgdorferi*

- Essentials of Diagnosis
  - Infective spirochete transmitted by infected deer tick (*Ixodes* species)
  - Incubation 3–30 days. Early symptoms are erythema chronicum migrans (macular erythema spreading from site of bite with central clearing or central edema and redness), fever, headache, myalgia, urticaria, and satellite rash
  - 50% develop later fever with migratory, monarticular, or pauciarticular arthritis of large joints
  - 20% develop neurologic symptoms—Bell's palsy, aseptic meningitis, polyradiculitis, peripheral neuritis, Guillain-Barré syndrome, encephalitis, ataxia, chorea
  - Clinical diagnosis. Testing may show ↑WBC and erythrocyte sedimentation rate (ESR), positive IgM cryoglobulins, CSF with lymphocytic pleocytosis and ↑protein, and joint fluid pleocytosis
  - Serologic diagnosis by ELISA and confirmatory immunoblot or rising IgG antibody titers done in an experienced laboratory

- Differential Diagnosis
  - False-positive serologic tests for Lyme are common in syphilis, HIV, leptospirosis
  - Rash may resemble pityriasis, erythema multiforme, drug eruption, erythema nodosum
  - Arthritis may resemble juvenile rheumatoid arthritis (JRA); reactive, septic, or leukemic arthritis; reactive effusion from contiguous osteomyelitis; rheumatic fever; systemic lupus erythematous (SLE), or Henoch-Schönlein purpura (HSP)
  - Neurologic signs may suggest—Bell's palsy, viral or parainfectious meningoencephalitis, lead poisoning, psychosomatic illness, chronic fatigue syndrome

- Treatment
  - Use tick repellent and avoid endemic areas. Wear long sleeves/pants and check frequently for ticks
  - Early infection—use amoxicillin, erythromycin, cefuroxime, doxycycline (in older children) 14–21 days
  - Treat arthritis with amoxicillin or doxycycline for 4 weeks
  - Persistent arthritis treated with parenteral ceftriaxone or penicillin G
  - Bell's palsy—oral antibiotics listed above for 3–4 weeks
  - No Lyme vaccine approved for use in children

- Pearl

Lyme disease is not a proven cause of chronic fatigue syndrome.

Relapsing Fever—*Borrelia hermsii*

- ## Essentials of Diagnosis
  - Spirochete transmitted by body louse (*Pediculus humanus*—epidemic) and soft-bodied ticks (genus *Ornithodoros*—endemic in western United States)
  - Ticks feed at night and only remain attached 5–20 minutes. Patients rarely remember having been bitten
  - After a 4–18-day incubation, fever, chills, nausea, emesis, headache, myalgia, arthralgia, trunk and extremity rash, bronchitis, dry cough
  - Symptoms improve in 3–5 days but relapse at 1–2-week intervals
  - Other complications during relapses—hepatitis, splenomegaly, iridocyclitis, facial palsy, optic atrophy, anemia, pneumonia, nephritis, myocarditis, endocarditis, seizures
  - Proteinuria, high WBC; in 70% of febrile patients, spirochetes found on dark field examination of blood smear or on thick and thin smears stained with Wright, Giemsa, or acridine orange stains
  - Tick-borne disease may relapse five to six times. Louse-borne disease generally relapses once. Relapses are progressively less severe

- ## Differential Diagnosis
  - Other infections—malaria, leptospirosis, dengue, typhus, rat-bite fever, Colorado tick fever, Rocky Mountain spotted fever
  - Collagen vascular diseases
  - Malignancy especially acute lymphoblastic leukemia (ALL), may present with recurrent fevers
  - Fever of unknown origin

- ## Treatment
  - Antibiotics ameliorate the initial attack and prevent relapses
  - Starting antibiotics after fever resolves reduces risk of Jarisch-Herxheimer reaction caused by sudden endotoxin release
  - Standard-dose penicillin or erythromycin for 10 days in children <8 years
  - Older children may receive doxycycline

- ## Pearl
Rarely, relapsing fever is passed transplacentally to the fetus from an infected mother.

Plague—*Yersinia pestis*

- **Essentials of Diagnosis**
  - Acute infection by gram-negative bacillus transmitted to humans by fleas from infected rodents or by droplet from infected human
  - *Bubonic plague*—sudden high fever, chills, headache, emesis, delirium. Regional nodes (buboes) suppurate and drain after 1 week. Endotoxin causes vascular necrosis, hemorrhage, myocarditis, and shock. Sepsis, meningitis, and pneumonia occur
  - *Septicemic plague*—initial presentation with sepsis
  - *Pneumonic plague*—inhaled *Yersinia pestis* causes primary pneumonia. Fever, cough, dyspnea, bloody sputum. GI symptoms sometimes prominent
  - Lymph node aspirate, sputum, blood all yield organisms. Fluorescent antibody or PCR is faster and very specific

- **Differential Diagnosis**
  - Septic phase may suggest meningococcemia, sepsis, rickettsioses
  - Bubonic form suggests tularemia, anthrax, cat scratch, streptococcal adenitis, and cellulitis
  - Gastroenteritis and appendicitis

- **Treatment**
  - Control rat population and fleas. Domestic animals may contact infected animals and acquire fleas
  - Don't handle rats, mice, prairie dogs, ground squirrels, chipmunks dead or alive in endemic areas (arid south west)
  - Strict droplet isolation of patients until antibiotics in use for 48 hours
  - Streptomycin IM for 7–10 days is effective
  - Doxycycline in older children with mild disease. Gentamycin, tetracycline, and chloramphenicol also effective

- **Pearl**

In New Mexico, mortality of all patients with septicemic plague is 70%. Mortality of pneumonic plague is 50–60%. Mortality of bubonic form is low when recognized and treated.

27

Tularemia—*Francisella tularensis*

- ## Essentials of Diagnosis
  - Gram-negative bacterium acquired from contact with infected animals (mainly wild rabbits). Other sources—ticks, domestic dogs and cats, infected blood or tissue, aerosolized infected material, fleas, contaminated meat or water
  - Ulceroglandular type accounts for 60% of childhood tularemia—pruritic red papule at entry site ulcerates painlessly. Tender, fluctuant regional nodes develop with high fever, chills, weakness, emesis
  - Other presentations show isolated pneumonia, adenopathy, tonsillitis, or oral ulcers, all with chills and fever
  - Recover *Francisella tularensis* from ulcers, nodes, sputum. Immunofluorescent staining also diagnostic. Agglutinin titers >1:16 indicate infection

- ## Differential Diagnosis
  - Typhoid, brucellosis, miliary tuberculosis (TB), Rocky Mountain spotted fever, mononucleosis
  - Pneumonic form resembles atypical or mycotic pneumonitis
  - Ulceroglandular type resembles pyoderma from staphylococcus, streptococcus, plague, anthrax, and cat scratch
  - Oropharyngeal type resembles streptococcal and diphtheritic pharyngitis, mononucleosis, herpangina, and other viral pharyngitides

- ## Treatment
  - Excellent prognosis if treated
  - Protect children from tick, flea, and deer fly bites
  - Be very careful in dressing and handling wild rabbits
  - Gentamycin, amikacin, and streptomycin are efficacious.
  - Doxycycline, chloramphenicol, and ceftriaxone associated with relapses
  - Clean skin lesions and leave open. Incise and drain lymph nodes if necessary

- ## Pearl

Warn your laboratory when you send specimens from suspected tularemia cases. Airborne transmission risk is very high and laboratory personnel must take extra precautions when handling these cultures.

27

Whooping Cough—*Bordetella pertussis*

- **Essentials of Diagnosis**
  - Acute highly contagious respiratory infection with severe bronchitis
  - Increasing incidence in the United States because of waning immunity 5–10 years after primary vaccination
  - Catarrhal phase—insidious-onset rhinitis, sneezing and irritative cough, slight fever
  - Paroxysmal phase—cough occurs in paroxysms followed by loud inspiratory "whoop," emesis, sweating cyanosis, exhaustion, conjunctival hemorrhages, epistaxis. Phase may last 4 weeks and worsen or recur with later viral respiratory infections
  - WBC 20,000–30,000/μL with 70–80% lymphocytes
  - Secondary bacterial pneumonia and atelectasis occur. Death results from inanition, pulmonary hypertension, post-tussive apnea, seizures with hypoxic brain injury, toxic encephalopathy
  - Sputum cultures positive only during catarrhal phase. PCR detection is more rapid and sensitive. Chest x-ray shows thickened bronchi and "shaggy" heart border

- **Differential Diagnosis**
  - *Bordetella parapertussis* causes a milder whooping cough
  - Bacterial, tuberculous, chlamydial, or viral pneumonia
  - Cystic fibrosis
  - Foreign body aspiration
  - Adenoviruses and respiratory syncytial virus (RSV) may cause paroxysmal cough and lymphocytosis
  - Leukemia, lymphoma may be suggested by high WBC

- **Treatment**
  - Active immunization in infancy. Booster vaccination between 11 and 18 years recommended
  - Isolate hospitalized patients. Careful cardiorespiratory monitoring especially in young infants. Aggressive nutritional support
  - Treat family and hospital contacts with azithromycin or erythromycin
  - Erythromycin, azithromycin, and clarithromycin may be effective during catarrhal phase
  - Corticosteroids and albuterol may reduce severity of paroxysms

27

- **Pearl**

Beware, aerosolized respiratory treatments may actually precipitate paroxysms of coughing.

Psittacosis—*Chlamydia psittaci*

- **Essentials of Diagnosis**
  - Variable presentation, usually mild in children. Inhaled organisms from feces or nasal discharge of infected parrot, parakeet, cockatoo, duck, hen, pigeon, turkey, sea gull. Bird may not appear sick
  - Rapid or insidious-onset fever, chills, severe headache, meningeal signs, backache, myalgia, dry cough
  - Pneumonia, splenomegaly, facial rose spots (Horder spots), epistaxis, meningismus, conjunctivitis, constipation, diarrhea, abdominal pain
  - Rare complications—myocarditis, endocarditis, hepatitis, pancreatitis, secondary bacterial pneumonia
  - Leukopenia with left shift, proteinuria, elevated liver functions
  - Organism can be isolated from blood and sputum after inoculation into mice but culturing is dangerous to laboratory personnel
  - Fourfold rise in complement fixation titers or single titer >1:32 are the usual diagnostic tests. PCR available

- **Differential Diagnosis**
  - *Mycoplasma pneumoniae* and *Chlamydia pneumoniae* infection
  - Tuberculosis, legionnaire disease, Hanta virus, and other pneumonias
  - With systemic involvement, differential includes typhoid, brucellosis, Q fever, tularemia, rheumatic fever, rheumatoid arthritis, autoimmune disorders

- **Treatment**
  - Doxycycline for 14 days after defervescence in patients >8 years old
  - Alternative therapy for younger children—erythromycin, azithromycin, or clarithromycin
  - Tetracycline or chloramphenicol are effective but rarely used
  - Isolation of patient recommended

- **Pearl**

Don't give mouth-to-mouth resuscitation to a sick parrot, or any parrot for that matter!

27

Legionella—*Legionella pneumophila*

- **Essentials of Diagnosis**
  - Pontiac fever—self-limited mild, flu-like illness of healthy adults with fever, headache, myalgia, and arthritis. Lungs unaffected
  - Legionnaire disease—acute, severe, rapidly progressing pneumonia of older adults with fever, diarrhea, lethargy, irritability, tremor, and delirium
  - Bacillus acquired by inhalation from water sources—faucets, showers, sprays, cooling towers, heat exchangers. Not spread person to person
  - Bacteria engulfed by macrophages. T-cell function necessary for intracellular killing
  - ↑WBC, patchy lung consolidation. Sputum (buffered charcoal yeast medium required) positive in 70–80%. Direct fluorescent antibody or sputum positive in 50–70% but 95% specific. Urine immunoassay very sensitive and specific

- **Differential Diagnosis**
  - Other severe bacterial and viral pneumonia
  - Mycoplasma and fungal pneumonia may be difficult to differentiate in immunocompromised patients

- **Treatment**
  - Prevent infections—monitor and periodically clean equipment in sprayers, cooling towers, heat exchangers by hyperchlorination and/or superheating of water supply
  - Intensive supportive care may be required including mechanical ventilation
  - Azithromycin is drug of choice. Rifampin is added in severe cases
  - Ciprofloxacin and levofloxacin effective in adults but not approved for children

- **Pearl**

Legionnaire disease is rare in healthy children. It is highly fatal in immunocompromised children with hematogenous spread from lungs causing sepsis, pericarditis, myocarditis, and focal renal infections.

Gonorrhea—*Neisseria gonorrhoeae*

- **Essentials of Diagnosis**
  - Gram-negative diplococcus may be transmitted sexually or non-sexually. Ratio of asymptomatic to symptomatic infection in adolescents and adults is 3–4:1 in females and 1:1 in males
  - Males develop urethral discharge and dysuria. Prepubertal girls develop vulvovaginitis. Postpubertal girls develop cervicitis, foul vaginal discharge, dysuria, dyspareunia
  - Other sites of infection include pharynx, rectum, conjunctiva (newborns or self-inoculation from eye rubbing), salpingitis
  - Salpingitis is a result of endometrial infection at onset of menses. May progress to peritonitis, perihepatitis, mono or polyarthritis, tenosynovitis, papulo-pustular dermatitis of extremities, endocarditis, and meningitis
  - Culture of fluid from vagina, urethra, pharynx, anus, joints, CSF, or pustule shows gram-negative diplococci. Smears may show gram-negative intracellular organisms

- **Differential Diagnosis**
  - Nongonococcal urethritis due to *Clamydia trachomatis* in males
  - Vulvovaginitis in prepubertal females—Shigella, GAS, Candida, *Herpes simplex*, trichomonas, pin worms, or foreign body
  - Cervicitis in postpubertal females—Candida, *Herpes simplex,* trichomonas, intrauterine device (IUD), other foreign body
  - Salpingitis—must be differentiated from appendicitis, urinary tract infection (UTI), ectopic pregnancy, endometriosis, ovarian cyst or torsion
  - Disseminated gonorrhea—differentiate from meningococcemia, rheumatic fever, HSP, JRA, SLE, leptospirosis, secondary syphilis, serum sickness, hepatitis, endocarditis

- **Treatment**
  - Preventative measures include sex education, condom use, treatment of contacts
  - IM ceftriaxone, PO cefixime, PO ciprofloxacin, PO ofloxacin, PO levofloxacin are effective single-dose options for local infection
  - Doxycycline, azithromycin recommended until *C trachomatis* ruled out
  - Other single-dose therapy for local infection includes parenteral ceftizoxime, cefotaxime, cefotetan
  - Pelvic inflammatory disease (PID) and other disseminated infections require longer term therapy

- **Pearl**

N gonorrhoeae *vulvovaginitis in a prepubertal female should be treated as strong evidence of sexual contact or abuse.*

27

Meningococcal Meningitis/Meningococcemia—
Neisseria meningitides

- **Essentials of Diagnosis**
  - Gram-negative cocci (major groups A, B, C, Y, and W-135) may be carried asymptomatically in upper respiratory tract
  - Group B accounts for 33% of outbreaks, C: 25%, Y: 25%, and W-135: 15%
  - Meningococcemia—upper respiratory infection (URI) prodrome followed by fever, headache, nausea, toxicity and hypotension, rapidly progressing purpura/petechiae with DIC, massive skin/mucosal hemorrhage, and shock
  - Chronic meningococcemia—episodic fever, arthralgia, petechiae and splenomegaly most common in adults
  - Meningitis—Headache, nausea, meningismus, stupor, abnormal CSF
  - WBC variable, platelets low even without DIC, CSF >1000 WBC/µL with ↑protein and gram-negative intracellular diplococci
  - Patients with defects in complement, particularly late components (C6, 7, 8, 9) are at ↑risk for meningococcal infection particularly group A

- **Differential Diagnosis**
  - Septicemia—*Haemophilus influenzae, Streptococcus pneumoniae,* GAS, and other bacteria may cause meningococcemia-like syndrome
  - Similar rash may occur in enteroviral infection, HSP, Rocky Mountain spotted fever, endocarditis, leptospirosis, rickettsial diseases, thrombocytopenia, or platelet dysfunction
  - In children, meningococcal meningitis must be differentiated by culture from other pathogens, mainly *H influenza, S pneumoniae,* mycobacteria, enteroviruses
  - Unusual organisms may cause meningitis in neonates and patients with immunosuppression

- **Treatment**
  - Quadrivalent polysaccharide or meningococcal conjugate vaccines licensed for use in children >11 years. Especially useful in outbreaks, patients with asplenia and travelers to endemic areas
  - Use rifampin to treat household, daycare, and hospital contacts
  - Immediate broad-spectrum IV antibiotics to child with fever, purpura, or any signs of meningococcemia
  - Penicillin G, cefotaxime or ceftriaxone for proven infection. Treat septic shock and DIC.

- **Pearl**

Survival in meningococcemia with meningitis is usually better than isolated meningococcemia.

27

Chlamydia—*Chlamydia trachomatis*

- **Essentials of Diagnosis**
  - Most common cause of sexually transmitted infection in the United States
  - Obligate intracellular bacterium replicates in host epithelia
  - Symptoms in females—dysuria, urethritis, vaginal discharge, cervicitis, PID
  - Symptoms in males—dysuria, urethritis, epididymitis, urethral discharge
  - 75% of females and 70% of males with Chlamydia are asymptomatic
  - PCR on vaginal or urethral discharge is most sensitive test. ELISA or direct fluorescent antibody tests are adequate
  - Reiter syndrome occasionally occurs in males with urethritis-causing sacroiliitis, low back pain, polyarthritis, mucocutaneous lesions, and conjunctivitis

- **Differential Diagnosis**
  - Gonorrhea
  - UTI
  - Other vaginal infections—trichomonas, candida, bacterial vaginosis

- **Treatment**
  - Symptomatic and asymptomatic patients and their contacts require treatment
  - Azithromycin 1 g PO single dose, erythromycin 500 mg PO qid for 7 days or doxycycline
  - Recheck after 3 months. Reinfection is common

- **Pearl**

Previously, patients with gonorrhea have been treated simultaneously for Chlamydia because of the common association of these infections. With more sensitive tests for Chlamydia, however, the Centers for Disease Control and Prevention (CDC) suggests that treatment for coinfection is not necessary.

27

Congenital Syphilis—*Treponema pallidum*

■ Essentials of Diagnosis

- Newborns may be asymptomatic or have jaundice, anemia, $\pm$ thrombocytopenia, hepatosplenomegaly, nucleated red blood cells (RBCs), meningitis
- Infants later develop mucocutaneous lesions, weak arms/legs, adenopathy, hepatosplenomegaly, rhinitis, anemia, rash on body, palms and soles, and orifices
- Children develop perioral scars, depressed nasal bridge, hydrocephalus, frontal bone periostitis, notched central incisors (Hutchinson's teeth), lobulated molar cusps (mulberry molars)
- Late complications—interstitial keratitis, chorioretinitis, meningovascular disease with mental retardation, spasticity deafness, speech defects. Tibial periostitis, knee effusions, gummas of nasal septum, palate, long bones, and subcutaneous tissue
- Diagnosis suggested when serial measurement infant VDRL titer does not decrease or increases over the first 3 months. CSF VDRL may be positive
- Spirochetes on darkfield examination of skin, nasal, or mucous membrane exudate are diagnostic
- Bony lesions almost diagnostic—metaphyseal lucencies, periostitis, wide zone of provisional calcification, bilateral tibial osteomyelitis with medial metaphysical fractures

■ Differential Diagnosis

- Neonates—sepsis, congestive heart failure, congenital rubella, toxoplasmosis, disseminated *Herpes simplex*, CMV, hemolytic disease
- Infants—brachial plexus injury, poliomyelitis, osteomyelitis, septic arthritis, coryza from viral infection, scabies, diaper rash
- Children—interstitial keratitis and bone lesions of TB, other causes of mental retardation, arthritis, spasticity, hyperactivity

■ Treatment

- IV crystalline penicillin G or IM procaine penicillin daily for 10 days. Erythromycin or tetracycline in allergic infants
- If mother has been inadequately treated, treat the neonate with single-dose penicillin G benzathine IM even if complete evaluation is negative
- If mother has been inadequately treated and neonate has any abnormality in physical examination, CSF, CSF VDRL, bone films, or fourfold increase in VDRL titer, give IV penicillin G for 10 days
- Follow-up of all at risk infants to detect signs of late infection

■ Pearl

If the mother's VDRL is positive and her history of treatment is unclear it is appropriate to treat the neonate as if he/she is potentially infected.

27

28

Viral and Rickettsial Infections

28

Poliomyelitis—(Enterovirus)

- ## Essentials of Diagnosis
  - 90–95% of cases are subclinical. 5% are symptomatic with fever, myalgia, sore throat, and headache. 1–3% have aseptic meningitis
  - Paralytic polio occurs when there is meningitis with fever, myalgia, anxiety, loss of reflexes, asymmetric flaccid paralysis (especially proximal muscles of legs). Sensory function preserved
  - Bulbar polio causes dysphagia, dysarthria, constipation, urinary retention, and cardiorespiratory collapse
  - Cerebrospinal fluid (CSF) shows mild ↑lymphocytes and protein. Poliovirus is isolated from throat and rectum but not CSF. Paired serology helpful

- ## Differential Diagnosis
  - Other viral meningitis caused by mumps, herpes, cytomegalovirus (CMV), adenovirus, human immunodeficiency virus (HIV), Epstein-Barr virus (EBV), influenza, West Nile, lymphocytic choriomeningitis virus
  - Parainfectious encephalopathy from cat scratch, *Mycoplasma pneumoniae*, Lyme disease, leptospirosis, and rickettsial disease
  - Postinfectious syndromes—Guillain-Barré is an ascending symmetric paralysis and sensory loss. No CSF pleocytosis
  - Pseudoparalysis due to pain or weakness caused by bone or joint disease
  - Toxin-mediated paralysis—botulism, tick paralysis

- ## Treatment
  - Prevent disease by immunization with inactivated polio vaccine
  - Supportive treatment especially for respiratory weakness
  - Intubation/tracheostomy, bladder catheter, tube feeding may be required
  - Postpolio paralysis is mild in 30%, permanent in 15%. Physical therapy may be required

- ## Pearl
  Immunodeficiency and underimmunization are the major causes of paralytic polio in the United States today. Vaccine-associated paralytic polio has been nearly eliminated by the use of inactivated vaccine.

28

Chicken Pox (Varicella zoster)

- ■ Essentials of Diagnosis
  - • Primary infection with chicken pox confers lifelong immunity
  - • Chicken pox—10–21-day incubation; scattered pruritic red macules and papules progress to vesicles, pustules, and crusting in 5–6 days; variable fever and systemic symptoms
  - • Virus remain latent in sensory ganglia upon resolution of acute disease
  - • Late reactivation occurs in 15–20% of patients. Vesicles appear in dermatome distribution usually truncal or cranial
  - • Complications—pneumonia, secondary bacterial infection (group A β-streptococcus [GAS] or staphylococcus), Reye syndrome, autoimmune thrombocytopenia or disseminated intravascular coagulation (DIC) causing hemorrhagic varicella
  - • Usually a clinical diagnosis. Virus can be identified by fluorescent-antibody stain of a lesion or rapid viral culture

- ■ Differential Diagnosis
  - • Similar vesicular rashes seen in coxsackievirus, impetigo, papular urticaria, scabies, parapsoriasis, rickettsial pox, dermatitis herpetiformis, folliculitis
  - • Linear eruption of *Herpes simplex*
  - • Contact dermatitis from poison ivy, poison oak, metal allergy

- ■ Treatment
  - • Live attenuated varicella vaccine is a routine childhood immunization and can be given as postexposure prophylaxis in high-risk cases
  - • Supportive treatment sufficient for most infections
  - • Acyclovir (better for *Herpes simplex*) can be used in immunosupressed patients and at risk neonates
  - • Varicella immune globulin not effective in established infection but can be given postexposure to high-risk patients

- ■ Pearl

Those at highest risk for reactivation of zoster include the elderly, the immunosupressed, children with chicken pox in infancy, and children born to mothers with chicken pox during pregnancy.

Roseola Infantum (Human Herpes Viruses [HHV] 6 and 7)

- **Essentials of Diagnosis**
  - Abrupt-onset fever up to 40.5°C with mild illness lasting up to 8 days
  - When fever ceases (1–2 days), an evanescent red macular non-pruritic rash (exanthem subitum) appears on body and spreads peripherally
  - Children 6–36 months most often affected
  - Mild pharyngitis, diarrhea, adenopathy, and rarely, febrile seizure
  - Usually a clinical diagnosis—CSF and blood cultures negative

- **Differential Diagnosis**
  - High fever requires consideration of serious bacterial infection. The relative well being of patients with HHV 6 and 7 is a distinguishing factor
  - Drug allergy

- **Treatment**
  - Benign condition except in immunocompromised patients. No therapy needed
  - Fever control, especially in those with history of febrile seizure
  - Careful monitoring for serious disease until clinical pattern is clear

- **Pearl**

A bulging fontanelle is seen in 25% of infants with HHV 6 and raises the possibility of meningitis until the characteristic rash occurs.

Infectious Mononucleosis—(Epstein-Barr Virus)

- **Essentials of Diagnosis**
  - Most common syndrome associated with EBV. Transmitted in saliva
  - Incubation 1–2 months, malaise, and anorexia for 1–2 days, then fever, exudative pharyngitis, enlarged lymph nodes, splenomegaly (50–75%) hepatomegaly (30%) with hepatitis, rash
  - ↓WBC early with atypical lymphocytes accounting for 10% of white cells
  - Positive heterophile antibodies (Mono spot test) in 90% of older children but unreliable in children <5 years
  - Measure immunoglobulin M (IgM) antibody to viral capsid (VCA) when diagnosis in doubt

- **Differential Diagnosis**
  - CMV mononucleosis syndrome
  - Pharyngitis—GAS, primary herpes simplex
  - Viral hepatitis A, B, or C
  - Kawasaki syndrome
  - Serum sickness
  - Other febrile infections with atypical lymphocytosis—initial HIV infection, rubella, adenovirus, toxoplasmosis

- **Treatment**
  - Fluid and nutrition support, antipyretics
  - Use corticosteroids if extreme hypertrophy of pharyngeal lymphoid tissue threatens to obstruct the airway
  - Patients with extreme splenic enlargement are at risk for rupture. No contact sports for 6–8 weeks
  - In immunocompromised patients with chronic EBV infection, treat with acyclovir, valacyclovir, penciclovir, ganciclovir, or foscarnet

- **Pearl**

If you put your febrile patient with tonsillitis on penicillin or ampicillin and he/she develops a macular, scarlatiniform, or urticarial rash, you are almost certainly dealing with a case of infectious mononucleosis.

Rotavirus

- **Essentials of Diagnosis**
  - RNA virus occurs in summer outbreaks
  - Most common cause of viral gastroenteritis in infants <2 years worldwide. 50,000 hospitalizations per year in the United States in children <5 years
  - ~90% of children have serologic evidence of rotavirus infection by age 5 years
  - Symptoms mild fever, malaise, anorexia, and emesis followed in 24–48 hours by watery diarrhea. Spontaneous resolution in 4–5 days
  - Stool sodium concentration is usually <20 meq/L
  - Diagnostic tests not needed in typical cases. Fluorescent-antibody stain or electron microscopy of stool is diagnostic
  - ↑morbidity and mortality in premature infants and term infants <3–6 months, malnutrition, immunodeficiency, poor access to clean water and medical care

- **Differential Diagnosis**
  - Other enteric viruses—intestinal adenovirus, coronavirus, norovirus
  - Other infections causing watery diarrhea—cryptosporidium, *Aeromonas hydrophilia*, Giardia, *Vibrio cholera*, enterotoxigenic *Escherichia coli,* salmonella, Yersinia
  - Drugs and toxins—laxatives, osmotic agents, antibiotics, food-borne staphylococcal toxin
  - Antibiotic-related diarrhea—onset not usually so acute

- **Treatment**
  - Pentavalent human-bovine reassortant vaccine is available. 3-dose regimen to start by 6–12 weeks of age
  - Most healthy infants only require attention to adequate fluid intake during acute stage
  - Prepared electrolyte solutions (Pedialyte) can replace milk intake for 24–48 hours during diarrhea. The 3% glucose in Pedialyte stimulates salt and water resorption and the Na content is appropriate for fecal salt losses
  - Breast-fed infants can continue to breast feed with added Pedialyte solution for thirst
  - Diarrhea causing hypernatremia and dehydration may require intravenous therapy and medical supervision

- **Pearl**

Rotavirus infection confers immunity to a subsequent infection in <50% of cases.

28

West Nile Encephalitis—(Flavivirus)

- ■ Essentials of Diagnosis
  - First described in 1999; now found in >160 bird species in the United States
  - Many infections asymptomatic. About 20% cause headache, fever, retro-orbital pain, nausea, emesis, lymphadenopathy, maculopapular rash
  - Meningitis/encephalitis occurs in <1% of patients, and 10% of these cases are fatal
  - Risk for severe disease increased by age >50 years and immune compromise
  - Distinguishing features—polio-like flaccid paralysis, movement disorder, brainstem symptoms, polyneuropathy, optic neuritis, muscle weakness, hyporeflexia, facial palsy
  - Diagnosis by IgM antibody or polymerase chain reaction in CSF or rising serum antibody titers

- ■ Differential Diagnosis
  - Differential is the same as listed for polio

- ■ Treatment
  - Supportive therapy only
  - Therapy with specific immune globulin is being studied but not available for routine use

- ■ Pearl

Person-to-person spread does not occur. Direct contact with infected birds or bite of infected mosquito vector is the most common route of infection. Organism can also be spread through donated organs, blood transfusion, breast milk, and transplacentally.

28

Dengue Fever—(Flavivirus)

- ■ Essentials of Diagnosis
  - • Person-to-person transmission by Aedes mosquito vector
  - • Incubation 4–14 days. Biphasic symptoms with first stage lasting 3–4 days, short remission, then recurrence for a second 1–2-day phase
  - • Fever, headache, myalgia joint, bone/retro-ocular pain, myalgia, maculopapular or petechial rash sparing palms and soles (50%), adenopathy
  - • Meningoencephalitis occurs in 5–10% of childhood infections
  - • Many cases acquired during travel in Caribbean, Asia, Central and South America
  - • Leukopenia and thrombocytopenia common. Diagnose by viral culture of plasma, IgM specific ELISA, rise in standard antibody titer, PCR

- ■ Differential Diagnosis
  - • Infections with similar features—malaria, typhoid fever, leptospirosis, measles, EBV, influenza, borreliosis enteroviruses, acute HIV infection
  - • Other viral exanthems
  - • An illness starting 2 weeks after the end of the trip or that lasts longer than 2 weeks is not dengue

- ■ Treatment
  - • Oral replacement of fluids loss from diarrhea and emesis
  - • Analgesics for pain. Do not use drugs which impair platelet function (aspirin)
  - • No specific antibiotic therapy

- ■ Pearl

Dengue hemorrhagic fever—thrombocytopenia, bleeding, hypoalbuminemia, ascites, and pleural effusion—occurs when persons with previous dengue fever become infected with another serotype of the virus. This antigen-antibody–mediated syndrome carries high mortality.

28

Erythema Infectiosum—(Human Parvovirus B19)

- ■ Essentials of Diagnosis
  - • Mild flu-like symptoms followed in 1 week by fiery red, maculopapular then coalescing lesions on face with "slapped cheek" appearance
  - • Rash spreads to forehead, chin, behind ears, and then to extensor surfaces, trunk, neck, and buttocks. Circumoral, palmar, and plantar sparing
  - • Central clearing of rash leaves a lacey pattern with fine desquamation. Rash recurs with irritation, heat, sunlight, and stress
  - • This is usually a clinical diagnosis. IgM and IgG antibody tests available
  - • Pure red cell aplasia, leukopenia, pancytopenia, idiopathic thrombocytopenic purpura, hemophagocytic syndrome may follow infection, especially in immunosupressed patients
  - • Arthritis follows infection in 10%
  - • Intrauterine infection may cause fetal anemia, hydrops, and fetal death

- ■ Differential Diagnosis
  - • Immunization against measles and rubella may be followed by similar rash
  - • Malar rash of systemic lupus erythematosus (SLE) or early rubella may be similar
  - • Rashes of enterovirus infection or scarlet fever have similar features, but patients are sicker
  - • Drug reactions cause similar rash and arthritis
  - • Postinfectious arthritis may mimic juvenile rheumatoid arthritis (JRA) or rheumatic fever

- ■ Treatment
  - • Benign illness in immunocompetent individuals
  - • Patients with aplastic crises may need transfusion
  - • Careful monitoring of fetus for hydrops in maternal infection
  - • High-dose intravenous immunoglobulin (IVIG) has cleared viremia and resulted in marrow recovery in some cases of prolonged aplasia

- ■ Pearl

The rash in erythema infectiosum is an immune response to the virus. Patient is viremic and contagious prior to but not after the onset of rash.

Measles—(Rubeola Virus)

- **Essentials of Diagnosis**
  - Attack rate high. Incubation 10–14 days. Spread via respiratory secretions
  - Fever, lethargy, sneezing, eyelid edema, coryza, photophobia, and dry cough
  - Red facial maculopapular coalescing rash starts at peak of respiratory symptoms spreading to trunk and extremities. Gone in 6 days
  - White macules on buccal mucosa opposite the lower molars (Koplik spots) are pathognomonic
  - Lymphopenia with ↓total WBC. IgM antibody present 3 days after onset of rash. PCR of oropharyngeal secretions or urine detects virus during incubation
  - Complications—DIC, myocarditis, hepatitis, reactivation of tuberculosis, fatal pneumonia, croup, encephalitis (1–3%), and late subacute sclerosing panencephalitis (SSPE)

- **Differential Diagnosis**
  - Infections causing red macular rash—adenovirus, rubella, scarlet fever, roseola, parvovirus, leptospirosis, ehrlichiosis, Rocky Mountain spotted fever
  - Toxin-mediated rash—staphylococcal scalded skin, toxic shock syndrome, erythema multiforme, Stevens-Johnson syndrome
  - Kawasaki disease
  - Drug allergy

- **Treatment**
  - Spontaneous recovery in 7–10 days. Supportive care only
  - Active immunization with measles-mumps-rubella vaccine (MMR) prevents disease. First dose at 12–15 months. Second dose at 4–6 years
  - Measles vaccination within 3 days of exposure may prevent disease in immunocompromised children. Ribavirin may attenuate illness
  - Treat superimposed bacterial infections promptly
  - Intrathecal interferon-α has been used in SSPE
  - Supplemental vitamin A may attenuate illness in very malnourished patients

- **Pearl**

MMR vaccination should not be withheld for concurrent mild illness, TB, breast feeding, or for immunosupressed contacts. Immunization is recommended for HIV-infected children with >15% CD4 cells.

28

Rubella—(Rubella Virus)

- **Essentials of Diagnosis**
  - Incubation 14–21 days. Spread in respiratory secretions
  - Nonspecific respiratory prodrome with posterior auricular and occipital adenopathy followed by maculopapular facial rash that spreads to body and disappears in 3 days
  - Rare complications of acute infection—postinfectious polyarthralgia, arthritis, SSPE
  - Maternal infection in first trimester causes congenital defects in 80% of infants—small for gestational age (SGA), pulmonary artery stenosis, patent ductus arteriosus (PDA), ventricular septal defect (VSD), cataracts, microphthalmia, retinitis, deafness, encephalitis, mental retardation, thrombocytopenia, hepatitis, osteomyelitis
  - So-called "blueberry muffin" rash of intrauterine infection is either purpura (↓platelets) or cutaneous nests of extramedullary hematopiesis
  - Infants with intrauterine infection have low platelets, hepatitis, hemolytic anemia, high rubella IgM antibodies and may shed virus for months

- **Differential Diagnosis**
  - Rash may resemble scarlet fever, erythema infectiosum, rubeola
  - Other causes of arthritis and encephalitis
  - Other intrauterine viral infections—CMV, toxoplasmosis, herpes
  - Septicemia with DIC in the newborn

- **Treatment**
  - No treatment needed for acute infection
  - Rubella vaccination should be given at 12 months with booster at 12 years
  - Routine pregnancy screening for rubella
  - Seronegative pregnant women should be immunized after delivery
  - Documented infection or seroconversion in the first trimester requires counseling about risks to fetus
  - Pregnant, nonimmune women exposed to rubella may receive IVIG within 48 hours of exposure

- **Pearl**

If it were not teratogenic, rubella infections would be of little clinical importance. If rubella occurs after the fifth month of pregnancy, only 5% of infants are affected.

28

Hantavirus—(Bunyavirus)

- ■ Essentials of Diagnosis
  - Hantavirus cardiopulmonary syndrome is acquired from exposure to the habitat of the deer mouse and other rodent reservoirs. No insect vector
  - Incubation 2–3 weeks. Sudden-onset fever, back, hip and leg pain, chills, headache, nausea and vomiting lasting 1–10 days
  - Dyspnea, tachypnea, pulmonary capillary leak, hypotension, hypoxemia, pulmonary edema, myocardial dysfunction, ↓cardiac output, and ↑systemic vascular resistance develop rapidly after prodrome
  - Fatality rate may be as high as 50%
  - ↑WBC with left shift, ↓platelets, hemoconcentration, ↑lactate dehydrogenase (LDH), serum IgM ELISA positive early in illness.
  - Diagnosis also made by tissue stain or PCR. Chest x-ray shows pulmonary edema and pleural effusions

- ■ Differential Diagnosis
  - Bacterial infections—legionella, plague, tularemia, mycoplasma, psittacosis
  - Viral pneumonia—severe acute respiratory syndrome (SARS)
  - Acute respiratory distress syndrome
  - Cardiac failure, myocarditis

- ■ Treatment
  - Ribavirin is effective in other bunyavirus infections and may be helpful when given early in cardiopulmonary syndrome
  - Oxygen, diuretics, mechanical ventilation, inotropic medications. Monitor central venous pressure and do not overload with fluid
  - Extracorporeal membrane oxygenation has been used in some cases of respiratory failure
  - Isolation not required. Person-to-person transmission does not occur

- ■ Pearl

Unexplained pulmonary edema in a previously healthy person from an endemic area should immediately raise the possibility of hantavirus cardiopulmonary syndrome. Ask about rodent exposure.

28

Rabies—(Rabies Virus)

- ■ Essentials of Diagnosis
  - • 40% infection rate after bite by rabid animal. Risk of infection increased with multiple bites, head and hand bites, significant salivary contamination, delay in wound cleansing
  - • Virus carried in saliva of many mammals—bats, dogs, cats, raccoons, skunks, foxes. Urban animals rarely carry rabies
  - • Incubation usually <90 days but reported up to 1 year
  - • Paresthesias in bite area with progressive limb and facial weakness in 30%
  - • Most patients develop anxiety, irritability, fever, confusion, combativeness, muscle spasms (especially pharyngeal) delirium, seizures, coma, and death
  - • Rabies antigen detected in corneal scrapings or tissue from brain or skin. Classic Negri cytoplasmic inclusions in brain tissue not always seen. CSF normal
  - • Infection in suspect animals confirmed by fluorescent-antibody stain on brain tissue

- ■ Differential Diagnosis
  - • Parainfectious encephalopathy
  - • Viral encephalopathy—Herpes simplex, mosquito-borne viral encephalitides
  - • Postinfectious neuropathy—Guillain-Barré syndrome

- ■ Treatment
  - • Vaccinate domestic animals
  - • Survival is rare in documented cases
  - • Prophylaxis of exposed individuals—immune globulin

- ■ Pearl

In contrast to dogs and other mammals, rabies may not cause obvious disease in the bat. Treat any bat as potentially rabid. Aerosolized feces and saliva in bat caves may contain sufficient virus to cause human disease.

Severe Acute Respiratory Syndrome (SARS)—(Coronavirus)

- **Essentials of Diagnosis**
  - Atypical pneumonia first seen in Asia in 2002
  - Fever, malaise, chills, headache, myalgia, diarrhea, coryza, dyspnea, and cough with progression over 2 weeks to fatal respiratory failure in 10–15%
  - Leukopenia, lymphopenia, thrombocytopenia, ↑LDH, ↑serum glutamic-oxaloacetic/glutamic-pyruvic transaminase (SGOT/PT), ↑creatine kinase (CPK)
  - Virus isolated from sputum, saliva, urine, and feces. PCR provides rapid diagnosis
  - Chest x-ray shows ground glass opacities or focal consolidation that becomes severe and bilateral

- **Differential Diagnosis**
  - Other atypical pneumonia—Q fever, *Legionella, Clamydophila psittaci*, influenza virus, and other viruses
  - *Mycoplasma* and *Chlamydia* pneumonias are preceded by more prominent coryza and sore throat than SARS

- **Treatment**
  - Prevention by surveillance and quarantine. Spread within hospitals is a major source of new infections
  - Only therapy at present is supportive
  - SARS-specific immunoglobulin is under study

- **Pearl**

The few children with documented SARS have had less severe disease with fewer chest radiographic abnormalities than adult cases.

Acquired Immunodeficiency Syndrome (AIDS)— (Human Immunodeficiency Virus [HIV])

■ Essentials of Diagnosis
- Transmitted via sexual contact, contaminated blood products, transplacentally
- HIV replicates in lymphoid tissue with loss of CD4 T-helper lymphocytes
- Virus causes flu-like illness initially with fever, fatigue, malaise, pharyngitis. Other symptoms include oral ulcers, genital ulcers, macular rash, mild meningitis/encephalopathy, candida esophagitis
- Infection becomes latent (months to years). Viral numbers kept low by adequate T-cell function. AIDS occurs when CD4 cell production is inadequate to prevent virus replication
- AIDS—progressive humoral and T-cell immune dysfunction allows opportunistic
- Low CD4 count is often the first indication of AIDS. HIV antibodies are not diagnostic in newborns because of transplacental maternal antibodies. HIV PCR is diagnostic at any age

■ Differential diagnosis
- Any B, T or combined immunodeficiency
- Organ diseases that may mimic the initial HIV infection— pneumonitis, hepatitis, encephalitis, nephritis,
- Mononucleosis due to CMV or EBV
- Primary malignancies may mimic malignancies associated with HIV—non-Hodgkin lymphoma, cervical carcinoma, Kaposi sarcoma (rare in children)

■ Treatment
- Suppress viral replication to preserve CD4 lymphocyte function
  - Nucleoside/nucleotide reverse transcriptase inhibitors to terminate chain of HIV DNA
  - Non-nucleoside reverse transcriptase inhibitors to stop HIV DNA synthesis
  - Protease inhibitors to produce noninfectious virions
  - Fusion inhibitos to prevent viral entry into cells
- Immunize patients with good CD4 counts
- Aggressively diagnose and treat intercurrent infection
- Antibiotic prophylasis for potential infections
- Monitor and support nutrition and growth

28

■ Pearl
Children have a remarkable ability to restore normal CD4 T-cell counts, even when treatment is started at an advanced stage of HIV infection.

Ehrlichiosis—*Ehrlichia sennetsu, Ehrlichia chaffeensis, Ehrlichia phagocytophilia, Ehrlichia equi*

- ■ Essentials of Diagnosis
  - Rickettsia—*Ehrlichia sennetsu* causes mononucleosis-like illness in Japan and Malaysia
  - In United States, *Ehrlichia chaffeensis* is found in wild rodents, deer, sheep and spread by a tick vector. *Ehrlichia phagocytophilia* and *Ehrlichia equi* also cause disease in the United States
  - *E chaffeensis* invades monocytes. Intracytoplasmic inclusions seen on H and E stain of blood. *E phagocytophilia* and *E equi* invade granulocytes
  - Fever, headache, gastrointestinal (GI) symptoms, distal limb edema, photophobia, conjunctivitis, myalgia, arthralgia, meningitis, hepatitis, pneumonitis, renal failure, adenopathy
  - Rash occurs in 30% of *E chaffeensis* and 10 % of *E phagocytophilia* and *E equi* infections.
  - Pancytopenia, DIC, immunofluorescent-antibody stain available at Centers for Disease Control and Prevention (CDC)

- ■ Differential Diagnosis
  - Fever of unknown origin
  - Septic or toxic shock
  - Other rickettsial infections—Rocky Mountain spotted fever
  - Viral and bacterial infections—Colorado tick fever, leptospirosis, Lyme disease, relapsing fever, EBV, CMV, viral hepatitis
  - Kawasaki disease
  - SLE
  - Leukemia

- ■ Treatment
  - Disease may last several weeks before spontaneous resolution
  - Doxycycline is treatment of choice for 7–10 days
  - Mortality <3% but higher in patients with immune compromise

- ■ Pearl

Rocky Mountain spotted fever and human monocytic ehrlichiosis are both spread by lone star tick. Lyme disease and human granulocytic ehrlichiosis are spread by the deer tick. Dual infections can result from a single bite.

28

Rocky Mountain Spotted Fever—*Rickettsia rickettsii*

- **Essentials of Diagnosis**
  - Dog and rodent reservoirs with lone star tick vector
  - Incubation period is 3–12 days
  - High fever, myalgia, headache, photophobia, emesis, diarrhea, conjunctivitis, splenomegaly, meningismus, irritability, and confusion
  - Rash occurs in ~90% by about day 3 of symptoms. Macules and papules start on palms, soles and extremities become petechial and spread centrally
  - Laboratory tests reflect vasculitis—↓platelets, hematuria, hyponatremia, abnormal liver functions
  - Mild ↑CSF white cells. Indirect fluorescent or latex agglutination antibodies positive by 7 days. Fluorescent-antibody stain of skin lesions is positive earlier

- **Differential Diagnosis**
  - Bacterial diseases—meningococcemia, other bacterial meningitis, staphylococcal sepsis, scarlet fever, leptospirosis, gonococcemia, endocarditis
  - Viral diseases—enteroviral infection, Colorado tick fever, measles
  - Rickettsial diseases—ehrlichiosis, murine typhus, Q fever
  - Kawasaki disease

- **Treatment**
  - Tick attachment lasting >6 hours is needed to spread infection. Frequent "tick checks" can reduce risk of infection
  - Antibiotics must be started early to be effective. Treat on suspicion in endemic areas
  - Doxycycline is treatment of choice regardless of age. Treat for 2–3 days after resolution of fever (minimum 10 days)
  - Death (5–7%) results from vasculitis of brain, heart, and lungs. Early antibiotic therapy may prevent morbidity

- **Pearl**

Rocky Mountain spotted fever is rare in the Rocky Mountains. It is much more common on the eastern seaboard of the United States. Most cases in the Rocky Mountain region are in patients who have recently traveled back east.

28

Q Fever—*Coxiella burnetti*

- **Essentials of Diagnosis**
  - Transmitted by aerosol inhalation from birth tissues and feces of sheep, goats, cattle, chickens, rodents. Unpasteurized milk of infected animals transmits rickettsia
  - Incubation 0–30 days. Chills, fever, headache, myalgia, weight loss, hepatosplenomegaly
  - Pneumonia prominent in 50%—chest pain, cough, with few findings on auscultation, segmental infiltrates on x-ray but rare consolidation or effusion
  - ↓WBC with left shift, ↓platelet count. Complement fixing antibody rise during infection is diagnostic. ELISA and PCR also available for acute phase diagnosis
  - Infection may become chronic causing granulomatous hepatitis; osteomyelitis; and/or culture negative endocarditis of aortic, mitral, or tricuspid valves

- **Differential Diagnosis**
  - Atypical pneumonias due to *M pneumoniae*, viruses, *Legionella*, *Chlamydia pneumoniae*
  - Viral hepatitis, chronic autoimmune hepatitis
  - Brucellosis
  - Other causes of culture negative endocarditis

- **Treatment**
  - Illness typically lasts 1–2 weeks without therapy. Tetracycline, doxycycline therapy may shorten symptomatic illness
  - Quinolones also effective acutely for older children
  - Mortality from culture negative endocarditis approaches 50%

- **Pearl**

Children with Q fever are usually less sick than adults.

28

29

Parasitic Infections

29

Malaria—*Plasmodium vivax, Plasmodium falciparum, Plasmodium ovale, Plasmodium malariae*

- **Essentials of Diagnosis**
  - Protozoa transmitted person to person by anopheline mosquito
  - Inoculated sporozoites infect hepatocytes. Merozoites enter circulation from liver and infect red blood cells (RBCs) causing hemolytic crises every 48–72 hours
  - Congenital and transfusion-associated infections do not have a hepatic stage
  - Symptoms vary by species, strain, and host immunity
  - Infants—fever, irritability, emesis, jaundice, splenomegaly
  - Older children—fever, headache, backache, chills myalgia, fatigue with well periods between attacks
  - Complications (*Plasmodium falciparum* only)—small vessel thrombosis with tissue ischemia, cerebral infection, seizures, respiratory failure, renal impairment, bleeding, shock
  - Plasmodia are identified by anatomic features visible on Giemsa stained thick and thin blood smears

- **Differential Diagnosis**
  - Infections causing relapsing fevers—borreliosis, brucellosis, serial common infections, rat bite fever
  - Other causes of relapsing fever—Hodgkin lymphoma, leukemia, rheumatoid arthritis, inflammatory bowel disease, systemic lupus erythematosus (SLE), other autoimmune disorders
  - High fever and headache—influenza, *Mycoplasma pneumoniae,* enteroviral infection, sinusitis, meningitis, enteric fever, tuberculosis (TB), occult bacteremia
  - Fever, headache, and jaundice—leptospirosis, yellow fever

- **Treatment**
  - Prophylaxis—chloroquine (5 mg/kg once weekly up to 300 mg) for chloroquine-sensitive *P falciparum* and all other *Plasmodium* species
  - Prophylaxis for chloroquine-resistant strains—weekly mefloquine (except children <15 kg), daily doxycycline (in children >8 years), or daily atovaquone/proguanil
  - Treat active infection with chloroquine. For resistant strains or infections from areas with resistant strains, use quinine with pyrimethamine/sulfadoxine, tetracycline, doxycycline, or clindamycin
  - Monitor for dehydration, hypoglycemia, anemia, seizures, pulmonary edema, and renal failure
  - Exchange transfusion may be required if parasitemia is >15%

- **Pearl**

29

It is thought that sickle cell disease persists in the African population despite its lethality because heterozygotes are resistant to malaria.

Toxoplasmosis—*Toxoplasma gondii*

- **Essentials of Diagnosis**
  - Ova in feces or tissue cysts from infected mammals (especially cats) and birds invade human intestinal cells after ingestion
  - Infected cells lyse and infection spreads to adjacent tissues and blood
  - Acquired infection is symptomatic in 10–20% usually causing adenopathy without fever. May cause syndrome of fever, fatigue, malaise, myalgia, hepatitis, lymphopenia, chorioretinitis
  - Intrauterine infection may cause miscarriage, prematurity, stillbirth, fever, microcephaly, hepatitis, chorioretinitis, seizures, cerebral calcification, pneumonitis, thrombocytopenia, hemolytic anemia
  - Toxoplasmosis is common in human immunodeficiency virus (HIV) patients. Simultaneous fetal infection with both toxoplasmosis and HIV is common
  - *Toxoplasma gondii* or its DNA is found in blood, body fluids, placenta, or fetal tissues. Rising immunoglobulin (IgG) antibodies (Sabin-Feldman dye test) and other antibody tests are also diagnostic

- **Differential Diagnosis**
  - Infectious mono syndromes resembling acquired toxo—CMV, EBV
  - Intrauterine infections resembling toxo—CMV, rubella, syphilis,
  - Neonatal infection resembling toxo—group B streptococcus, Listeria, and other bacteria
  - Erythroblastosis fetalis, severe ABO incompatibility, other hemolytic diseases resemble congenital toxo

- **Treatment**
  - Good hand washing prevents infection
  - Serologic screening of pregnant women in high prevalence areas. Treat documented infection in pregnant women with spiramycin
  - Treat congenital infection with 6 months pyrimethamine/sulfadiazine followed by 6 weeks spiramycin alternating with 4 weeks pyrimethamine/sulfadiazine for the next 6 months
  - Antibiotics do not reverse congenital central nervous system (CNS) damage but decrease late sequelae
  - Mild acquired disease is often not treated due serious complications of therapy—bone marrow failure, gastrointestinal (GI) upset, allergic reactions
  - In chorioretinitis, pyrimethamine/sulfadiazine for 4 weeks with a short course of corticosteroid

- **Pearl**

29

Immunocompromised patients (HIV, lymphoma, leukemia, organ transplant) are at highest risk for severe toxoplasmosis—encephalitis, chorioretinitis, myocarditis, pneumonitis, and relapsing disease.

Amebiasis—*Entamoeba histolytica*

- **Essentials of Diagnosis**
  - Fecal-oral transmission often from asymptomatic carriers
  - Infection causes acute colitis with bloody stool, fever, abdominal pain, and tenesmus
  - Rarely, colitis is fulminant causing death
  - Chronic infection is indolent, with recurrent bouts of diarrhea, pain, and rectal bleeding. Ameba often localized to the cecum or rectum
  - Complications—intestinal perforation, peritonitis, perianal ulcers, liver, lung, or cerebral abscess
  - Diagnosis by histologic examination of stool or biopsy of colon ulcers

- **Differential Diagnosis**
  - Other acute colon infections—Shigella, salmonella, campy-lobacter, *Escherichia coli* 0157:H7, pseudomembranous entero-colitis of *Clostridium dificille, Neisseria gonorrhoeae*
  - Inflammatory bowel disease—especially ulcerative colitis
  - Rectal bleeding from polyps, allergy, fissure, bleeding disorders

- **Treatment**
  - GI infection responds well to iodoquinol but side effects common
  - Paromomycin or diloxanide furoate generally effective for GI infection
  - Extraintestinal disease requires metronidazole or tinidazole
  - Large abscesses require surgical drainage
  - Drink bottled or boiled water, cook fruits and vegetables in endemic areas

- **Pearl**

Entamoeba coli, Dientaboeba fragilis, *and* Endolimax nana *are common stool commensal organisms. They rarely cause disease but are sometimes treated in patients with mild chronic diarrhea when no other cause is found.*

29

Giardiasis—*Giardia lamblia*

- **Essentials of Diagnosis**
  - Intestinal protozoan. Fecal-oral spread in contaminated water. Day care center outbreaks are common
  - Parasite attaches to small bowel mucosa, blocking nutrient absorption
  - Incubation 1–2 weeks followed by acute-onset nausea, foul, greasy diarrhea, flatulence, abdominal pain, striking weight loss
  - Urticaria, arthritis, biliary tract disease, and constipation occasionally seen
  - Protracted intestinal shedding with intermittent symptoms is common
  - Increased risk of infection in IgA deficiency and other immunodeficiency syndromes (HIV)
  - Diagnosis by *Giardia* cysts or *Giardia* antigen in stool. Trophozoites can be seen in duodenal aspirate or mucosal biopsy

- **Differential Diagnosis**
  - Acute small bowel viral infection—rotavirus, intestinal adenovirus
  - Other small bowel parasites—cyclospora, cryptosporidium especially in immunodeficient individuals
  - Malabsorption syndromes—celiac disease, lactase deficiency
  - Malignancy is suggested by dramatic weight loss and malaise

- **Treatment**
  - Prevention of giardiasis requires proper maintenance of water purification systems, careful hygiene in day care centers and universal precautions around active cases
  - Metronidazole or nitazoxanide are drugs of choice
  - Treatment failures may respond to furazolidone or albendazole

- **Pearl**

Nothing smells as bad as the stool of a patient with active Giardia *infection. It's almost diagnostic.*

Visceral Larva Migrans—*Toxocara canis*, *Toxocara cati*

- ■ Essentials of Diagnosis
  - Dogs or cats infected with ascarids shed eggs in feces
  - Ingestion of eggs does not always cause disease
  - Disease occurs when larvae penetrate the intestine and migrate to liver, lungs, or eyes where they incite a granulomatous reaction as they die
  - Symptoms—anorexia, fever, fatigue, pallor, abdominal distension, hepatomegaly, seizures, myocarditis, encephalitis
  - Laboratory—dramatic eosinophilia up to 60–70%. Positive *Toxocara* ELISA is diagnostic
  - Ocular larva migrans—*Toxocara* causes unilateral posterior or peripheral inflammatory mass in older children. Presents with strabismus
  - Ocular larva migrans usually does not have eosinophilia. Antibody titers low in serum but high in ocular vitreous and aqueous fluid

- ■ Differential Diagnosis
  - Other diseases with eosinophilia—trichinosis, eosinophilic leukemia, collagen vascular disease, strongyloidiasis, ascariasis, tropical eosinophilia, allergies
  - Other diseases causing seizures, enlarged liver, pneumonitis, and cough—the tip-off is eosinophilia

- ■ Treatment
  - Prevent pica. It is the most common cause of this infection
  - Hand washing after handling soil frequented by dogs and cats
  - De-worm dogs and cats with *Toxocara*
  - Most patients recover spontaneously, but disease can last 6 months
  - In patients with brain, heart, eye, or lung disease—thiabendazole, diethylcarbmazine, albendazole, or mebendazole are used
  - Corticosteroids used to treat marked inflammation especially of lung and eye

- ■ Pearl

Prevalence of seropositivity to Toxocara *in the United States ranges from 2.8% in unselected populations to 54% in rural areas of the south.*

29

Cestodes—*Taenia saginata, Taenia solium*

- ■ Essentials of Diagnosis
  - Beef tapeworm (*Taenia saginata*) cysts in muscle transmitted to beef-eating humans cause taeniasis
  - *T saginata* cysts mature in the GI tract to adult tapeworms. Proglottids of mature worms shed in feces
  - Taeniasis may cause chronic abdominal pain and weight loss. Large parasite load may obstruct the intestine
  - Humans can be the intermediate host for *Taenia solium*. Larvae released from eggs ingested by humans encyst in human muscle, brain, and eye (cysticercosis). Most cysts cause no symptoms
  - In cysticercosis, cysts cause late-appearing brain mass, seizures, headache hydrocephalus, meningitis, retinal detachment, and uveitis
  - Diagnosis to taeniasis rests on finding *T saginata* eggs or proglottids in feces or perianal skin
  - In cysticercosis, CT scan of the brain may reveal cysts. ELISA antibody titers to *T solium* positive in 98% of patient sera and 75% of patient CSF

- ■ Differential Diagnosis
  - Seizure disorder
  - Bacterial or viral meningitis/encephalitis
  - Brain tumor
  - Chronic headache
  - Chronic abdominal pain
  - Failure to thrive

- ■ Treatment
  - Beef and pork inspection, proper cooking of meat, washing of vegetables and fruits, treatment of carriers, and prohibition of "night soil" as fertilizer has almost eliminated cestode infestation in the United States
  - Prognosis for *T saginata* infestation good. Praziquantel and albendazole are both effective
  - Treat cysticercal meningitis or encephalitis with praziquantel or albendazole to eliminate cysts and ameliorate symptoms
  - Death of *T solium* larvae during antibiotic treatment may cause edema and exacerbate cerebral symptoms. Dexamethasone helps with this complication

- ■ Pearl

T saginata *used to be recognized as a cause of human vitamin B_{12} deficiency. The organisms compete with the host for dietary B_{12} and if the parasites load is big enough it can deprive the host.*

29

Trichomoniasis—*Trichomonas vaginalis*

- ■ Essentials of Diagnosis
  - Protozoan flagellate causes vaginitis in 50% of infected women
  - Vaginitis symptoms—green-gray, malodorous, frothy discharge; dysuria; postcoital bleeding; and dyspareunia
  - Pelvic examination reveals vulvar edema and cervical friability
  - 50% of infected males have urethritis causing discharge and dysuria
  - Organisms are seen on microscopic examination of vaginal/urethral discharge, cervical Pap smear, urinalysis. PCR, culture, and antigen detection are diagnostic but rarely needed

- ■ Differential Diagnosis
  - Candidal vulvovaginitis
  - Nonbacterial vaginosis
  - Sexually transmitted diseases causing vaginitis/cervicitis/urethritis—*N gonorrhoeae, Herpes simplex, Chlamydia, Mycoplasma genitalium*
  - Vaginal foreign body and locally irritating vaginal douche

- ■ Treatment
  - Identify and treat sexual contacts. Reinfection is common
  - Screen and treat pregnant women with infection
  - Drug of choice is oral metronidazole 7 days, vaginal gel for 5 days (.75% metronidazole or 2% clindamycin)
  - Single-dose 2 g metronidazole is also effective

- ■ Pearl

Studies show that women with trichomoniasis during pregnancy have an increased risk of premature labor and low-birth-weight infants.

Cryptosporidiosis—*Cryptosporidium parvum*

- ■ Essentials of Diagnosis
  - • Intracellular protozoan multiplies in respiratory and intestinal epithelial cells. Acquired from contaminated water or contact with infected animals and humans
  - • Mainly a disease of patients with humoral or cellular immune defects
  - • Usual course is self-limited watery diarrhea lasting 2–26 days. Children <2 years more susceptible than older children
  - • Immunodeficient patients can develop chronic diarrhea, cholecystitis, pancreatitis, hepatitis, and pneumonia
  - • Organism identified by ELISA or PCR in stool or tissue biopsies

- ■ Differential Diagnosis
  - • Other watery diarrhea syndromes—viral gastroenteritis, *Giardia,* secretory tumors, enterotoxin-secreting *E coli,* cholera
  - • Infections causing watery diarrhea in immunodeficient patients— *Aeromonas hydrophilia, Cyclospora, Isospora belli, Giardia*

- ■ Treatment
  - • Immunocompetent or temporary immunodeficiency—use nitazoxanide, antidiarrheal agents, and hydration
  - • Re-establishing immunocompetence leads to resolution of infestation
  - • Immunodeficient patients may require intensive fluid and intravenous nutrition support
  - • Immunodeficient patients may be treated with nitazoxanide, paromomycin/azithromycin, rifabutin, or hyperimmune bovine colostrum
  - • Octreotide acetate (somatostatin analogue) sometimes reduces massive secretory diarrhea

- ■ Pearl

When water purification plants fail, the incidence of simultaneous Cryptosporidium *and* Giardia *infestations increases in immunodeficient patients.*

Pinworms—*Enterobius vermicularis*

- **Essentials of Diagnosis**
  - Small nematode (5–10 mm long) lives in the colon. Eggs deposited on the perianal skin usually at night
  - Major symptom is intense anal pruritis
  - Scratching contaminates the fingers allowing transmission to contacts and autoinfection. Transmission in contaminated fomites is common
  - Migration of worms to vagina and urethra may cause vaginitis and urinary tract infection
  - Worms can be seen on the perianal skin while the child is sleeping
  - Eggs may be obtained for microscopic identification on a piece of transparent tape pressed to the child's anus in the morning

- **Differential Diagnosis**
  - Pruritus ani
  - Perianal streptococcus infection
  - Nonspecific vaginitis
  - Urinary tract infection

- **Treatment**
  - Launder bedsheets and night clothes frequently
  - Keep hands and nails clean. Prevent scratching by wearing underwear to bed
  - Check and treat all affected family members at the same time
  - Pyrantel pamoate single does (11 mg/kg) is effective. Single-dose mebendazole and albendazole also effective
  - Reinfection at school from untreated classmates is common

- **Pearl**

Parents freak out over this common harmless infection. My old parasitology professor, Dr Harold Brown, always advised parents that "pinworms are found even in the seats of the mighty," meaning that even the cleanest child from the most immaculate home gets pinworms.

29

Ascariasis—*Ascaris lumbricoides*

- **Essentials of Diagnosis**
  - Fecal-oral spread of ova from human to human
  - Swallowed ova hatch in intestine. Larvae penetrate intestine, enter venous system, travel to lungs, are coughed up, and swallowed. Larvae mature in the intestine
  - Many infestations are asymptomatic. Severe infestations cause pain, weight loss, anorexia, diarrhea, vomiting, and rarely intestinal perforation or obstruction of small bowel, bile ducts or appendix
  - Larvae migrating through the lungs may cause eosinophilic pneumonia (Löffler syndrome)
  - Ova can be seen by microscopic examination of stool. Ascarid worms as long as 10 cm are sometimes passed in stool

- **Differential Diagnosis**
  - Acute and chronic GI infection
  - Recurrent abdominal pain of childhood
  - Gall bladder and biliary disease

- **Treatment**
  - Ascariasis is usually self-limited because the adult worms live <1 year. Since adult worms lay 1000 eggs per day, it is preferable to treat all cases
  - Mebendazole, pyrantel pamoate, albendazole are highly effective
  - In cases of intestinal or biliary obstruction, use piperazine because it narcotizes worms and helps relieve obstruction
  - Surgical removal of obstructing ascaris worms from intestine or biliary tract is sometimes required

- **Pearl**

Freezing weather kills ascaris ova in the soil preventing endemic infestation in nontropical areas.

30

Fungal Infections

30

Blastomycosis—*Blastomyces dermatitidis*

- ■ Essentials of Diagnosis
  - Soil fungus found primarily in Mississippi and Ohio River valleys, Great Lakes, and states of southeastern/south-central United States
  - Inhalation of spores by healthy individuals causes self-limited pneumonia with noncaseating granulomata. Most cases asymptomatic
  - Dissemination first causes ulcerative or warty skin lesions with later spread to bones, prostate, testes, larynx, lymph nodes, kidneys, and brain
  - Immunodeficient patients at highest risk for chronic pneumonia and disseminated disease
  - Diagnosis by culture or visualization of fungus in sputum, lung biopsy. Antibody tests available
  - Extensive radiographic evaluation in suspected disseminated infections to identify all sites of infection

- ■ Differential Diagnosis
  - Primary pulmonary infection resembles acute viral, bacterial, or mycoplasmal pneumonitis
  - Chronic pneumonia resembles histoplasmosis, tuberculosis, and coccidiomycosis but caseating granulomas are typical of these infections
  - Disseminated disease resembles bacterial infections of bone, central nervous system (CNS), and other organs

- ■ Treatment
  - No treatment for mild pulmonary or skin blastomycosis
  - Amphotericin B for life-threatening infection in immunocompromised patients or CNS infection
  - Itraconazole and ketoconazole for less severe infections. Bone infection requires up to 1 year of therapy
  - Surgery to remove devitalized bone, drain abscess, or remove area of resistant pulmonary infection

- ■ Pearl

Alveolar macrophages inhibit the transformation of the inhaled conidial form of Blastomycosis into its invasive yeast form. This is the basis for the resistance to infection in healthy individuals.

Coccidiomycosis—*Coccidioides immitis*

- **Essentials of Diagnosis**
  - Dimorphic fungus endemic in west Texas, southern New Mexico, Arizona and California, and northern Mexico
  - Infection after inhalation or inoculation of spores. No human-to-human transmission
  - >50% of primary infections are asymptomatic
  - Symptomatic primary disease may be mild (fever and arthralgia) or severe (influenza-like illness with fever, nonproductive cough, severe pleurisy, myalgia, arthralgia, headache, night sweats, anorexia)
  - 10% of infected children have indurated ulcers at inoculation site, contiguous tissue infection, regional adenopathy, erythema nodosum or multiforme
  - Disseminated disease occurs in neonates but is rare in children. Sites of dissemination are meninges, single bone or joint, kidney, lung
  - Diagnosis made by identifying endospore-containing spherules in sputum, pus, cerebrospinal fluid (CSF), or biopsy. CSF shows ↑protein, ↓glucose, and mononuclear cells (70% with eosinophils). Antibodies (precipitins) appear by 2–3 weeks
  - 50% of symptomatic cases have infiltrates and hilar adenopathy on chest x-ray

- **Differential Diagnosis**
  - Primary lung infection resembles viral, bacterial, or mycoplasma pneumonia
  - Subacute presentation resembles TB, histoplasmosis, blastomycosis
  - Chronic lung or disseminated disease resembles cancer, TB, other fungal infections

- **Treatment**
  - No treatment for mild pulmonary disease in normal hosts
  - Amphotericin B for patients with prolonged fever, weight loss, severe pneumonia, or any form of disseminated disease
  - Amphotericin B for high-risk groups—neonates, immunosuppressed patients, pregnant women, and patients with high antibody titers
  - Fluconazole or itraconazole preferred for less severe disease and meningitis
  - Lifelong itraconazole after meningitis prevents relapse
  - Surgical excision of pulmonary cavities, pulmonary abscess, draining nodes, cutaneous sinus tracts and bone

- **Pearl**
Erythema nodosum or erythema multiforme in a child with coccidiomycosis is a favorable sign indicating a good immune response to the organism with probable clearing of infection.

30

Histoplasmosis—*Histoplasma capsulatum*

- Essentials of Diagnosis
  - Fungus endemic in east/central United States, Mexico, and South America. Bat and bird feces contaminate soil with spores which are inhaled by humans
  - Infection occurs in >66% of children in endemic areas. Most are asymptomatic causing scattered pulmonary calcifications
  - Acute lung infection—influenza-like illness with fever, myalgia, arthralgia, cough, weight loss, night sweats, pleurisy
  - Dissemination occurs mainly in immunocompromised patients and involves the reticuloendothelial system causing hepatosplenomegaly, anemia, fever, bone marrow failure. Mortality very high
  - Eye, brain, heart valves, pericardium, intestine, skin, adrenals can be affected in disseminated disease
  - Organism visible by microscopy in macrophages but not sputum, urine, or CSF. Cultures yield organisms in 1–6 weeks. Histoplasma antigen in sputum, urine, blood, CSF is the fastest and most sensitive test

- Differential Diagnosis
  - Chest x-ray of patient with asymptomatic lung infection resembles TB
  - Acute pneumonia resembles viral infections, TB, coccidiomycosis, blastomycosis
  - Systemic disease resembles disseminated fungal or mycobacterial infection, leukemia, histiocytosis, or cancer

- Treatment
  - No treatment for mild infections
  - Amphotericin B for severe or protracted pulmonary disease, disseminated disease, children <1 year
  - Itraconazole for milder disease and after initial favorable response to amphotericin B

- Pearl

Of the 3 most common fungi in the United States that cause disease in normal hosts (Coccidioides, Histoplasma, *and* Blastomyces); Histoplasma *is the one most likely to reactivate if the individual later becomes immunosuppressed.*

Pneumocystis—*Pneumocystis jiroveci*

- ■ Essentials of Diagnosis
  - • Classified as a fungus by structural characteristics, this organism responds to antiprotozoals and folic acid antagonists
  - • Ubiquitous pathogen spread via inhalation from environment or person to person
  - • Primary infection rarely causes disease in healthy hosts or at most mild, afebrile pneumonia
  - • Reactivation or new exposure causes severe lung infection in patients with T-cell dysfunction, eg, HIV, corticosteroids, neonates, severe malnutrition, hematologic malignancy, chemotherapy, organ transplant
  - • At-risk patients develop fever tachypnea, dyspnea, nonproductive cough with rapid progression to respiratory failure if untreated

- ■ Differential Diagnosis
  - • In immunocompetent infants, primary pneumocystis infection resembles *Chlamydia trachomatis* pneumonia
  - • Differential in immunocompromised children—influenza, respiratory syncytial virus, CMV, adenovirus, bacterial and fungal pneumonias
  - • Noninfectious diseases with hypoxia and tachypnea—pulmonary embolus, pulmonary hemorrhage, congestive heart failure, lymphoid interstitial pneumonitis, pneumothorax

- ■ Treatment
  - • Prophylax all patients with T-cell dysfunction using trimethoprim-sulfamethoxazole 3 days/week
  - • Prophylax newborns of mothers with HIV starting at 6 weeks and continue until infection has been ruled out
  - • Acquired infection—treat with oxygen, nutritional support, trimethoprim-sulfamethoxazole intravenously for 3 weeks
  - • Use methylprednisolone in HIV patients with severe pneumonia during the first 5 days of therapy
  - • Pentamidine isethionate for patients intolerant to trimethoprim-sulfamethoxazole

- ■ Pearl

Tachypnea, dyspnea, and hypoxemia out of proportion to auscultatory and x-ray findings in a patient with abnormal T-cell immunity is Pneumocystis *until proven otherwise.*

Index